WELLNESS NURSING: CONCEPTS, THEORY, RESEARCH, AND PRACTICE

Carolyn Chambers Clark, A.R.N.P., Ed.D., is a Fellow of the American Academy of Nursing. She is a prolific contributor to nursing literature. Her most recent book is *Enhancing Wellness: A Guide for Self-Care* (Springer, 1981). She is on the editorial board of *The Journal of Holistic Nursing* and *Women's Health Care International*. She founded The Wellness Institute, edits and publishes *The Wellness Newsletter*, and serves as a wellness consultant.

WELLNESS NURSING:
Concepts, Theory, Research, and Practice

Carolyn Chambers Clark
A.R.N.P., Ed.D., F.A.A.N.

SPRINGER PUBLISHING COMPANY
New York

Springer Publishing Company, Inc.
536 Broadway
New York, NY 10012

86 87 88 89 90 / 5 4 3 2 1

Library of Congress Cataloging-in-Publication Data

Clark, Carolyn Chambers.
  Wellness nursing.

  Includes bibliographies and index.
  1. Health promotion.   2. Health education.
3. Nursing.   I. Title.   [DNLM: 1. Health
Promotion—nurses' instruction.   2. Patient
Education—nurses' instruction.   WY 87 C592w]
RT90.3.C48   1985   613'.07'1   86-13856
ISBN 0-8261-5150-7 (soft)

Printed in the United States of America

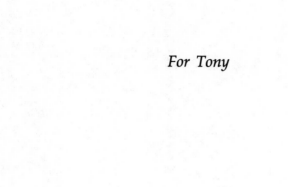

For Tony

CONTENTS

Preface   xi
List of Illustrations   xiii
List of Tables   xiv

1   Introduction to Wellness Theory   1
Wellness Nursing Defined   1
The Importance of Arriving at a Stated Purpose for
   Nursing Through Wellness Theory   5
Societal Factors Supporting the Use of Wellness
   Nursing Theory and Practice   8
Definition of Terms and Their Relevance to
   Wellness Theory   11
Assumptions Underlying the Wellness Model   14
Boundaries of Wellness Theory   14
Integrative Learning Experiences   15

2   Beginning to Move Toward Wellness   20
Differentiation of Self   20
Value Clarification   26
Centering   28
Facilitating Movement Toward Wellness   30
Integrative Learning Experiences   53

3   Positive Relationship Building   58
Empathy   58
Assertiveness   62
Integrative Learning Experiences   78

4   Stress Management   81
Assessing Stress Symptoms and Stress
   Management Skills   81

Stress Management Interventions 85
Coping Skills Procedures 100
Integrative Learning Experiences 107

5 Nutritional Wellness **113**
Food and Wellness 113
Guidelines for Reading Nutritional Information 115
Food Myths 115
Suggested Dietary Goals 116
Vitamins and Minerals 119
Nutrients for Prevention 122
Drug–Nutrient Interactions 151
Weight Maintenance 152
Integrative Learning Experiences 160

6 Exercise and Movement **167**
Some Theoretical Frameworks for Fitness 167
Assessing Fitness 177
Fitness Interventions 185
Exercise for Special Populations 194
Overcoming Obstacles to Exercise 199
Body/Mind Interactions and Fitness 200
Integrative Learning Experiences 202

7 Self-Care, Touch, and Wellness **205**
Theoretical Frameworks for Touch and Healing 205
Self-Care Assessments 214
Touch and Healing Assessments 216
Smoking Cessation: A Self-Care Intervention 233
Touch and Healing Interventions 235
Integrative Learning Experiences 255

8 Environmental Wellness **258**
Environmental Factors Influencing Wellness 258
Assessing Environmental Wellness 268
Environmental Interventions 272
Integrative Learning Experiences 280

9 Community Wellness Programs **283**
Justification for Community Wellness Programs 283
Assessing Wellness Program Needs 285
A Survey of Wellness Programs in Industry, Hospitals,
and Clinics 290
Some Federally Funded Community Wellness
Programs 291
Planning and Implementing Wellness Programs 294

Evaluation of Wellness Programs 307
Integrative Learning Experiences 313

10 **Research and Wellness Theory** **315**
The Content of Nursing Research 315
Turning Illness-Oriented Research Questions into
Wellness-Oriented Ones 316
Research Procedures for Holistic, Complex
Processes 320
Research Providing Support for Wellness Theory 326
Developing Relationship Statements and Testing
Theoretical Relationships 329
Integrative Learning Experiences 332

Epilogue: In Search of Wellness Nursing Practice **334**

A Note on Nursing Diagnosis and Wellness **337**

Index **341**

PREFACE

Any new theory is first attacked as absurd; then it is admitted to be true, but insignificant; finally—it seems to be important, so important that its adversaries claim that they themselves discovered it!

Henry James

This book shares some of the ideas I have about what wellness is, how it provides a framework for change, and how we can change ourselves and facilitate wellness in others. Many of the interventions are new to nursing practitioners; others have been alluded to in the literature or are practiced by a small minority of nurses. I believe all add a different and needed dimension to nursing practice. I have apprenticed myself to expert practitioners in many areas to learn approaches which I believe every nurse must master to participate in an integrated wellness practice. Each of these approaches appears in the book with suggestions for use with self, peers, and clients. Most, if not all, interventions can be completed by the client or the client and a peer who has mastered the procedure. A major emphasis of wellness nursing practice is assisting the client to be independent and able to provide self-care measures to enhance wellness.

The idea of health promotion is not a new one in nursing, but the idea that the client is the expert in his or her own wellness *is*. Giving up the expert role (at least in the traditional sense) to work on one's own wellness, to role model wellness for clients, and to allow clients to make their own informed decisions (even when we disagree with their choices) is difficult but challenging. Nurses *and* clients are responsible for keeping up-to-date on the constantly changing information sources relevant to wellness; nurses are not the dispensers of information, they are the teachers of clients about how to access information systems, and the recipients of knowledge from clients.

Another theme (or paradox) pervading this book is the essential uniqueness, yet similarity of nurses and clients. We're all on the journey to wellness together—no one totally lacking it and no one totally attaining it, but all managing a brief glimpse of total wellness potential. Students, teachers, nursing practitioners, and clients are all learners and teachers of one another.

Another theme is the importance of self-awareness and planned interventions in each wellness dimension. Nutritional wellness, fitness/movement maximization, stress management, positive relationships, coherent beliefs, and environmental sensitivity interact to provide purposeful movement toward wellness.

Strong societal forces support the wellness movement which has proven itself to be more than a fad. I am confident that nurses will become leaders in this movement, and will seize the first available opportunity to start wellness nursing practices in schools, hospitals, industry, and communities.

"Integrative Learning Experiences" at the end of each chapter have been developed to provide a challenge both to the novice and expert practitioner; many can be used as they are with clients, or they can be adapted for use. It is suggested that the nurse try out each experience prior to using it with clients. Case studies provide a focus for discussion and a synthesis of information. Table 23 (p. 108) provides a format for the nursing process in wellness nursing and includes suggestions for evaluating nursing interventions. These evaluation suggestions can be used by students, peers, or faculty members.

As you read through the book and complete the learning exercises, remember to be easy on yourself. You are a unique being; give yourself understanding, nurturance, and time to blossom.

CAROLYN CHAMBERS CLARK
St. Petersburg, Florida

LIST OF ILLUSTRATIONS

Figure

1	Intersystems wellness nursing model	4
2	Whole person wellness	6
3	Getting to your ideal weight	159
4	Common areas of holding	174
5	The lateral line and compensated balance	174
6	An overburdened individual	174
7	Bowing backward and forward	174
8	Knees	174
9	Feet	175
10	Tight pelvis and "normal" pelvis	175
11	"Normal" pelvis and retracted pelvis	175
12	Progression of top to bottom trapped energy	175
13	Metacarpal–phalangeal extension	182
14	Foot reflexology points	232
15	Sun salutation	242
16	Integrating and relaxing the brain	247
17	Back massage	248
18	Preventive acupressure	249
19	Overall balancing: ear acupressure	250
20	Acupressure for neck and shoulder releases	251
21	Variables facilitating and preventing nursing students from engaging in wellness behaviors	330

LIST OF TABLES

Table

1 Comparison of Traditional Nursing Process and Wellness Nursing Process | 2

2 Comparison of Health and Wellness: Process and Product | 3

3 Comparison of Wellness Nursing and Health Education | 7

4 Examples of Behaviors that Can and Cannot be Counted | 32

5 Reinforcers for One Student | 33

6 A Behavioral Contract for Mr. & Mrs. Sconce | 35

7 Wellness Self-Assessment | 36

8 The Clark Health/Wellness Belief Scale | 40

9 Relaxation Exercises | 44

10 Using Imagery to Solve Problems | 46

11 Using Imagery to Prepare for an Upcoming Situation | 46

12 Using Imagery to Enhance Healing | 47

13 Using Imagery to Decrease Painful or Negative Feelings | 48

14 Levels of Empathy | 59

15 Assertiveness Assessments | 65

16 Self-Instructions for Overcoming Hidden Agendas | 78

17 Assessing and Reducing Stressful Life Changes | 83

18 Stress Symptom Assessment | 83

19	Basic Instructions for Self-Hypnosis	91
20	Coaching Clients in Self-Hypnosis	91
21	Refuting Irrational Ideas	100
22	Time Management Assessment	103
23	Nursing Process in Promoting Wellness	108
24	Signs of Balanced Eating	114
25	What Does Your Body Need?	114
26	The Low Salt Controversy	120
27	Vitamin Functions, Deficiency Symptoms and Food Sources	123
28	RDAs of Vitamins; Reasons Supplementation May Be Needed	128
29	Reference to Minerals, RDAs Functions, Sources and Factors Leading to Insufficient Uptake	131
30	Wellness Enhancing Foods	136
31	Does Vegetarianism Protect Against Chronic Disease?	140
32	Drug-Induced Nutrient Malabsorption	153
33	Structural Assessments	179
34	Developmental Movement Interventions	186
35	Choosing a Shoe for Running or Walking	190
36	Keeping your Back Fit	191
37	Flexibility Exercises	193
38	Exercises for Bedridden Clients	195
39	Directions for Breast Self-Examination	215
40	Directions for Examining Some of the Lymph Nodes	216
41	Directions for Examining the Abdomen of Another Person	217
42	Directions for Two Methods of Examining the Thyroid Gland	218
43	Fitness Record	219
44	Communicating About Our Sexual Experiences	223
45	Vaginal Self-Examination	224
46	Detection Tests and Preventive Measures for Major Illnesses	225
47	Questionable Screening Procedures	230
48	Smoking Cessation Suggestions	233

49 Massage   244
50 Breath for Unity   273
51 Protection from Environmental Influences   274
52 Use of Color to Heal   279
53 Community Assessment   287
54 Examples of Quality of Life Responses and
    Wellness Dimensions   331

1

INTRODUCTION TO WELLNESS THEORY

This chapter discusses the following topics:

- The definition of wellness nursing
- The importance of arriving at a stated purpose for nursing through wellness theory
- Societal factors supporting the use of wellness nursing theory and practice
- Definition of terms and their relevance to wellness theory
- Assumptions underlying the wellness model
- Boundaries of wellness theory

One purpose of this book is to provide evidence for using wellness as the guiding purpose for nursing practice. To do this, the parameters of wellness must be defined.

WELLNESS NURSING DEFINED

Wellness Nursing is focused on a joint assessment of client needs; application of theory; facilitation of whole person healing and self-healing/self-care measures; and joint evaluation of client movement toward wellness. Nurse–client interactions are based on the (apparent) paradox, "You alone do it, but you don't do it alone. There is no wellness practitioner but you, the individual person" (Pilch, p. 18). Thus, the nurse is not the person who stands back, assesses, plans, and evaluates,

Table 1. Comparison of Traditional Nursing Process and Wellness Nursing Process

Traditional nursing process	Wellness nursing process
Assess client	Model integrates whole person wellness for the client
	Teach client self-assessment procedures
Diagnose	Assess unique learning needs based on client belief systems
Set goals	Teach client to set wellness goals meaningful to him or her
Develop nursing care plan	Client develops plan of action with nurse facilitator and takes responsibility for carrying it out
Carry out nursing interventions	Teach client self-care and self-healing measures consistent with client beliefs
Evaluate results	Teach client to self-evaluate results

but a *facilitator* who teaches clients how to self-assess, decide on wellness goals, plan on actions to meet those goals, and self-evaluate success.

Wellness nursing deals with how the flow of energy between subsystems of mind/body/spirit is interrupted or blocked and how the flow of energy is reopened or rechanneled. The nurse facilitates the removal of obstacles to energy flow among subsystems, resulting in enhanced well-being and self-actualization of potentials.

The *wellness model* has implications for the nursing process. Table 1 examines these differences. Two essential behaviors of the nurse in a wellness model are role model and facilitator. Behaviors such as assessing, diagnosing, goal-setting and evaluating become less and less important as the nurse strives to teach *the client* to take responsibility for self-assessment, self-care, and self-evaluation.

Although this may seem a radical departure from traditional nursing practice, exploration proves this conclusion invalid. The systematic approach to problem solving remains intact; there is still an assessment, use of data base, intervention, and evaluation. What changes is *who* performs the steps in the procedure; in the traditional nursing model, the nurse performs many of the steps; in the wellness model, the client or the nurse and client collaborate to perform the steps.

Motivation is intrinsic to the model; the client is the one who chooses a goal of meaning to him or her; compliance becomes irrelevant because the client is responsible for decisions. The process of moving toward wellness is more important than the product, wellness. Table 2 com-

Table 2. Comparison of Health and Wellness: Process and Product

Wellness	Health
A *process* of moving toward greater awareness of oneself and the environment leading toward ever-increasing planned interactions with the dimensions of nutrition, fitness, stress, environment, interpersonal relationships and self-care responsibility.	A *state;* either it exists or it does not. Occurs throughout life between periods of illness and disease.
A *positive* striving; no guilt involved since the important factor is striving, not attainment.	*Guilt* or negative associations may be attached to not being able to measure up to states attained by others or prescribed by others.
Unique to the individual.	*An average;* primarily associated with the absence of disease.
Purposeful in direction, working to become the best one can be.	Thought to be severely *restricted* by factors such as age, race, genetics, etc.
The individual self-assesses the need for a wellness goal; the wellness practitioner acts as a facilitator for learning and change; individuals striving toward wellness may be medically uninteresting.	*An expert is consulted* and asked to provide an evaluation and prescription for what is needed to attain health.
Can be ill and still have wellness if there is a life purpose, and a deep appreciation for and joy of living.	*Illness and health are oppositional states.*

pares health and wellness in terms of process and product. Using the model may require that the nurse take on a different frame of reference. Ensuring that the patient does what is "good" for him or her becomes facilitating movement toward a goal chosen by the client. Such a change may require a change in belief systems by the nurse; therefore, the model suggests that nurses (as whole persons) also examine their belief systems for consistency, especially in terms of the model. Additionally, the model requires that nurses also be engaged in moving toward wellness by choosing, facilitating, and evaluating their own movement toward wellness goals.

Figure 1 exemplifies nurse–client interactions from a wellness perspective. In this model, both nurse and client are complete systems that interact within themselves [inputs, throughputs (activities within the system), and outputs], and interact with each other (intersystems) across interfaces to achieve jointly planned and achieved goals and feelings of well-being.

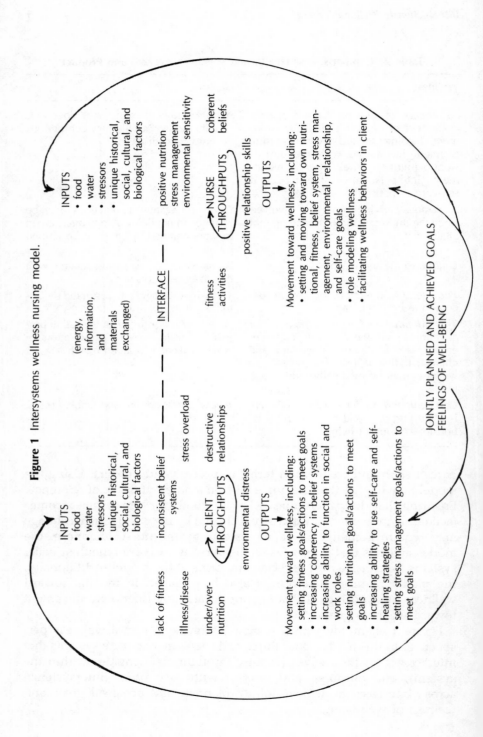

Figure 1 Intersystems wellness nursing model.

Figure 2 shows the relationships between biological, historical, social, and cultural factors, environment, and the whole person. The whole person evolves toward wellness by learning to:

- manage life experiences
- seek out challenges
- relate to others in a flexible, differentiated, assertive manner
- use self-care strategies
- examine and readjust beliefs and practices into an integrated, goal-directed whole
- develop coping strategies that produce success

During the evolutionary process of moving toward wellness, whole persons interact with stressors in a more rational, efficient way by perceiving and managing situations differently. Biological, historical, social and cultural factors can also be affected (and affect whole persons) in the process: for example, childhood perceptions that affect adult behaviors can be reevaluated and readjusted in adulthood; the immune system (genetic given) can be strengthened (or weakened) by using (or not using) self-care strategies. Table 3 identifies differences between wellness nursing practice and health education.

THE IMPORTANCE OF ARRIVING AT A STATED PURPOSE FOR NURSING THROUGH WELLNESS THEORY

If nursing is to seize control of its practice, a theory base is necessary. Theory can provide professional autonomy and a power base. Wellness theory may be the theoretical base that can unite nurses in their practice. Nurses have always said that their practice was based on health promotion, yet many of the terms used and practices observed are based on medical terms and practices and are disease-focused. Wellness nursing theory can support nursing practice that is consistently focused on health promotion. It can also increase cohesiveness among nurses by providing a broad base for practice. It can be argued that the profession that possesses theoretical knowledge about wellness is most likely to provide wellness-enhancing services for clients. As knowledge about wellness accrues in nursing, nurses will value their knowledge and find access to resources such as money, space, and people more readily. Additionally, arguments over the purpose of nursing would become less predominant and cohesiveness within the profession would increase.

Nurses who use a wellness theory base are on firmer ground when

Figure 2 Whole person wellness.

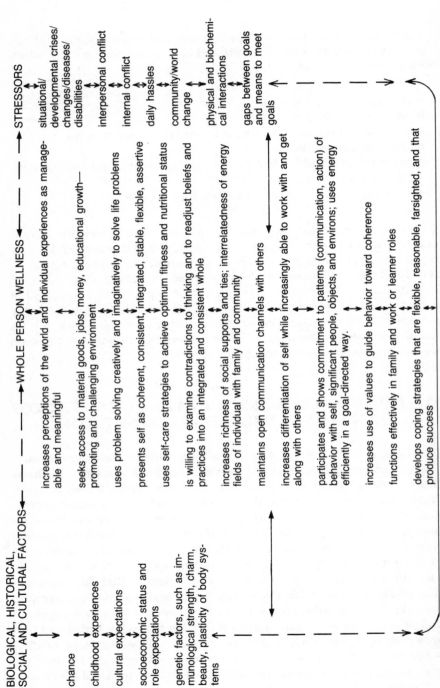

Source: This figure suggested by the work of Ahmed and Coehlho (*Toward a New Definition of Health*, Plenum, New York, 1979); Antonovsky (*Health, Stress and Coping*, Jossey Bass, San Francisco, 1979); and Dunn (*High Level Wellness*, Beatty, Arlington, VA, 1961.)

Table 3. Comparison of Wellness Nursing and Health Education

Wellness nursing	Health education
Concerned primarily with the quality of life and moving toward higher levels of wellness.	Emphasizes the prevention of disease through personal behavior change that reduces mortality or morbidity.
Focuses on the multidimensional, holistic nature of persons by focusing on life style rather than problem behaviors or risk factors, unless identified by the client as goals.	Seeks to reduce risk behavior, e.g., smoking.
Seeks to develop further self-development and self-actualization in all populations.	Focused on populations at risk.
Seeks to *teach* clients to: • set own wellness goals • locate own resources • plan own wellness activities • evaluate movement toward wellness • set new wellness goals	Provides information and motivation for behavior change based on educator's knowledge and goals.

Suggested by R. Petosa, "Wellness: An Emerging Opportunity for Health Education," *Health Education*, October/November, 1984, pp. 37–39.

their ideas are challenged (Chinn & Jacobs, 1983, p. 7). Imagine a physician who questions the nurse's use of imagery or affirmation for pain reduction. If the nurse's answer contains a rationale based on theory, the physician will be more apt to listen and may even defer to the nurse to handle clients with pain in the future. Without theory, nurses are on shaky ground when breaking away from the medical model and the tradition of following physician's orders.

Lack of coherence of purpose is everywhere in the literature and in real life situations. Nurses have difficulty agreeing on what it is we are about and how to arrive at an agreed upon purpose. Wellness theory can help nurses decide whether their purpose is (1) health restoration, (2) health maintenance, or (3) wellness.

On an even more basic level, perhaps, is the potential effect wellness theory and its application can have on nurses as human beings, and therefore on the quality of practice. O'Connor (1982) found that nursing leaders from many areas of practice who participated in her study were *most ineffective* (by self-report) in the following areas:

• communications, especially assertive communications
• management practices such as using authority to solve problems

- self-esteem
- interactions with nurse superiors and peers

Many, if not all, of these behaviors have correlations with and relevance for wellness. High self-esteem is basic to the other ineffective leader behaviors, just as it is to engaging in wellness behavior (Faber & Reinhardt, 1982; Schafer, 1979). A wellness orientation could be very useful for nurses who choose not to be wellness practitioners *per se*, but who need to enhance their leadership potential.

When nurses become wellness role models and take action to move toward wellness in their own lives, not only will they be a visible encouragement to clients and consumers, but they will have a greater potential for being effective leaders.

SOCIETAL FACTORS SUPPORTING THE USE OF WELLNESS NURSING THEORY AND PRACTICE

Convergence of nursing practice toward wellness theory will also result in a more relevant response to societal demands. There is growing disillusion with medical care as the treatment of choice for many. Consumers are becoming increasingly aware of the effect of life style on well-being and level of wellness. Self-care is deeply rooted in cultural tradition. Surveys indicate that more than 75% of all symptoms today are treated without professional assistance. The self-care movement is shifting the locus of decision making away from professional dominance and toward consumers (Barry et al., 1983).

A shift in the allocation of governmental funds and services is another sign that prevention and health promotion are of importance. For example, the Public Health Service has an Assistant Secretary for Disease Prevention and Health Promotion and a Director, Office of Health Information, Health Promotion, and Physical Fitness and Sports Medicine. The Centers for Disease Control (Atlanta, Georgia) have a relatively new Center for Health Promotion and Education and a Center for Prevention Services. The National Institute of Mental Health established a Center for Work and Mental Health in 1980; its work is to develop and test interventions aimed at improving productivity, job satisfaction, and health by reducing or preventing one or another form of stress in the workplace. The National Cancer Institute is beginning to focus on prevention; for example, in 1983 it announced requests for research grant applications for the Use of Self Help Strategies in Smoking Prevention and Cessation and Longitudinal Evaluation of School-Based Smoking Prevention Programs (NIH Guide for Grants and Contracts, July 15,

1983). In June of 1983, the National Center for Health Services Research announced its number one area of program interest as Health Promotion and Disease Prevention (NCHSR Program Notes, 1983). In 1984, a number of National Institutes solicited research related to the prevention and treatment of obesity. The National Cancer Institute requested grant proposals on the mechanisms by which overnutrition and obesity increase the risk of developing cancer, and on behavioral strategies to reduce dietary fat intake and their application to large population groups. The National Institute of Arthritis, Diabetes, and Digestive and Kidney Diseases requested applications related to the effect of mild exercise on appetite and its relationship to weight control. The National Institute of Child Health and Human Development was looking for behavioral intervention strategies to treat obesity in infancy, childhood, and adolescence (NIH Guide for Grants and Contracts, March 30, 1984). In 1982, The National Institute of Mental Health announced applications for the support of Preventive Intervention Research Centers to conduct research aimed at the prevention of mental illness (Special Research Grant Announcement, April, 1982). The National Institute on Aging has called for research to examine specific changes in life style or behavior that maintain health or prevent particular diseases; for ways of converting awareness of healthful practices into sustained behaviors; and for ways of coping with stress, ranging from "daily hassles" to life-threatening events (NIH Guide for Grants and Contracts, June 17, 1983). The National Heart, Lung, and Blood Institute, Preventive Cardiology Branch has encouraged grant proposals addressing the "identification of precursors and determinants of the development and maintenance of behaviors in children and adolescents conducive to cardiovascular health—sound nutrition, nonsmoking, physical activity, and other areas" (NIH Guide for Grants and Contracts, January 28, 1983).

Governmental funding is not the only kind of funding available for a change in lifestyle. For example, the Puget Sound Health Systems Agency of Seattle received a grant of $406,932 from the W.K. Kellogg Foundation to encourage local companies to promote healthier lifestyles at the workplace (News Release, Puget Sound Health Systems Agency, June 2, 1982).

Insurance companies have responded to accumulating evidence that lifestyle is the key to well-being and wellness by offering reduced premiums to nonsmokers and to those engaging in fitness programs. The Stay Well program offered by Blue Shield of California pays members to stay healthy by rewarding their policyholders with up to $500 if they do not use insurance coverage. The ideal is to have insurance reimbursement for wellness activities; however, providers are reluctant to pay until there is conclusive evidence that a specific weight loss or exercise program is appropriate for reimbursement. To date, some health insurance policies reimburse for health promotion services if ordered by a physician (Hosokawa, 1984). As more nurses qualify for third party reimbursement, they will be in a better position to be reimbursed for wellness nursing activities.

"Employee medical costs in American companies are rising so fast— 20% a year, compounded—that within eight years they will offset after-tax profits in the average large corporation" (Daniel, 1985). Because of this problem, many companies have begun to establish wellness programs for employees because these programs save money. Herzlinger, a professor of business administration at Harvard's Business School, counsels that business must "Go far beyond their largely token programs in disease prevention and health promotion into massive, action-oriented education for employees, their families and communities" (Daniel, 1985).

Herzlinger cautions that "Band-Aid" responses like Diagnostic Related Groups (DRGs) will simply inflate charges.

> You know, DRG's were tested in New Jersey, and the federal government wants to get out of the experiment there—chiefly because DRG's don't work . . . Heart disease costs us $65 billion a year. Add in cancer and arteriosclerosis and by conservative estimate the country spends $160 billion a year on disease highly correlated with life style. (Daniel, 1985)

Even the American Hospital Association (AHA) has jumped on the wellness band wagon. In 1978, the AHA created the Center for Health Promotion. By 1982, a representative of the AHA reported receiving 60 to 90 requests/month from hospitals for assistance in developing health promotion/wellness programs for businesses.

There is increasing evidence that educational, organizational, and environmental interventions can be effective in keeping people well and in preventing many chronic diseases. Wellness is also important in containing medical costs, in guiding consumers to use the health care system appropriately, to take a more active role in their own wellness, and to know what they are paying for when they receive medical and nursing services. If nursing can respond to the challenge, wellness may indeed be the focus of practice in the 1990s.

Despite the paucity of degree programs in wellness nursing, many nurses are functioning in roles as wellness facilitators, but without an adequate theory base. One of the problems in nursing education is that at the first level degree, there is barely sufficient time to learn the basics of illness nursing. By the time a nurse enters a master's degree program, a specialty area is chosen and wellness may not be a focus. Instead, the nurse may focus on mental health (of adults, children, or families), adult health, family nurse practitioner skills, etc. Probably the best place to learn wellness nursing at a basic (generalist) level is in an upper division baccalaureate nursing program or graduate program because students have already mastered illness nursing and are ready to learn new wellness skills and theory. As wellness nursing becomes more prevalent, nursing educators may begin to reduce the content in illness nursing in first degree nursing programs and focus on wellness concerns. Education for wellness nursing practice at an advanced and specialized level with clients and larger systems would occur at the graduate level.

DEFINITION OF TERMS AND THEIR RELEVANCE TO WELLNESS THEORY

Concepts can range from the empirical to the highly abstract (Chinn & Jacobs, 1983, p. 53). For example, height and weight are directly observable, and thus are relatively empirical concepts. Wellness cannot be directly observed and it is a relatively abstract concept; it must be inferred from other more observable concepts. Wellness is so abstract that it can be thought of as a *construct* (because it is constructed from multiple sources).

A primary purpose of this chapter is to develop a systematic view of the concepts and interrelationships among them so that eventually this view can be used to describe, explain, predict, and/or control nursing practice.

The model for nursing practice used in this book is a systems model: it is an organized set of dynamically interrelated parts. *Systems* exchange information, matter, and energy at the interface between systems. A homeodynamic state is developed from the interaction of elements within and between system(s). A variety of identifiable role patterns are developed from these interactions, including the individual or whole person, the family, the group, the community, and the organization. Systems have the inherent potential for change, which is actualized as interactions with the environment take place (Chin, 1961).

In the model, *whole persons* are conceptualized as energy systems of mind/body/spirit moving in a spiraling course through time and space from conception to infinity. Whole persons are in constant change as they move between and within dimensions toward and away from illness, disease, aggressive acts, and withdrawal. The spiral movement continues through time and space as whole persons evolve toward high level wellness and self-actualization. Whole persons are believed to have innate self-healing and self-repair abilities which may lie dormant or become blocked in the process of interrelating with the environment. Nurses and clients are examples of whole person systems; both can become *integrated* whole persons as they move toward wellness.

As a whole person, the nurse is also in constant flux between the dimensions of wellness. The nurse's role in assisting the client toward wellness is to:

- be an effective role model for wellness
- facilitate consistent client involvement in the assessment, implementation, and evaluation of wellness goals
- teach clients to perceive life experiences as manageable and meaningful by increasing self-responsibility and commitment to self-care
- teach and facilitate client self-care strategies to enhance fitness, nutritional status, stress management, positive relationship building, coherent belief systems, and their environment
- facilitate client creative problem solving to enhance wellness
- facilitate client assertive behavior
- teach clients effective communication skills
- assist clients to differentiate themselves from the nurse and significant others
- facilitate richness of client social supports
- facilitate effective learner, family, and work role behaviors in clients

Whole persons are in constant flux between fitness and lack of fitness; over/undernutrition; positive and negative/destructive relationships and positive, satisfying ones; stress management and stress overload/deprivation; clear life purpose, consistent belief systems, commitment to self-care and "giving up," inconsistent belief systems, lack of commitment to self-care; environmental distress/unawareness and environmental sensitivity/comfort. Each of these dimensions will be discussed in detail in subsequent chapters.

Wellness is a process of moving toward greater awareness of and satisfaction from engaging in activities that move the whole person toward fitness, positive nutrition, positive relationships, stress management, clear life purpose, consistent belief systems, commitment to self-care, and environmental sensitivity/comfort. The wellness process can be pursued by clients to prevent illness, facilitate rehabilitation, or enhance the quality of life and more fully actualize potential when ill, dying, or overcoming disability.

Differentiation of self is an important concept in the model; actualization of this concept enables a clear boundary development between the emotional and intellectual subsystems of a whole person, leading to enhanced problem-solving ability, flexibility in behavior, intimacy in relationships, and a higher level of wellness. *Pseudo-self*, or that which has not been processed through a value clarification process, is the part of a whole person at the whim of the emotional system of others and leads to manipulation of the whole person. *Solid self* increases as a consistency between beliefs, feelings, and actions is actualized through the value clarification process (Bowen, 1975). The value clarification process and its relationship to wellness are presented in detail in Chapter 2.

Environment is external to whole persons; it is a changing field that is continuous and contiguous with whole persons. Environment can be modified by whole persons as well as modify whole persons.

Self-care can be defined as those activities and programs whole persons perform for themselves. Dorothea Orem, a nurse theorist, includes the activities individuals personally initiate and perform on their own behalf in her definition of self-care (1980). Orem's concepts are of interest in wellness nursing as building blocks. However, in her framework, clients are viewed as "patients" (implying a dependent status), and there is no discussion of the *collaborative* efforts of nurse and client in the movement toward wellness, nor of the dynamic interchange of energies between client and nurse. For example, the energy exchanges at nurse and client interfaces are important to wellness nursing. Additionally, Orem seems primarily concerned with conforming to what is "normal" and resisting hazards to life and well-being than to self-actualization of nurse and client. Barry et al. (1979, p. 5) contend that *self-care* has been unclearly defined and can include such divergent activities and programs as:

- learning experiences teaching clients how to diagnose and treat common ailments
- groups which help consumers modify their lifestyles toward positive nutrition and to smoking and alcohol cessation
- teaching the chronically ill how to manage their conditions without the continual care of a physician or nurse
- lay-initiated clinics, especially women's clinics
- non-Western or otherwise nontraditional techniques, such as yoga, biofeedback, meditation, accupressure, and Tai-Chi

The wellness model presented in this book provides a middle ground definition of self-care; to the far right are those self-care programs which are initiated and developed within the nursing profession; at the other extreme are self-care activities developed in lieu of nursing services. In the model presented, the nurse is involved in self-care activities, but the decisions about goals, actions, and evaluation are the client's.

ASSUMPTIONS UNDERLYING THE WELLNESS MODEL

The wellness nursing model has been developed based on the following assumptions about whole persons, who:

- are capable of self-assessing their own wellness needs
- are capable of taking action to meet their wellness goals
- are capable of evaluating their progress toward wellness
- are in the process of moving toward wellness
- are capable of displaying characteristics of wellness even when ill, disabled, or dying
- have innate self-healing processes which can be activated to enhance wellness
- can learn to move to a higher level of wellness when facilitated by nurses well-grounded in wellness theory and practice
- can learn from modeling, clearly structured goals, means to meet those goals, and peer support.

BOUNDARIES OF WELLNESS THEORY

The boundary lines of a theory or model suggest that they are concerned with a particular area of inquiry, in this case, the intra- and interaction of the whole person and environment. *Boundaries* may be influenced to some extent by the restrictions of nurse attitudes and moral and cognitive complexity attainment.

According to Joyce and Weil (1972), a person at a high level of *cognitive complexity* is able to negotiate rules and take responsibility for his or her own learning and structure. Kohlberg (1975) speaks to the issue of moral development. Nurses must be at a high level of moral development in order to negotiate contracts with clients and respect the dignity of individuals. Although many nurses and nursing students may not have attained this level of functioning, moral reasoning and cognitive complexity can be influenced in the direction of higher levels by exposing people to them. As nurses are exposed to the next higher stage of reasoning, contradictions to the current level of reasoning can be identified in the value clarification process, discussed in Chapter 2.

Wellness theory is not restricted by level of health. Wellness theory is appropriate to persons who are ill, disabled, dying, or relatively well.

Wellness theory is not restricted by age or setting. School programs focusing on wellness and the knowledge of one's body are now being developed for very young children. Nurses who work with families in community settings can also affect the wellness of newborns and even fetuses by facilitating parent wellness.

This chapter has provided a conceptual basis for wellness nursing practice. Chapters 2 and 3 are transitional chapters; they are designed primarily to assist nurses to enhance their level of wellness and positive role model status. "Integrative Learning Experiences" at the end of this chapter and other chapters provide other avenues for enhancing wellness; some are most useful for nurses, while others can be used, or adapted for use, with clients.

Integrative Learning Experiences can assist you in putting into practice the concepts described in each chapter. Completing the experiences can help you move toward wellness; the process will also assist in understanding the process clients will need to pass through to move toward wellness. Once you have completed the experiences you can adapt them for use with clients. Beginning level experiences are most appropriate for the beginning wellness practitioner, e.g., B.S.N. students and practitioners who are relatively unfamiliar with wellness practice. Advanced level experiences are most appropriate for more advanced wellness practitioners, e.g., graduate students who are proficient in basic wellness nursing skills and advanced wellness practitioners.

INTEGRATIVE LEARNING EXPERIENCES

1. Set aside a notebook for journal writing. Always date your entries and write nonjudgmentally. After finishing an entry, read what was recorded and write any additional thoughts, avoiding judging what has been written. Use the following statements to explore wellness and you.
   A. Wellness is related to your purpose in life. Explore your life goal, your reason for living.
   B. Wellness is related to your idea of life's authentically satisfying and fulfilling human pleasures. Which of life's pleasures do you deny yourself? Cherish? Which ones give you the most pleasure? How do you get fun out of living? What else could you do to get more fun out of living? Do you want to get more fun out of living?
   C. Wellness hinges on your freedom to determine the course of your life; who runs your life? Are you able to make a free decision? Would you like to be freer? What is getting in your way of being freer? How can you overcome that obstacle?
   D. Wellness is related to your motivation. Explore how you get yourself started in wellness behaviors, how you keep it going, what you need from others to keep it going, and how you can

get what you need. Does your religion encourage you to practice wellness? What does your religion say about the body,
about relationships, etc.? How could you relate your religious
beliefs to wellness so they could provide support for practicing
wellness? Do you want to?

E. Wellness requires change. Explore how comfortable you are
with change in your life. Where in or on your body do you
locate your wellness and worseness? Does this change? Could
it? Under what conditions? What threatens your level of wellness, what lowers its level and what enhances it? What can you
do to enhance it? Write down wellness teachings from your
sacred literature; are these teachings reflected in your day-to-
day life? What changes would enhance these reflections? Do
you want to change them?

F. Wellness often depends on getting support for wellness behaviors. Discuss who has helped you move toward wellness
and the specifics of what that person or persons did to help.

G. Wellness may depend on reworking painful feelings and experiences so well-being can exist. How have you reworked painful feelings? What else could you do to rework them? Are you
ready to?

H. Wellness is related to integrating attachment to others with
separateness and differentiation of self. Do you "belong" to too
many others or things? Are you detached, engaged, seeking,
plugged-in, rooted, tied at the umbilical cord to someone or
something? Are you happy with your degree of attachment?
What would you want to change? How could you go about
changing? What is your index of separateness or differentiation? Do you have time and space for yourself? Do you want
more? How can you get it? Do you allow your inner world time
and space for imagination, fun, fantasy? Would you like to
allow it more? How can you? What do you need and how can
you get there? Are you ready to begin?

I. Wellness is related to a high degree of self-esteem. How have
you defined yourself till now? Are you comfortable with this
definition? Do you want to change it? What prevents you? How
can you overcome this?

J. Wellness depends on positive relationships with others. As
you write, it may become clear to you that you have specific
unfinished business with one or more other people in your life.
Write a dialogue with one or more of them about the unfinished business. When you are finished, reread the dialogue
and see what insights you have. Finally, decide whether you

want to open a dialogue with the person in real life. If so, set a time and place for doing so.

K. Wellness is related to your level of fitness; write about your fitness level.

L. Wellness is related to what you take into your body—food, chemicals, liquids, cigarette smoke, etc. Write about your level of nutrition.

M. Wellness is related to your environment; write about what in your environment affects you positively and negatively.

N. Wellness is related to your ability to stand up for your rights and assert yourself. Write about your level of assertiveness.

O. Wellness is related to your ability to manage stress; write about your stress management needs and skills.

P. Wellness is related to "quality of life." What specific things do you think increase your quality of life? What can you do to enhance your quality of living? What things can others do to enhance your quality of living? Are you ready to enhance your quality of living?

Write in your journal at least once a week. As you work, identify wellness goals for yourself. Prioritize them, choosing a goal that is attainable and that you are sure you are ready to pursue. Be sure your goal is specific and written in behavioral terms (e.g., practice assertive skill of broken record with Ms. Jones in clinical conference at least twice a week).

Find a peer at work (if possible) or someone you can talk to on the phone whenever it is necessary to obtain support and facilitation; writing notes to one another has also been shown effective. This person will be your peer facilitator.

- Write in your journal weekly about your movement toward wellness and your relationships with your peer facilitator.
- Choose one specific wellness goal and write it in behavioral terms in your journal. Examine your readiness and motivation for choosing that goal. If you are not ready to work on the goal or are motivated to work on it because you think you "should" rather than because you want to, choose another goal.
- Write down four specific actions (using behavioral indicants) you plan to take to meet your wellness goal.
- Discuss your goal with your peer facilitator; be sure your goal is appropriate for you and specific enough.
- Write in your journal about ways you might try to sabotage yourself from attaining your goal; write down observable actions you will take to make sure you avoid sabotaging yourself.

• Write down any questions you have or assistance you want from your peer facilitator and share this information with him or her. Be sure to make a specific plan to meet, talk on the telephone or write to one another weekly so you can attain your goal.
• Each week, write in your journal concerning progress made, how your peer has been helpful or unhelpful and share the information with your peer facilitator each week.

(This exercise was developed by adapting material from the following sources: Pilch, John J. *Wellness, Your Invitation to a Full Life.* Minneapolis, MN: Winston Press, 1981; and Progoff, Ira. *At a Journal Workshop, The Basic Text and Guide for Using the Intensive Journal.* New York: Dialogue House Library, 1975; and empirical experiences teaching nurses to develop personal wellness goals.)

2. Identify a situation when you felt challenged by a physician. Close your eyes and imagine yourself handling the interaction by remaining relaxed and confident, and giving a rationale for your nursing actions based on a wellness conceptual model.

3. Write in your journal about your feelings and thoughts about seizing control of nursing practice.

4. Write in your journal about your current or potential status as a wellness role model. What would you have to do to be one? In what ways are you already?

5. Brainstorm with your peer facilitator about how nursing can get "a piece of the funding action," or with a client about how consumers can have a greater voice in funding decisions.

6. Write a critique of the wellness model presented in this chapter, including ideas about how concepts need further refinement, etc. Make some efforts at refining the model.

7. Compare and contrast your ideas about self care with those presented in this chapter. What would you have to do to accept the concept as presented here?

REFERENCES

Barry, P., et al. (1979). *Self-Care Programs: Their Role and Potential.* Chapel Hill, NC: The University of North Carolina.
Bowen, M. (1975). *Family Theory in Clinical Practice.* New York: Jason Aronson.
Chinn, R. (1961). The utility of systems models and developmental models for practitioners. In *The Planning of Change*, Bennis, W., Benne, K., and Chin, R. Eds. New York: Holt, Rinehart and Winston.

Chinn, P., and Jacobs, M. (1983). *Theory and Nursing, A Systematic Approach.* St. Louis: C.V. Mosby.

Daniel, J. (1985). Health costs: why the blue chips see red. *American Health* (January/February). 4(1):74–89.

Faber, M., and Reinhardt, A. (1982). *Promoting Health Through Risk Reduction.* New York: Macmillan.

Hosokawa, M. (1984). Insurance incentives for health promotion. *Health Education* (October/November):9–12.

Joyce, B., and Weil, M. (1972). *Models of Teaching.* Englewood Cliffs, NJ: Prentice-Hall.

Kohlberg, L. (1975). The cognitive-developmental approach to moral education. *Phi Delta Kappan* 56(10):670–677.

NCHSR Program Notes (1983). Rockville, MD: National Center for Health Services Research, June.

News Release (1982). Seattle, WA: Puget Sound Health Systems Agency, June 2.

NIH Guide for Grants and Contracts (1983 and 1984). Washington, D.C.

O'Connor, A. (1982). Educating nursing's leaders: agenda for action. *Nursing Leadership* (December) 5(4):4–8.

Orem, D. (1980). *Nursing: Concepts of Practice.* New York: McGraw-Hill, pp. 42–47.

Pilch, J. (1981). *Wellness: Your Invitation to a Full Life.* Minneapolis, MN: Winston Press.

Schafer, R. (1979). The self-concept factor in diet selection and quality. *Journal of Nutrition Education* 11:37–39.

2

BEGINNING TO MOVE
TOWARD WELLNESS

This chapter explores the following topics and their relationship to wellness:

- Differentiation of self
- Value clarification
- Centering
- Facilitating movement toward wellness

As role models for wellness, nurses learn to differentiate intellectual from emotional systems and take on a wellness value system. Theory and procedures for accomplishing this task, suggestions for use with clients, and additional procedures for facilitating client wellness are presented in this chapter.

DIFFERENTIATION OF SELF

Bowen suggests there are emotional and intellectual systems in the brain; these two centers are probably connected by neural tracts, but there is variation among people in the connections. At a low level of differentiation the *intellectual* center (which allows people to think about their lives and plan and control their behavior) is not well differentiated from the *emotional* center. At a high level of differentiation, the intellectual center is well developed and screens stimuli from the emotional center. People who are less well differentiated have a high level of fusion between their emotional and intellectual systems, with the latter controlling decisions and behavior (Bowen, 1978).

Bowen uses the term *differentiation* to refer to the degree to which the intellectual system is differentiated from the emotional system as well as to explain the extent to which people are differentiated from each other in their emotional relationship system. (Miller, 1982, p. 19)

Although Bowen considers people to be on a continuum from low level differentiation to high level differentiation, it may be more useful to consider people as moving back and forth between various levels, depending on the amount of anxiety they are experiencing; high levels of anxiety short circuit the intellectual system and lead to overly emotional responses. For example, when experiencing anxiety, nurses may over-react to a situation; their emotional systems take precedence over their intellectual systems and perceptions, and self-talk similar to the following might occur: "Oh, oh, time to panic!" or "I can't handle this, I'd better get out of here" or "How dare she say that!"

If nurses are at a higher level of differentiation, the intellectual system screens noxious stimuli, and thoughts and perceptions may be more like the following: "Keep calm," "I can handle this," "What am I getting so excited about? This isn't the end of the world; I can handle this."

It is clear that responding at a lower level of differentiation is more likely to be associated with increased stress, fatigue and burnout; thus, measures to enhance relaxation and decrease stress can enhance level of differentiation, e.g., centering and measures discussed in Chapters 3, 4, and 5.

Some signs that are associated with low level differentiation during stressful situations with clients include increased blood pressure, pulse, and respiration, and decreased ability to focus on the work at hand. (Physiological correlates of high anxiety and lack of the relaxation response have been known for many years. See Peplau, 1952; Selye, 1956, 1974; Simmons, 1950; and Wolff, 1953, among many others.)

CASE STUDY: *Staff Nurse Mary S. Demonstrates a Low Level*
of Differentiation

Mary S., an experienced staff nurse on ICU, was working with Mr. White, who was hospitalized on that unit. His family was visiting at the time and the physician was also in attendance. Suddenly, a new staff nurse appeared in the room, marched up to Mary S., and stated very loudly: "What are you doing!? You're doing that wrong! Let me show you how to do it right!" Mary S. turned beet red, experienced rage sufficient to trigger murder, and asked the other nurse to step outside. What happened next remains censored. Had Mary S. remained differentiated, she would have been able to perceive that the new graduate was seeking to meet her own needs, albeit in a somewhat hostile manner. Instead, Mary S. responded to the comment in an emotionally overreactive way and experienced increased stress.

CASE STUDY: *Staff Nurse Mary S. Moves to a Higher Level*
of Differentiation
Mary S. brought the above example to class the following evening and was
able to identify how angry she had become and how the anger was blocking
her from collaborating with the new staff nurse. The class was able to help
Mary see how her anger had led to an undifferentiated response, and suggested she go out and hit a tennis ball (her favorite sport) until her anger had
been dissipated. They also suggested she write in her wellness journal and
explore her anger more deeply. The next week Mary S. came to the seminar all
smiles and reported that the staff nurse had "pulled a similar maneuver, but I
remained calm and introduced her to the physician as 'our new staff nurse,
Ms. Whitney.' " The class applauded and congratulated Mary on her movement toward wellness.

When families demonstrate a *low level of differentiation*, there is a
tendency for two or more family members to act (emotionally) as one.
They may have difficulty differentiating their feelings and show anger
(or other feelings) if another family member does, or try to live through
one another by controlling life choices or events. Bowen refers to this
phenomenon as "fusion" (1978). A family with a high level of fusion
does not permit self-actualization in individuals. Nurses using a wellness framework for practice seek to increase differentiation of self in
themselves and in their clients.

Becoming differentiated is a lifelong process requiring commitment
and ongoing evaluation of movement. Bowen notes that the more differentiated one is, the more *solid self* one has:

The solid self is made up of clearly defined beliefs, opinions, convictions,
and life principles. These are incorporated into self from one's own life
experiences by a process of intellectual reasoning and careful considering of
the alternatives involved in each choice. In making a choice, one becomes
responsible for self and the consequences. Each belief and life principle is
consistent with all the others, and self will take action on the principles even
in situations of high anxiety and duress. (1978, p. 365)

In family systems theory, the ability to make a responsible decision or
choice is called the "I position." The pseudo-self has not been acquired
through conscious consideration; people who have more pseudo- than
solid self guide their reactions by emotional shifts in their relationships,
and may see others only as resources for meeting their needs (Miller,
1982, p. 20).

Bowen developed a profile of differentiation from low (basing decisions on feeling responses, being comfortable and loved, and reducing
anxiety) to high. At the low level of differentiation, chronic dysfunction,

high dependency on others, living by moving from one crisis to another, and institutionalization are found.

At the *moderate level of differentiation*, people are more able to function (as in work settings), but life pursuits are focused on relationship systems. Pleasing the teacher or the boss or gaining relationship status from one who knows is more important than learning subject matter or the quality or value of the work itself. Pseudo-self may be large; principles and beliefs may be a helter skelter assortment of ideas collected under the pressure of pleasing others. "They may master academic knowledge, but they are unable to use this knowledge in intense relationships" (Miller, 1982, p. 21). Some characteristic behaviors noted in people at a moderate level of differentiation include the tendency to be a rebel or a disciple, to search for the perfect relationship and to fuse or distance oneself emotionally (due to increased anxiety about intimacy) when a relationship is found.

The *moderate to good level of differentiation* is characterized by the ability to make decisions not dominated by the emotions; although outbursts may occur, during periods of calm the ability to reason is used to develop principles and beliefs that are then used to overcome automatic, emotional responses in situations of high anxiety; lives are orderly because there is energy available to plan; relationships are freer because solid self does not fuse with the self of the other person and create anxiety; marriage is a functional partnership; intimacy is possible because fear of loss of self is not a threat; all family members take responsibility for their behavior and decisions rather than blaming one another for their failures or crediting one another for successes; there is no need to attack one another's beliefs or principles; people are able to develop life goals based on their own interests, not someone else's (Miller, 1982, pp. 22–23).

The *highest level of differentiation* may be more hypothetical than real. At this level, people are the most free to engage in intense emotional responses because they are not compelled to react in a specific way; choice is available. There is the greatest freedom from automatic reactions and the least tension when relating with others (Miller, 1982, pp. 23–24). Nurses can encourage differentiation in themselves by learning and practicing centering, assertiveness, and stress reduction procedures; they can encourage differentiation to the client by teaching them these measures and encouraging them to use them.

Differentiation of self affects the ability to parent. Samaroff (1980) describes the differentiation of self in parenting from *symbiotic* (low differentiation) to *perspectivistic* (high differentiation):

1. *Symbiotic:* There is no separation of the other's responses from one's own, e.g., "You are angry because I am."
2. *Categorical:* Traits and characteristics of the child are viewed as separate from those of the parents, e.g., "The child is stubborn," "My boss is stupid," "The teacher is unfair."
3. *Compensating:* Traits are viewed as age-related, e.g., "The child is stubborn because he or she is a toddler," "Jane is rebellious because she is a teenager."
4. *Perspectivistic:* Behavior stems from individual experiences in specific environments, e.g., "Jeremy, perhaps you behaved that way because you were with friends who egged you on."

People who show lower levels of differentiation tend to get drawn into rigid three-person *triangles*.

A triangle works as follows: two people are involved in a relationship of emotional significance; anxiety or stress builds up between them; and another person, issue or object is pulled in to decrease discomfort. (Miller, 1982, p. 26)

Triangles occur in all families (and in other social and work situations in which there is high anxiety). In the less-differentiated family or person, triangles are more rigid and more automatic. Here are some typical triangles:

1. Husband and wife plan a vacation without their child; child becomes ill. More-differentiated couples can cope with conflicting demands and roles and will problem solve to meet all role relationships satisfactorily. Less-differentiated couples will sacrifice one role, usually the husband–wife one, to focus on the child.
2. Partners have an argument. In less-differentiated families, one partner may form a triangle by pulling in the child (and complaining or arguing with him or her), their job, or school ("And if you hadn't gone back to school, we wouldn't have this problem"), or some other object or person, including in-laws, alcohol, drugs, or food. In more-differentiated families, partners will stick to the issue of the argument and find a way to resolve it that suits both people.
3. A client is anxious about his or her ability to get answers from his or her physician and triangles in the nurse to talk to the doctor. Variants on this triangle are 1) a nurse who questions her ability and triangles in the physician, and 2) a physician who questions his ability to talk with the client—about the impending death of a client or other highly charged issues—and triangles in the nurse to do his talking for him.

4. There is a change in a work or school system, such as the hiring or firing of a new boss or the introduction of a new procedure, such as primary nursing accreditation, or a new curriculum without sufficient collaboration with those involved. As stress in the work or school system increases, others (usually those with less power) are triangled in; students may be criticized, nurses' aides scapegoated; nurses may triangle in physicians when uncomfortable about the client's reactions; supervisors may battle with one another, leaving the nurse in the middle; or stress may appear in the form of illness in an important system member.

CASE STUDY: *Low Level of Differentiation in the White Family*
Ms. White lives with her two children, Jeremy, aged 1, and Jessica, aged 2 months. Birth control methods were explained to Ms. White after her last pregnancy, but she feels like a "somebody" when she invests love in caring for her children, and so became pregnant again. She is constantly with the children and anticipates their every need, frequently assuming their feelings; for example, she covered Jessica's head with a towel one day, "because she was angry with me." Whenever Jeremy tries to assert his independence, his mother starts talking about Jessica.

CASE STUDY: *A Nurse with a Moderate Level of Differentiation*
Nancy K. is working toward her baccalaureate degree in nursing. She has been married for 10 years, but feels isolated from her husband: "I always expected Joe would be my knight in shining armor, but now I'm not so sure he is." Nancy and Joe have two teenage daughters who are "going through that rebellious stage." Nancy was devastated at school the other day when she got a paper back with a C on it, and she exclaimed: "How could I get a C when I worked so hard and learned so much doing it! Can't I ever please that teacher?"

CASE STUDY: *A Family at a Good Level of Differentiation*
The Mays have encountered many stressors lately, and they have been arguing more often than usual, but when the storm is over, they are able to think and talk about the issues and to come to an understanding. The parents, Barb and Jo May, have a close relationship and they go to dinner and dancing once a week and take the children on a weekend trip every week. All three children are responsible for specific chores and are expected to develop their own life interests. Every Wednesday evening, the Mays have a family meeting to share problems and achievements, and to disagree with each other without attacking. The family members describe themselves as "happy" and they have few colds and other illnesses.

In addition to understanding what issues trigger anxiety in specific situations, it is important to maintain an "I" position or a good level of differentiation of self. There are a number of measures that nurses can take to increase their level of differentiation, including value clarification and centering.

VALUE CLARIFICATION

Value clarification can assist nurses and clients to develop larger portions of solid self, and thus become more differentiated. The steps of value clarification and their attendant processes are the following (Raths et al., 1966, pp. 63–65; Kirschenbaum and Simon, 1974, pp. 264–266; Kirschenbaum, 1975, pp. 102–104).

Prizing

1. Prizing and cherishing. At this step in the process, nurses learn to set priorities, become aware of what they are for or against, begin to trust their inner experiences and feelings, and examine why they feel as they do.
2. Clearly communicating one's values and actively listening to others'.

Choosing

1. Choosing freely by examining values others have imposed on them.
2. Choosing thoughtfully between alternatives by examining the process by which they choose, and considering the possible consequences of each choice.

Acting

1. Trying out the value choice includes developing a plan of action and trying it out; contracts to act may be drawn up between the nurse and self or others.
2. Evaluating what happened when action was taken and making plans to reinforce actions that support their values. (Integrated Learning Experiences, Beginning Level, p. 54, Nos. 6–11, provide value clarification experiences for each value clarification process; they can be adapted for use with clients.)

CASE STUDY: *Clarifying Values about Assertiveness Issues*
All students in the nursing seminar were asked to bring an assertiveness issue that they wanted to work on to class. (Choosing freely) The instructor helped each student discuss why he or she might want or not want to be assertive in a situation brought to class. (Prizing and Cherishing; Examining alternatives and consequences of action) Students selected another student to pair up so as to practice role playing the assertiveness situation. Some students decided to contract with one another to try out the situation in real life and to receive

positive reinforcement from one another for doing so. (Trying out; contracting; reinforcing change). All students were encouraged to try their new assertive behaviors out in real life situations and to report back to the class by evaluating their performance. (Evaluating)

CASE STUDY: *Assisting a Client to Clarify His Values*

Theresa F., a community health nursing student, was working with Mr. Thomas, who was recovering from a myocardial infarct. Mr. Thomas was overweight and smoked a pack of cigarettes a day. Although Theresa's first impulse was to tell him to quit smoking and lose weight, she restrained herself and decided to try value clarification instead. One of their conversations follows:

NURSE: What kinds of things about yourself are you most concerned about?

CLIENT: I'm afraid I'll have another heart attack. (choosing freely)

NURSE: Anything else? (encouraging choosing from alternatives)

CLIENT: My wife's nagging; she's always trying to get me to stay on a diet, but at the same time, she bakes cakes and pies!

NURSE: Perhaps we should get your wife in here too to work on this. (Goes out and brings wife into the room.)
Your husband was just telling me about your concerns about his staying on a diet.

WIFE: The doctor told him to lose weight and I try, but he's always sneaking goodies.

NURSE: Are you interested in losing weight, Mr. Thomas?

CLIENT: Well, if it would make my wife happy . . .

NURSE: I'm wondering what would make you happy.

CLIENT: Not having a heart attack again.

NURSE: What do you know about preventing a heart attack?

CLIENT: The doctor says losing weight, exercising regularly, and stopping smoking, but it seems like a lot to me.

NURSE: What if you could choose one of those to begin with; which would it be?

CLIENT: Exercising. I've always been active in construction and baseball until this heart attack laid me low.

NURSE: Suppose we find an exercise plan for you and your wife agrees to exercise with you? How does that sound?

CLIENT: Sounds good to me, but can you get her to stop nagging me?

NURSE: I can teach you both how to support each other without nagging. We can start by using assertiveness skills such as "I" messages and other communication skills that have been found useful by some of my other clients. How does the plan sound to you, Mrs. Thomas?

WIFE: O.K. I guess.

(Discussion continues as nurse proceeds through rest of value clarification processes and makes plans with the couple to try out new behaviors and evaluate them.)

CENTERING

Centering refers to

finding within oneself an inner reference of stability . . . a sense of self-relatedness that can be thought of as a place of inner being, a place of quietude within oneself where one can feel truly integrated, unified and focused. (Krieger, 1979, pp. 35–36)

Centering is a powerful, easily achieved skill for enhancing differentiation of self and thereby freeing nurses from becoming too personally identified with the client's life issues. When nurses are not centered, they are apt to feel fatigued, stressed, depressed, or angry when working with a client who displays these qualities. Centering allows the nurse to be separate from yet open to input from clients. By differentiating oneself from clients through the act of centering, many blocks to listening drop by the wayside, including:

- *Comparing* (only partially listening to clients because of trying to assess who is smarter, more competent, more emotionally healthy, or suffering more)
- *Mind Reading* (not paying attention to what is being communicated; trying to figure out what the client is *really* thinking and feeling, rather than listening closely to what is being said)
- *Rehearsing* (not listening because of rehearsing what to say next; some people rehearse whole chains of responses, e.g., "I'll say, then he'll say, then I'll say")
- *Filtering* (listening to only part of what is said, e.g., what will relieve the guilt, threat, or unpleasantness)
- *Judging* (not paying attention because the client's comments have already been labeled as stupid, nuts, or unqualified)
- *Dreaming* (not listening because the client says something that triggers a chain of private associations)
- *Identifying* (taking what the client says and referring it back to one's own experience, e.g., his pain reminds you of yours)
- *Advising* (not listening for a full expression of the issue, or acknowledging the other's pain prior to suggesting what one should do)
- *Sparring* (looking for ways to disagree, discount, or put down what the other person says)
- *Being Right* (unable to listen to criticism because mistakes cannot be acknowledged)
- *Derailing* (changing the subject when bored or uncomfortable; joking or quipping is a common derailing technique)
- *Placating* (agreeing with everything to be pleasant and nice)

(McKay, Davis, & Fanning, 1983, pp. 16–19)

As a center of stability is achieved through centering, these blocks to communication are not necessary and real listening can occur.

Centering can be achieved while standing or sitting, but beginning efforts produce the best results in a sitting position.

1. Sit in a comfortable chair with feet flat on the floor and hands resting quietly in your lap; close your eyes.
2. Check out your body for tension spots and relax these areas as you exhale.
3. Inhale easily, filling your body with relaxation.
4. Exhale, moving your breathing to your center, about the level of your navel.
5. Continue breathing in this manner until you feel calm, integrated, unified, and focused.
6. (Optional) Picture the body surrounded by a protective shield that allows positive energy in, but keeps negative energy out. The shield may be conceived as a color, light source, or spiritual sense.

Centering takes little time once the idea is mastered. Nurses have reported to the author the following ways of using centering:

- "I take a moment, go to the rest room, and get centered between clients."
- "I center myself as I'm walking down the hall on the way to my next client."
- "I center myself when I'm with the client; I ask the client to center herself or himself and we do it together. I find we both have a lot more energy to concentrate on the tasks ahead when we do."

Clients can also be taught to use centering. For example, they may find it helpful to use prior to any anxiety-provoking situation in the hospital, at home, in social situations, or at work. The steps in centering remain the same. Directions given for the nurse can be copied or adapted for use with clients.

CASE STUDY: *A New Director of Nursing*

Dr. Jones (R.N., Ph.D.) is the new director of nursing at Berrymount Hospital. The assistant director of nursing has recently started meeting with the nursing supervisors to determine how to punish the nurses' aides for their low level of functioning. Ed Bart, the clinical specialist in mental health nursing, has begun to teach classes on centering to all nursing personnel because he believes the nurses' aides are being triangled in by the assistant director to lower anxiety about the new director. He is determined that he will not add anxiety to the system and maintains an "I" position when at work. As Ed began working with the nursing personnel, he found the aides appeared less stressed and the nursing supervisors started to talk about plans for working more effectively with Dr. Jones. As the Assistant Director became curious about the approach and learned how to center, she was able to focus on the effect of the change on everyone's behavior rather than exaggerating the aides' behavior.

FACILITATING MOVEMENT TOWARD WELLNESS

Once nurses have attempted to raise their level of differentiation through centering and value clarification, they are ready to proceed with clients. Facilitating movement toward wellness with others includes the use of a number of approaches: evaluating the effect of change toward wellness, resistance to and readiness for change, and use of contracting, self-assessments, belief scales, imagery, structured relaxation, affirmation, and neurolinguistic programming.

Evaluating the Effect of the Proposed Change

Movement toward wellness requires change. One reason people resist change is because the new is unfamiliar. If movement toward wellness is viewed as a threat to current status, existing ways of life, job, or money, familiar habits, or autonomy or free will, resistance to change can be expected. When facilitating movement toward wellness, it is useful to ask the following questions:

- What other factors in the persons' life will be affected as a result of changing?
- What forces are operating to inhibit change at this time?
- What information or experiences must precede the change?
- What new procedures or experiences will need to be developed as a result of the change?
- Who is likely to suffer from the change?
- How will power, influence, custom, or life-style be affected by the change?
- How aware is the client of the need for change or of its purpose?
- Is the client sufficiently involved in planning for the change?
- What past experiences between the nurse and the client might be influencing resistance to change now?
- How open has the client been to the introduction of change in the past?

The best developed model for assessing readiness for change is the *Health Belief Model.* It is used to predict the likelihood that individuals will seek help or change behavior in order to avoid illness. The model asserts that even when individuals recognize personal susceptibility they will not take action unless they believe illness would bring serious physical or social repercussions. The Health Belief Model is based on the idea of avoiding negatively-valued outcomes or personal threats, such as illness disability, nonproductivity, discomfort, and death. It is questionable to what extent a model based on avoidance is adequate to explain self-actualization and maximalization of potential.

Pender (1982, p. 66) has developed a *Health Promotion Model* based on a synthesis of the wellness and health promotion literature. In Pender's Model, individual factors [importance of health/wellness, perceived control, desire for competence, self-awareness, self-esteem, definition of health (actualization vs. stabilization), perceived health status, and perceived benefits of health-promoting behaviors] interact with modifying factors (demographic variables such as age, race, sex, ethnicity, education, income), interpersonal variables (expectations of significant others, including health care professionals), situational variables (prior experience with health promotion and options available), perceived barriers (unavailability, cost, inconvenience, extent of life change required), and cues to action (advice from others, mass media, awareness of potential for change and growth) to influence the likelihood of behavior change.

A factor to assess when examining client responsibility is the level of dissatisfaction with current life style and the readiness for change. A client who is constantly slightly depressed and lacking in energy and who has tried all medical treatments may be dissatisfied enough to be ready to try jogging or another form of exercise as a treatment. Another client who has tried all the fad diets available in an effort to lose weight may be ready to try a long-term weight management program if it seems enticing and if support is provided. Another client who is in chronic pain that is not touched by strong medication may be willing to learn self-hypnosis as a last resort.

There may be a number of times clients are most open to taking responsibility for wellness. One is childhood. This is an age when beliefs about illness and wellness may not yet be well formed. It has been suggested that a major health education effort be mounted in the nation's school systems to enhance wellness (Conference on Future Directions in Health Care, 1975).

Another time of openness is the mid-life crisis, ages 35–45. At this time, people begin to see they are alone, mortal, and are searching for internal, not institutional, validation. It is a time when people can move out of roles defined by others and into their self-fulfillment (Sheehy, 1974).

There may be other times when people are open to taking responsibility for their wellness. Times of crisis are times when change is possible and clients may be more willing to accept responsibility or to try a change in life style.

Decreasing Resistance to Change

Once sources of resistance to change have been identified, steps can be taken to reduce it. If anxiety or threat are the source of resistance to change, clients can be taught to practice centering.

Resistance to change will be decreased if rewards for changing are given and problem solving is used. The first step in learning more effective behavior is to identify the behavior to be changed. Behavior is an action, not a feeling, attitude, or mood. Behaviors must be pinpointed and expressed in such a way that they can be counted. Table 4 shows examples of behaviors that can and cannot be counted.

Once the behavior is expressed in countable terms, *baseline data* can be gathered. These data consist of information gathered prior to treatment; the pinpointed behavior is counted or measured to see how often it occurs now. These data can be charted and hung in the client's home or elsewhere, and can be recorded on the treatment chart, in the client's journal, or wherever agreed upon. Data from this "before" or baseline phase can be used later to check progress toward the goal. There are a number of ways to count behavior: frequency, rate over time, or how long the behavior continues. The method used to count depends on the behavior. For example, the frequency method might be best for participating in relaxation exercises, the rate over time to measure weight gain or loss, and the duration method to measure jogging. A notebook, graph, chart, or journal can be used to gather baseline data.

Table 4. Examples of Behaviors That Can and Cannot Be Counted

Countable behaviors	Noncountable behaviors (general behaviors or internal states)
Jogging	Being neat
Brushing and flossing teeth	Being motivated
Drinking fluids	Being angry
Losing weight	Being depressed
Gaining weight	Feeling guilty
Smoking a cigarette	Improving communication
Practicing relaxation exercises	Being noncompliant
Attending yoga class	Grieving
Eating complex carbohydrates	Being hostile

The next step in increasing desirable behavior is to find out what is rewarding and depriving to the particular client. Table 5 shows reinforcers for a student who was chronically late to class. Clients, too, can be asked to make such a list. There are some nearly universal rewards such as attention, smiles, praise, and candy or other sweets. If the client is unable to state a reward, a universal reward can be used or the chart can be read to find hints. Of course, giving sweets to someone with diabetes or who wants to lose weight would be self-defeating. A reward cannot be used if control cannot be established over when the reinforcer is dispensed. For example, if a family lets a child watch TV whether or not the child participates in family meetings, watching TV cannot be used as a reward for the child's participation in family meetings. If the client is hospitalized, more rewards can be controlled. If the client is at home, fewer rewards are under nursing control. It is wise to enlist the aid of families, other personnel, and whoever it is who dispenses rewards; the best way to do this is to reward them for helping by giving them attention, not scolding them when they do not comply, and by using whatever other things seem to be rewarding to them. When operating from a wellness framework, keep in mind that self-modification or client choice in applying behavior modification principles and voluntary changes in selected aspects of their own behavior is the focus, not changing the behavior of others through the manipulation of rewards and punishments (Pender, 1985, p. 80).

In order to increase the occurrence of a goal-directed behavior, the reward must immediately follow movement toward that behavior. Giving the client words of praise 2 days after he or she walked around the block is less likely to increase walking behavior than praising right after the walk.

In some cases it may be unrealistic or impossible to provide the reinforcer immediately following the occurrence of the goal-directed behavior. In that case, a written contract, wall chart, token system, or some other method can be used to indicate a reward is due. For ex-

Table 5. Reinforcers for One Student

Positive, rewarding reinforcers	Negative, depriving reinforcers
Eating ice cream	Watching cartoons
Seeing a movie	Working overtime
Sleeping late on weekends	Being reminded that I'm late
Talking with other nurses	Doing dishes
Going dancing	Doing reports
Reading mysteries	Eating cottage cheese

ample, a wall chart could be used to show participation in planned exercise. A mark could be used to indicate 30 minutes of TV time or crossword puzzle work that could be collected that evening or on the weekend for each time 30 minutes of exercise is accomplished. Or, clients can be given tokens to indicate completion of a behavior; a specified number of tokens can be used to purchase a reward.

Some desired behaviors may occur at random or very rarely. In those cases, shaping techniques to reinforce approximations to the target behavior can be used. For example, telling the client the exact words to say and then praising the behavior, or asking the client to avoid smiling when talking are ways of *shaping behavior*. When shaping client behavior, nurses act as sculptors, helping clients to approximate the behavior that will be successful for them.

CASE STUDY: *Helping a Client Start an Exercise Program*

Mr. Sconce had just been discharged from the hospital and had been advised to begin an exercise program by his physician. The client revealed his anxiety about beginning such a program to the nurse, Ms. Joshua. The nurse began by listing the steps in an exercise program (learn how to take pulse, learn warm-up and cool down exercises, choose a suitable type of exercise, set up rewards and a way to chart movement toward exercise goal). Next, the nurse demonstrated the steps, ignoring any statements of fear of failure and praising any positive attempts. (The use of the negative reinforcer of not commenting verbally or nonverbally on fears will extinguish that behavior in time if used consistently.) Next, Ms. Joshua asked Mr. Sconce to copy what she did, and praised him for each step successfully completed. Ms. Joshua also enlisted Mrs. Sconce in the effort and both client and spouse soon were actively engaged in a walking program together. Ms. Joshua taught the Sconces how to make a contract with one another for changing behavior. Table 6 shows the contract the Sconces used.

Whether nurses work with clients, peers, family members, or self-contracts to achieve wellness goals, the *contracting process* remains the same:

1. *Mutual exploration of wellness interests.* Questions to ask include: Is this goal realistic for me now? Why is this goal being chosen now? Has this goal been chosen before and what were the results, things learned, barriers encountered? Does this goal have a high personal priority or was it chosen to please others? How appropriate is this goal now? How specifically written is the goal? Has only one goal been chosen?

NOTE: The more specific, realistic, appropriate, and attainable the goal, the more likely it is to be attained; be sure only one goal is worked on at a time.

Table 6. A Behavioral Contract for Mr. and Mrs. Sconce

Wellness Goal: To walk briskly for 30 minutes every day

I, Adolph Sconce, promise to walk briskly with Edith Sconce 30 minutes every day for a period of 2 weeks, whereupon Edith and I will treat ourselves to a movie. I understand that if I do not fulfill this contract, the designated reward (movie) will be withheld.

Signed: _____
                               (Client)

_____
(Facilitator)

_____
(Nurse)

_____
(Date)

2. *Identification of actions needed to accomplish the goal.* What countable behaviors are involved in meeting the goal? (The more clearly and specifically actions are stated, the easier it is to evaluate progress toward the goal.)

3. *Establishment of reward(s) for movement toward goal.* What is reinforcing and realistic as a reward?

4. *Division of responsibilities.* What responsibilities are involved? Who is responsible for which ones? What specific assistance will the facilitator give the other person?—e.g., encouragement, phone calls, assertive asking about how the wellness goal is going, weekly meetings to discuss the goal.

5. *Time limit.* What mutually agreed upon time limit is set to accomplish the goal and/or evaluate movement toward the goal?

6. *Evaluation of movement toward goal.* How will movement toward the goal be evaluated? By whom? When? What consequences will accrue as a result? What additional assistance does the goal writer need from the facilitator in order to move toward goal attainment? What barriers are interfering with movement toward the goal and how can they be surmounted?

7. *Modification, renegotiation, or termination of the contract.* If a goal is met, a new one is reset. If a goal proves inappropriate, a new goal is found.

Facilitators for wellness goals can be nurses, but they can also be peers, family members, other health professionals, or anyone who agrees to learn and follow the procedure for contracting. Self-contracting can also be used, but research and empirical knowledge have shown that people with low self-esteem or little perceived control over what happens to them may not take responsibility for carrying through on a contract (Pender, 1982, p. 190).

Table 7 shows possible wellness goals. This self-assessment can be used to assist in the choice of a wellness goal.

Table 7. Wellness Self-Assessment

Directions: Read the statements for each dimension of wellness; circle the number which most appropriately resembles the importance of each statement to you and your well-being and current interest in changing your life style as follows:

1. I am already doing this. (Congratulate yourself!)
2. This is very important to me and I want to change this behavior now.
3. This is important to me, but I'm not ready to change my behavior right now.
4. This is not important in my life right now.

Nutritional Wellness

I maximize local fresh fruits and uncooked vegetables in my eating plan.	1	2	3	4
I minimize the use of candy, sweets, sugar, and simple carbohydrates.	1	2	3	4
I eat whole foods rather than processed ones.	1	2	3	4
I avoid foods that have color, artificial flavor, or pre-servatives added.	1	2	3	4
I avoid coffee, tea, cola drinks, or other substances that are high in caffeine or other stimulants.	1	2	3	4
I eat high fiber foods daily.	1	2	3	4
I have a good appetite, but I eat sensible amounts of food.	1	2	3	4
I avoid crash diets.	1	2	3	4
I eat only when I am hungry and relaxed.	1	2	3	4
I drink sufficient water so my urine is light yellow.	1	2	3	4
I avoid foods high in saturated fat, such as beef, pork, lamb, soft cheeses, gravies, bakery items, fried foods, etc.	1	2	3	4
I use bottled water or an activated carbon filtration system to insure safe drinking water.	1	2	3	4

Fitness and Wellness

I weigh within 10% of my desired weight.	1	2	3	4
I walk, jog, or exercise vigorously for more than 20 minutes at least 3×/week.	1	2	3	4
I seem to digest my food well (no gas, bloating, etc.)	1	2	3	4
I do flexibility or stretching exercises daily and always prior to and following vigorous exercise.	1	2	3	4
I am satisfied with my sexual activities.	1	2	3	4

Table 7 *(continued)*

When I am ill, I'm resilient and recover easily.	1	2	3	4
When I look at myself nude, I feel good about what I see.	1	2	3	4
I use imagery to picture myself well and healthy every day.	1	2	3	4
I use affirmations and other self-healing measures when ill, injured, or to enhance my fitness.	1	2	3	4
I avoid smoking and smoke-filled places.	1	2	3	4
Stress and Wellness				
I sleep well.	1	2	3	4
I have a peaceful expectation about my death.	1	2	3	4
I live relatively free from disabling stress or painful, repetitive thoughts.	1	2	3	4
I laugh at myself occasionally, and I have a good sense of humor.	1	2	3	4
I use constructive ways of releasing my frustration and anger.	1	2	3	4
I feel good about myself and my accomplishments.	1	2	3	4
I assert myself to get what I need instead of feeling resentful toward others for taking advantage of or intimidating me.	1	2	3	4
I can relax my body and mind at will.	1	2	3	4
I feel accepting and calm about people or things I have lost through separation.	1	2	3	4
I get and give sufficient touch (hugs, etc.) daily.	1	2	3	4
Wellness Relationships and Beliefs				
I have at least one other person with whom I can discuss my innermost thoughts and feelings.	1	2	3	4
I keep myself open to new experiences.	1	2	3	4
I listen to others' words and the feelings behind the words.	1	2	3	4
What I believe, feel, and do are consistent.	1	2	3	4
I allow others to be themselves and to take responsibility for their thoughts, actions, and feelings.	1	2	3	4
I allow myself to be me.	1	2	3	4
I live with a sense of purpose.	1	2	3	4
Wellness and the Environment				
I have designed a wellness support network of friends, family, and peers.	1	2	3	4
I have designed my personal living, playing, and working environments to suit me.	1	2	3	4
I work in a place that provides adequate personal space, comfort, safety, direct sunlight, fresh air; and limited air, water, or material pollutants; or I use nutritional, exercise, or stress reduction measures to minimize negative effects.	1	2	3	4
I avoid cosmetics and hair dyes that contain harmful chemicals.	1	2	3	4
I avoid pesticides and the use of harmful household chemicals.	1	2	3	4

Table 7 *(continued)*

I avoid x-rays unless serious disease or injury is at stake, and I have dental x-rays for diagnostic purposes only every 3 to 5 years.	1	2	3	4
I wear a good sunscreen ointment when exposed to the sun.	1	2	3	4
I use the earth's resources wisely.	1	2	3	4
Commitment to Wellness				
I examine my values and actions to see that I am moving toward wellness.	1	2	3	4
I take responsibility for my thoughts, feelings, and actions.	1	2	3	4
I keep informed on the latest health/wellness knowledge rather than relying on experts to decide what is best for me.	1	2	3	4
I wear seat belts when driving and insist that others who drive with me also do so.	1	2	3	4
I ask pertinent questions and seek second opinions whenever someone advises me.	1	2	3	4
I know which chronic illnesses are prominent in my family and I take steps to avoid incurring these illnesses.	1	2	3	4
I work toward achieving a balance in all wellness dimensions in order to enhance my sense of well-being and satisfaction.	1	2	3	4

Using Self-Assessments to Promote Wellness

Self-assessments (such as Table 7) may be more appropriate to wellness facilitation than risk appraisals for several reasons. Self-assessments generally point the way to goals; they also may point out, and reinforce, positive behaviors. Since they are self-assessments, clients self-assess their wellness. The nurse may discuss the findings with the client or use them to assist clients to develop wellness goals, but the choice is the client's.

Health Hazard/Health Risk Appraisals (HHA/HRA) are focused on risks that may have negative effects on life outcomes; an individual's health-related behaviors and personal characteristics are compared by a professional to mortality statistics and epidemiologic data to estimate risk of dying versus the amount of that risk that could be eliminated if life style is changed. Often, a score is provided indicating risk and chance of death if the behavior is continued.

Based on a review of available studies and discussions with HHA/ HRA developers, Wagner et al. (1982) concluded that the scientific basis for them is problematic due to impreciseness in measurements and inaccuracies in client-supplied information. Also, beliefs in the ability of HHA/HRAs to motivate behavioral change cannot be substantiated from evidence; additionally, adverse effects have been noted. For example, depressive responses to life expectancy predictions have occurred. Another problem with HHA/HRAs is that they may be touted as behavioral change motivators in themselves; the relationship between facilitator and client has been demonstrated to be the crucial variable, not the sophistication of the assessment tool (for example, see the author's research reported earlier, pp. 326–328).

Finally, although self-assessments can be used to engender guilt, when used from a wellness perspective the object is not to shock or evoke guilt in the client, but rather to assist the client to decide whether change is a high priority for that client. Since risks are not stated in number or word form, the chances are that clients are probably less likely to respond negatively to self-assessments.

Client Assessment Questions that Can Assist in Movement Toward Wellness

A wellness framework implies that the responsibility for the client's body/mind/spirit resides with the client, unless there is a life threatening situation in which the client cannot decide. It also implies that a wellness goal chosen by the client may not have high priority for the nurse. For example, an obese client may have set a high priority on stress management, while the nurse thinks weight loss should be the first priority. A wellness framework assumes the client sets the goal, not the nurse.

Stepping out of the caretaking role may be difficult. However, consider the following. If the client takes self-responsibility for body/mind/ spirit in one small issue, the process has been learned and it can be transferred to other issues, including those of high priority for the nurse. Also, if the nurse is able to demonstrate how success in attaining (life) goals can be accomplished, trust can be established and the client is more apt to agree to pursue a wellness goal of agreed upon high priority.

Nurses may not be working in situations in which clients have a great deal of energy to invest in setting and striving toward wellness goals. For example, nurses working in acute care settings may wonder how wellness can be encouraged in their settings. A beginning step is to adapt nursing histories to fit a wellness framework. Some questions that could be asked of clients on admission are:

1. What are the symptoms *you* are concerned about?
2. What feelings and emotions are *you* concerned about?
3. What are the goals *you* would like to begin moving toward?

4. What are your strong points and special abilities?
5. What kind of help do you want from me?
6. What do *you* think is wrong with you?
7. Why do you think you are having this problem *now* in your life?
8. What does this disease (symptom, worry, etc.) mean in your life?
9. What would you have to give up or take on to get rid of this problem (disease, symptom, worry, etc.)?

The Wellness Belief Scale

Another measure nurses can use to facilitate wellness includes assisting clients to examine their wellness beliefs. Table 8 shows a *wellness belief scale*. The scale was modeled after Rotter's original work (1966) on *internal locus of control* or the degree to which people believe they have control over what happens to them. The purpose of the belief scale is to measure client responsibility for wellness, by measuring degree of internality. Those who score 21 are at a high point of internality. Beliefs about wellness can influence the degree to which people take responsibility for their wellness. Numerous studies support the idea that people with strong beliefs about their ability to control destiny are more likely to be alert to information in the environment, place greater value on skills or achievement rewards, be more concerned about this ability (especially if the ability is lacking), and be resistive to subtle attempts to influence them. Rotter referred to these two basic stances as internal- and external-orientation. For example, Brown et al. recently reported that people who believe they have little personal control over events that happen to them do not engage in health promotion activities (1983).

Table 8. The Clark Health/Wellness Belief Scale

These questions can be used to find out how different people feel about health and wellness. Each item consists of a pair of statements, a and b. Select the statement for each pair which you most strongly agree with or think is true, not the one you think you should choose. There are no right or wrong answers; this scale is a measure of what you believe. For some items, you may find you believe both statements or neither one. In such cases, be sure to select the one you most strongly believe by checking one "agree" for each number. Try not to be influenced by your previous choice.

AGREE

1. A. I carry the key to my own well-being in the way I choose to live.   _____
   B. Health and illness are both luck and beyond my control.   _____

2. A. Wellness is a lifelong effort.   _____
   B. If I wait, medical science will develop cures for all illnesses.   _____

3. A. It matters little whether my health care practitioner pursues wellness as long as he or she looks after mine.
   B. I think it's important to steer clear of health care practitioners who are not pursuing their own wellness by not smoking, by keeping their weight down, etc.

4. A. No matter how hard I try, I think I'll probably still get ill (won't be able to quit smoking or lose weight), so I might as well do what I want to do.
   B. I have faith in my ability to increase my wellness.

5. A. I think that if I'm going to be ill, I'm going to be ill.
   B. Trusting to fate about my wellness doesn't work. I find I have to take a definite course of action.

6. A. Staying well is a matter of hard work, and luck has little or nothing to do with it.
   B. Staying well is a matter of being born under the right condition and being in the right place at the right time.

7. A. Environmental factors have little effect on whether I get ill or not.
   B. Heredity plays a major role in whether I get ill or not.

8. A. I can influence governmental decisions about wellness.
   B. Politicians, business people, and scientific experts make the decisions about my wellness.

9. A. When I devise a wellness plan, I am pretty certain I can make it work.
   B. I don't make long-term wellness plans because I don't think they work.

10. A. Sometimes I don't think I can control my state of health.
    B. It is hard for me to believe that my state of health is always due to luck or chance.

11. A. I might as well decide my wellness goals by flipping a coin.
    B. Getting what I want in terms of wellness has little or nothing to do with luck.

12. A. With enough effort I think I can decrease the anti-wellness parts of my environment.
    B. I think it's difficult and perhaps impossible to decrease the anti-wellness factors in my environment.

13. A. A good health insurance plan ought to include incentives for staying well.
    B. A good health insurance plan should be inexpensive, covering catastrophes like chronic illnesses and heart attacks.

14. A. It doesn't really matter what I eat since wellness is unrelated to food.
    B. I should choose what I eat carefully, because it contributes to my wellness.

15. A. I should work at being physically and mentally fit because both contribute to my wellness and health.
    B. It doesn't matter whether I'm fit or not since wellness is due to luck and my doctor's prescription.

Table 8 *(continued)*

16.	A. Stress is due to factors beyond my control.	____
	B. I can learn to reduce my stress level and thereby be healthier.	____
17.	A. If I heal when I'm hurt or ill, it's because something outside me helped me to heal, like an antiseptic or medicine.	____
	B. I can learn to use my own healing potential and thereby enhance my wellness.	____
18.	A. I think it's important to stand up for my rights when I feel others are trampling on them.	____
	B. It doesn't pay to stand up to others since they don't listen anyway.	____
19.	A. I think it's important to question health care practitioners, lawyers, and anyone from whom I purchase a service because I share the responsibility for what happens to me.	____
	B. I assume doctors, lawyers, nurses, and other authorities know what I need better than I do.	____
20.	A. Meeting new friends is a matter of luck and being in the right place at the right time.	____
	B. Meeting new friends is up to me to go places, introduce myself, and suggest we spend time together.	____
21.	A. Pain is something that has to be endured and it will pass.	____
	B. When I am in pain, I can take action to reduce my pain.	____

People who are internally oriented are more likely to take responsibility for wellness; others are apt to let a health care practitioner or fate determine level of wellness. Most people fall along a continuum from externality (0 = take little responsibility for own wellness) to internality (21 = take a great deal of responsibility for own wellness).

Once the client completes the belief scale, a discussion about what the answers mean to the client can ensue. Writing down what is peripherally known can often clarify thoughts and feelings and can be the basis for change. When responses are discussed in a group, lively debates and (sometimes) changes in beliefs can occur.

Some research suggests that locus of control *(internality-externality)* can be changed. In one study, student counselors changed their locus of control from external to internal after becoming more aware of their muscles' activity by receiving electromyographic feedback (Scalese, 1978). This study suggests that learning to tune in to internal body processes increases the belief of control over one's own fate.

Coller (1977) reported that clients became more internal in their locus of control as a result of a specific kind of group counseling called the *EPIC model.* The EPIC groups followed six exercise units consisting of perception and feedback skill training; self-disclosure; self-explanation skill building; assessment and understanding of self; personal contracting for change and growth; development of programs for achieving personal growth; and achieving and assessing personal goals and growth. This research suggests that structured exercises that help clients focus on themselves, develop goals, and work toward them can increase internality.

A study by Rotter (1966) looked at the effect of training in success-oriented learning situations with preadolescents. He examined the idea that if people receive enough training in success-oriented learning situations to counteract their previous learning, they will begin to attribute successes and failures to their own behavior; in other words, they would become more internal. The results of the study were that externally-oriented individuals who were exposed to success at learning tasks did become more internally-oriented. It may be that nurses who expose clients to success at learning may affect their internality and their movement toward wellness in a positive way.

Relaxation Techniques

There are a number of techniques that can assist in relaxation and enhance change toward wellness. Relaxation of the muscles reduces pulse rate and blood pressure and decreases perspiration and respiration rates. The body responds to anxiety provoking thoughts and events with muscle tension. Physiological tension increases the subjective experience of anxiety. Muscle relaxation is incompatible with anxiety; learning to respond with one blocks the habit of responding with the other. Relaxation techniques have been found useful in the treatment of muscular tension, anxiety, insomnia, depression, fatigue, irritable bowel, muscle spasms, neck and back pain, high blood pressure, mild phobias, and stuttering (Davis, Eshelman, & McKay, 1982, p. 23). Most people do not realize which of their muscles are chronically tense nor think about how the constriction may be affecting their circulation, movement, or tendency to develop chronic illness or discomfort. Working while relaxed with a relaxed client also allows the nurse and client to be more open to one another, to listen, and to learn more easily. Kern and Stejskal (1983) found that relaxation in the classroom reduced students' anxiety and improved their learning and recall.

Relaxation is a skill requiring practice and daily sessions to achieve mastery. Table 9 presents several types of relaxation exercises.

Imagery

Everyone has had experiences with self-generated images: dreams, daydreams, and fantasies may contain strong images generated by the right

Table 9. Relaxation Exercises

Progressive Relaxation

1. Lie down in a comfortable spot or sit in a comfortable chair.
2. Close your eyes. Follow steps 3–10, tensing for 5–7 seconds and relaxing for 20–30 seconds. Allow yourself to deeply experience your bodily changes.
3. Tense all the muscles of your hands, forearms, and upper arms.
4. Let all the tension out of the muscles of your hands, forearms, and upper arms.
5. Tense all the muscles of your head, face, throat, and shoulders, including the forehead, cheeks, nose, eyes, jaw, lips, tongue, and neck.
6. Release all the tension in your head, face, throat, and shoulders.
7. Tense all the muscles in your chest, stomach, and lower back.
8. Release all the tension in your chest, stomach, and lower back.
9. Tense all the muscles in your thighs, buttocks, calves, and feet.
10. Release all the tension in your thighs, buttocks, calves, and feet.

Taking a Trip in Your Mind's Eye

1. Find a comfortable, quiet spot and assume a relaxed position.
2. Close your eyes.
3. Let your breathing begin to move lower in your body, moving toward your abdominal area. Each time you exhale, your breathing moves lower in your body toward your abdominal area.
4. Take yourself on a trip in your mind's eye to a place that is comfortable and relaxing, somewhere you have been or somewhere you would like to be. See all the sights associated with your quiet, relaxing place. Hear all the sounds associated with your quiet, relaxing place. Smell all the smells associated with your quiet, relaxing place. Taste any tastes associated with your quiet, relaxing place. Fully experience all the sensations associated with your quiet, relaxing place.
5. Totally immerse yourself in your quiet, relaxing place until you are ready to return, then gradually return from your trip, keeping the relaxation and calmness with you for as long as you wish. Then gradually open your eyes and resume your day.

Quick, Total Relaxing Exercise

1. Find a door with a strong door knob. Close the door tightly and grasp the door knob.
2. Place your feet shoulder distance apart, 2 to 3 feet from the doorknob, depending on the length of your body; the distance should be adequate to allow you to totally stretch out but not strain your body.
3. Let your body totally relax, and let your head drop toward your chest.
4. Hold this position until you feel your body relaxing; stand up, take a few deep breaths, and repeat steps 2–4.

Note: Relaxation tapes may be needed to learn the process since it is difficult to read while trying to learn to relax. For information regarding relaxation tapes and their use, write: THE WELLNESS NEWSLETTER, 3451 Central Ave., St. Petersburg, FL 33713.

side of the brain. Experiences in the present may evoke images of past experiences that were similar. Most children have a well-developed sense of imaging. As they age, their skills may lie dormant as the logical, rational side of their brains is used in schoolwork and linear thought processes.

Imagery is a powerful tool for self-use or for engaging the client in movement toward wellness. The power of the approach is derived from its right-brained source. The right brain, which controls the left side of the body, is primarily responsible for orientation in space, body image, artistic endeavor, and recognition of faces. The right hemisphere deals with visual, holistic, intuitive, nonlinear thought. The left side of the brain is involved with analytic, logical thinking, particularly verbal and mathematical functions (Ornstein, 1972, p. 52). Imagery or visualization allows direct access to the subconscious and the autonomic nervous system functions, bypassing the left brain and its tendency to try to solve problems through logical processing. Unfortunately, logical processing can go awry and lead to ruminating or repetitive worrying that increases stress. Imagery can cut through rumination to the essential core of issues and thus lead to effective problem solving, decreased anxiety in interpersonal situations, and increased healing potential.

Through imagery it is also possible to learn to control functions previously thought to be under involuntary control, such as body temperature and heart rate. The power of imagery goes far beyond controlling physiological responses.

Everyone has had some awareness of how the images and thoughts he holds in his mind can affect the world around him. Probably everyone has noticed that if he awakens cheerfully, with a positive image of himself and the coming day, that image will manifest itself in the external world. People he meets will also tend to be cheerful and happy, or will become so in the presence of his positive attitude. Events that draw his attention are likely to be positive, or he will tend to see something positive in them. (Samuels, 1975, p. 70)

Since imagery is a right-brain process, it is difficult to describe in a linear, left-brained written description. To grasp the power of imagery, it is necessary to try out different kinds of imagery exercises. Use Tables 10–13 to understand the process; if necessary adapt the exercise and read "yourself" instead of the word "client." Imagery can be used in a number of ways, including: (1) solve problems, Table 10; (2) prepare for upcoming situations, Table 11; (3) enhance healing, Table 12; (4) decrease the influence of negative feelings and relationships, Table 13.

Table 10. Using Imagery to Solve Problems

1. Find a quiet spot and sit in a relaxed position; close your eyes.
2. Clearly define the problem. Use 3–5 words to state the problem succinctly. If you are having difficulty defining the problem, picture yourself telling the problem to a friend.
3. Ask, "Am I ready to solve this problem?" and wait for an answer. If the answer is "yes," proceed to step three; if "no," choose another problem.
4. Place the clearly defined problem in a frame using your choice of color to create a border around the problem.
5. See the solution in a frame using your choice of (a different) color to create a border around the solution.

Table 11. Using Imagery to Prepare for an Upcoming Situation

1. Decide on an upcoming situation for practice. Choose a situation you are anxious about, one whose outcome you are worried about or need practice in handling.
2. Assume a comfortable position with body relaxed and eyes closed.
3. Use the contraction/relaxation exercise to attain relaxation.
4. Imagine yourself as the director of a movie that you are going to run in your mind's eye. As director, you can stop or start the movie at any point that discomfort occurs.
5. Begin the situation, imagining everything about the situation: what is said, what you feel, what the other person(s) in the situation say and do. When you notice yourself becoming uncomfortable, stop the movie in your mind and go back to focusing on relaxing your body. When relaxed again, begin the movie at a spot a little before you felt anxious. Continue the movie until you feel uncomfortable or displeased with what occurs and return to relaxing. Work back and forth between the movie in your mind and relaxing until you can complete the whole situation while remaining relaxed.

Note: Your mind does not differentiate between an *image* of a situation and the actual experience of being in the situation, so a great deal of learning can occur using imagery and it will be much easier to remain calm and relaxed in the real-life situation once you have used the movie of the mind technique.

CASE STUDY: *Assisting a Client with the Movie of the Mind Technique*

Sarah K., a recent college graduate, expressed her anxiety about confronting her boss about obtaining a pay raise. Don W., a staff nurse in the outpatient clinic, talked to Sarah about using imagery to prepare for the confrontation. Sarah agreed to try the technique. Don W. played a relaxation tape for Sarah K.; he asked the client to signal by raising the index finger of her right hand when she was relaxed. Don sat opposite Sarah and watched for the finger signal for relaxation; when Sarah raised her finger, Don asked her to imagine herself as the director of a movie with her as the star and her boss as the supporting actor. Sarah was asked to go on with the scene until she felt uncomfortable and then signal by raising the index finger of her left hand.

Don worked with Sarah in this manner until she opened her eyes and exclaimed: "I got through the whole situation without feeling fearful!" Don then asked her to continue the practice at home and told her she would notice that it became easier and easier to get through the scene and as that happened it would be even easier to talk to her boss about a raise.

Table 12. Using Imagery to Enhance Healing

Imagery can be used in two ways to enhance healing: through universal images or by using the opposite of the client's image of the injured area.

The following universal images can be used for:
Asthma or upper chest congestion: image of cool throat and warm chest
Hemorrhoids or anal pain: image of heavy, cool anus and warm pelvis
Itching or pain: image of coolness or picture an ice cube in the area
Low back pain: image of a heavy spine
Gynecological disorders: image of warm pelvis
Viruses: image of immune system (for example, white blood cells imagined as knights on horseback attacking the illness-producing cells and carrying them off to be excreted from the body)
Anger, resentment, etc.: image of peace, love, harmony
Headache: image of a hole in the head near the area of the headache; on exhalation of breath, imagine the pain going through the hole as a color
Chronic sinus problems: imagine tubes opening and draining, e.g., a sink unclogging in the area
Tense areas: imagine the muscles in the area getting wider and longer, unknotting or relaxing
Hot areas: imagine coolness, e.g., submersing the area in cool water
Moist areas: imagine the area becoming dry, e.g., a desert growing in the area
Dry areas: imagine the area becoming moist, e.g., a spring or fountain growing in the area
Fatigue: picture energy and vitality entering the area

CASE STUDY: *Helping a Client Develop a Healing Image*

Rebecca S., a student nurse, had just learned about the use of imagery to assist healing and wanted to try it out with a family member with low back pain due to tension and stress. She told her aunt about the method and her aunt soon agreed, stating, "These pain pills just don't work anymore and I'm at the end of my rope." Rebecca asked her aunt to close her eyes and listen to the relaxation tape she had brought. When the tape finished, Rebecca asked her aunt to keep her eyes closed and picture what her lower back looked like to her mind's eye. Her aunt reported that her lower back looked like, "Tight, twisted red hot ropes." Rebecca asked her aunt to imagine her lower back becoming relaxed and healthy. Her aunt opened her eyes after a few minutes and said, "I just imagined dumping ice cubes on those red hot ropes and untying the knots in the rope; now my back looks healthy and feels good." Rebecca suggested her aunt use imagery whenever she began to feel the pain return.

Table 13. Using Imagery to Decrease Painful or Negative Feelings

1. Help the client relax using either a taped relaxation exercise or instructions in Table 9.
2. Ask the client to picture the painful or negative feelings.
3. Ask the client to think of a container and picture it vividly.
4. Ask the client to put all the painful or negative feelings in the container, put a tight lid on it, and lock it tightly.
5. Ask the client to put the locked container in a place where it can no longer influence the client.
6. Ask the client to open her/his eyes when the task has been completed.
7. Ask the client to discuss what happened during the treatment.

Note: Clients may have difficulty with any of the following: finding the right container, keeping the lid on it, and putting it somewhere where it can no longer influence them. Often, clients will automatically recognize they are not yet ready to give up their painful or negative feelings when difficulty is encountered in the containerization process.

The nurse may wish to ask the client to verbalize the process by which healing was enhanced or may allow the client to complete the process without verbalizing unless he or she wishes to. The verbalization does not aid in the process for the client, but can give the nurse clues about the client's ability to visualize and further issues with which the nurse can be of assistance.

A major asset of imagery as a nursing intervention is that the client need not expose situations that may be anxiety-provoking or embarrassing, or discuss the process; this is a major advantage when using the approach in a group or when working with a client with whom a deep level of trust has not yet been established. Frequently showing the client that the nurse can be of assistance without establishing an intimate relationship can build trust. Additionally, imagery interventions allow the nurse to work with clients who are unable or unwilling to establish an open, working relationship with the nurse. Clinical outcomes show that imagery works best in nursing situations when the nurse gives the broadest directions, allowing clients to develop their own images.

Affirmations

An *affirmation* is a positive thought that you consciously choose to immerse in your consciousness to produce a desired result (Ray, 1976, p. 14). The following guidelines are suggested for use of affirmations:

- Provide a relaxing, sharing atmosphere. Consider using a relaxation exercise as a prelude to the affirmation process.
- Obtain information from the client about health issues he/she is concerned about.

- Dialogue with the client to see whether the affirmation is best stated in the attitude, feeling, or action mode. If affirmations are stated too quickly in the action mode, clients may be unable to benefit from them; ask the client, "Are you ready to start thinking about changing or are you ready to use affirmations to take action to change?" Sometimes clients may be unsure themselves and *think* they want to change, but may find during the affirmation process that they are not yet ready to change and are really at the contemplation stage; affirmations are useful for either stage, but should be stated in the appropriate way, e.g., "It's getting easier and easier to smoke 10 cigarettes a day" (behavior mode) vs. "It's getting easier and easier to *think* about smoking 10 cigarettes a day" (attitude mode).
- Assist the client to state the affirmation in his/her own words. Actively listen to the client until it is clear how an affirmation might be stated, but then keep checking with the client until it suits him or her. ("It sounds as if an affirmation for you might be, 'It's getting easier and easier to let go of my angry feelings toward Cora.' How does that sound to you?") Affirmations are best stated in the becoming mode, e.g., "It's getting easier and easier to . . ." or "I'm becoming more comfortable with the idea of . . ."
- Once an affirmation has been agreed upon, ask the client to write or say the affirmation 10 to 20 times each day while listening to one's inner, gut response to hearing it said or writing it. (Practice this process with the client at least once together. Ask the client to say the affirmation, then ask, "What is your reaction to hearing yourself say that?" Ask the client to say the affirmation again, and ask, "How does it sound this time?" Continue working with the client this way; clients usually begin by responding with inner responses such as, "I'll never be able to do it"; with repetition, their inner responses begin to move toward, "Maybe I can do it.")
- Clients can be advised to carry their chosen affirmation with them on a 3 × 5 card and place it in a brief case, purse, or car dashboard where it will be read throughout the day. Underscore how hearing oneself on tape, viewing oneself saying the affirmation, or writing and reading it back provides two kinds of feedback and thus is more powerful than simply saying the affirmation to oneself. Stress the importance of trying all methods of doing affirmations and choosing the best one for that individual client.
- Clients can record their affirmations and play them back or look in the mirror and say the affirmation until they see themselves saying it, maintaining good eye contact and having a relaxed expression.
- Clients can also practice with the nurse or with a supportive peer in the following way: Sitting across from one another, say the affirma-

tion to your partner until you are comfortable doing so. Ask for feedback from your partner after each statement or your affirmation, e.g., "Did I squirm, fidget, or was I unclear or contradictory in what I said and how I looked?" Next, have the partner say the affirmation to the client using the second person, e.g., "Sarah, you're finding it easier and easier to . . ."

- Provide, or have the client provide, an ongoing method of reinforcement for continuing the affirmation.
- Use affirmations to support other medical, nursing, or related therapies the client has chosen to participate in.
- Present affirmation as a new method that has proved useful for many clients with many different kinds of problems. Ask for the client's full participation in working with you to develop useful affirmations.
- Provide support if the client becomes frustrated, lacks skills, or expects too much, e.g., "This is difficult, but you *will* get it." "Keep trying, you're making progress." "Don't expect to change patterns you've taken years to develop overnight."

CASE STUDY: *Using affirmations*

Judy T., a nurse on a rehabilitation unit, asked John H., a client who was having difficulty following through with his exercise regime, if he wanted to try affirmations. He agreed and Judy T. proceeded to help John phrase an appropriate affirmation. At first it seemed he was ready to develop an affirmation to exercise; as they talked, it became clear he had not taken personal responsibility for exercise. They phrased the following affirmation, "I, John, am finding it easier and easier to accept the idea of exercising to get better." The first few times John repeated the affirmation, he seemed negative about accepting the idea; when he said it the fourth time, he smiled and said, "You know, maybe exercising would help!" John continued saying his affirmation and he carried the written form of it with him on a 3 × 5 card wherever he went; Judy observed him reading it several times during her shift. The following week, John said he had mastered the affirmation and was ready to develop an affirmation about exercising.

Neurolinguistic Programming

Neurolinguistic programming (NLP) is a useful way of establishing rapport with clients and assisting them to overcome parts of themselves that are resistive to the idea of wellness. NLP is a way of reframing information so it is more acceptable or helpful to the individual. *Reframing* is changing the frame from which events are perceived in order to change the meaning or the context. When meaning or context changes, responses and behaviors follow. Reframing is a powerful communication tool that can assist the nurse to enhance wellness. An assumption of

NLP is that no behavior is in and of itself useful. All behavior will be useful somewhere. Identifying *where* is context reframing.

Richard Bandler and John Grinder (1982), the originators of NLP provide examples of reframing that have been adapted for use in nursing:

- A nurse helps a father reframe a "stubborn" daughter to think of her as having a priceless gift that will protect her when others try to take advantage of her. (changing the context used to evaluate behavior)
- A nurse reframes the dreaded event of the client passing out in a shopping mall to a paradoxical prescription of, "Now I know this is an important thing for you to do; it's something that can help you. I want you to go out every day to a different mall and pass out." (changing the meaning of the behavior to a controlled event)
- A client who conceives of himself as "devious" is assisted by the nurse to rename the behavior as, "Your ability to be creatively constructive." (changing meaning of behavior)
- A student who dwells on how "greedy" for money she is is helped by the nurse to be greedy about learning about wellness. (changing context for behavior)
- A client who complains there were too many wellness workshops scheduled at once was told by the nurse, "I understand, but one of the nice things about it is it gives you extra practice in the decision-making process." (changing meaning of behavior)
- A client who complained wellness is too much work was told by the nurse, "It must make you feel really good about yourself to realize you have so much perseverance." (changing meaning)
- A client who was angrily yelling and complaining was told, "I want to tell you that I know you are angry; you look angry and you sound angry. One of the important things a person can do is know that he feels the feelings he has and can express them directly." (changing meaning)
- A client angry with her son calls him "stupid"; the nurse comments, "Some people use stupidity as a way to learn a tremendous amount. Some people use stupidity to get people to do things for them. That's pretty smart." (changing meaning)

In addition to reframing, the nurse can learn to speak the client's language by observing and responding to client *representational systems*. People link experience to sensory input and tend to recall information based on their preferred representational system. Hover (1983) points out there are no nurse–client communication failures or resistant clients, only inflexibility in the nurse. If the nurse is willing to try something new there are limitless possibilities for meaningful nurse–client interaction. Some ways to speak the client's language are:

1. *Listen to clients' word choices regarding sensory representation and use them too:*
   If clients say, "From my point of view . . .," or, "I can see . . .," use visual words like, "see," "observe," "view," or "focus" with the client.
   If clients use words such as "hear," "harmonize," or "sounds like . . .," use auditory language to match theirs.
   If clients use words such as, "I'm in touch with . . .," "I feel . . .," or "I'm pressured," use kinesthetic words like "sense," "feel," "touch," "texture," or "pressure."
2. *Observe client eye and breathing movements, validate your observations, and then use them to establish rapport and understanding.*

   - Clients who look up and to the left are often having a remembered (past) image. Check this out by saying, "I'm wondering if you're picturing something in your past."
   - Clients who look up and to the right are often having a constructured (future) image. Check this out by asking, "I wonder if you're seeing something that could happen in your future."
   - Clients who look down and to the left are often hearing a remembered voice. Check this out by saying, "I'm wondering if you're hearing someone's voice from the past."
   - Clients who look to mid-right are often hearing a constructed auditory experience, such as making up a song. Check this out by saying, "I'm wondering if you're hearing how something might sound."
   - Clients who look down and to the right are often reliving a kinesthetic, olfactory or gustatory experience. Check this out by saying, "I'm wondering if you're recalling a feeling experience."

Asking clients to describe a recent good experience or tell you what they do well and then ask them how they know they do it well will elicit additional information about their representational system.

When the nurse observes and matches client verbal predicates (see, hear, feel, smell, taste) and nonverbal cues (breathing rate, voice tone, posture or gestures), rapport can be established rather quickly. Clients can also be taught to speak each other's language and gain enhanced rapport with family members, friends, coworkers, peers, etc.

Example

RUTH: I resent you leaving all your dishes in the sink after you cook those disgusting vegetarian meals.

NURSE: When you see that stuff, what does it remind you of?

RUTH: I see the whole house a mess. It's overwhelming.

NURSE: Robert, what do you feel overwhelmed about in this relationship?

ROBERT: I worry about Ruth's smoking. I know I can't do anything to make her quit, but I think I should be able to.

NURSE: So when Ruth sees the dishes in the sink she feels just as helpless and overwhelmed as you do, Robert, about Ruth's smoking.

RUTH: I never knew you felt that way.

ROBERT: Me either.

In NLP, *anchors* are sensory experiences that help the client organize experience. For example, if the client is very depressed and does not seem to have the energy to complete the agreed upon exercise program, the nurse can help develop an anchor. The following steps can be used:

1. Assist the client to attain a relaxed state by using one of the structured relaxation exercises.
2. Ask the client to "Picture a time in your life when you had a lot of energy and enthusiasm. Signal me by raising your right index finger when you have it vividly in your mind's eye."
3. When the client signals, tap lightly on the top of his or her shoulder. This will anchor the experience and make it easily accessible in the future when those feelings need to be called forth. The client or nurse or a trusted other person can be taught to tap lightly on that spot to elicit the energy and enthusiasm needed.

The purpose of NLP is to assist clients to feel better about themselves, organize internal information in a more congruent fashion, and break out of the boundaries of their self-restricting behavior. As such, NLP is a creative addition to wellness nursing practice.

The reader is referred to the following sources for additional information on NLP by Bandler and Grinder and published by Real People Press, Moab, Utah: *Frogs Into Princes, Trance-Formations, Reframing.*

INTEGRATIVE LEARNING EXPERIENCES

Beginning Level

1. Write in your journal about your experiences with the following:

A. comparing	E. judging	I. sparring
B. mind reading	F. dreaming	J. being right
C. rehearsing	G. identifying	K. derailing
D. filtering	H. advising	L. placating

2. Practice the following exercise with a nursing peer:

   A. Ask your peer to talk with you for 3 minutes about an event that happened recently that has personal significance for your peer.
   B. At the end of 3 minutes, make some notes about what you heard, noticed, and how you felt.
   C. Now, center yourself; when ready, ask your peer to talk with you for 3 more minutes about the chosen event.
   D. Write down (and then discuss with your peer) any differences noted in you, her or him, or what was heard.

3. Practice centering until you have mastered it. Try it out in several nurse–client situations and write in your journal about the results, including 1A–1L.
4. Identify your level of differentiation in various nurse–client situations and devise a plan for moving to a higher level of differentiation.
5. Identify triangles you engage in and develop a plan for taking the "I" position more frequently.
6. Write in your journal about what is important to you as a nurse; set priorities and communicate the essence of what you've written with at least one other person.
7. Write in your journal about values your parents, teachers, peers, or significant others have taught you; examine each and choose freely those you totally agree with. Devise a plan for reducing the importance of values not freely chosen, e.g., use the information in Table 13.
8. Consider all possible consequences of your value choices.
9. Devise a plan for trying out your value choice. Consider writing a self-contract to implement your value choices.
10. Evaluate what happened when you tried out your value choice. Note any inconsistencies between affirmed values and actions; make plans to reinforce actions that will support prized values.
11. Identify a situation that you think requires change. Write down all the possible resistances to change in that situation. Devise a plan for reducing resistance to change.
12. Identify a client you are working with and draw up a behavioral contract. Try out the approach and write about your experience in your journal.

13. Identify a problem you wish to solve; use the steps in Table 10 to solve it.
14. Try out the problem solving steps in Table 10 with a peer; one of you act as a nurse, the other as a client. Discuss what happened and any learning that occurred. Identify how you might apply the procedure with clients.
15. Try out the problem solving steps in Table 10 with a client who needs to solve a problem or make a decision. Write about the results in your journal.
16. Identify an upcoming situation that you feel apprehensive about. Use the steps in Table 11 to assist you to perform competently in the situation. Write about your experience in your journal.
17. Work with a peer who has an upcoming anxiety-provoking situation. Take the nurse's role in replicating the situation in Table 11. Write in your journal about the experience.
18. Work with a real-life client who has an upcoming anxiety-provoking situation using the information in Table 11. Write in your journal about your findings.
19. Use the information in Table 12 to enhance healing in yourself.
20. Help a peer devise a healing image for an identified problem. Write in your journal about your findings.
21. Help a client devise a healing image for an identified problem. Write in your journal about your findings.
22. Use the information in Table 13 and information on NLP to decrease the influence of negative feelings in your life. Write in your journal about the experience.
23. Take the nurse's role with a peer and use the information in Table 13 to assist him or her to decrease the influence of negative feelings. Write in your journal about the experience.
24. Use the information in Table 13 to assist a client to decrease the influence of negative feelings. Write in your journal about your findings.
25. Identify a situation in your life that could be helped by using affirmations. Devise an affirmation and write about the results in your journal.
26. Work with a peer to help him or her develop a useful affirmation and practice it until it has become integrated with the person (as evidenced by comments such as "I can . . ." or "It is getting easier . . ." or "I believe it").
27. Work with a client using affirmations. Describe the experience in your journal including any learning that occurred, obstacles and how you overcame them or could overcome them, and successes.

Advanced Level

1. Complete 1-27 above if not already completed.
2. Teach a client how to center.
3. Teach a client how to identify triangles that may produce difficulty.
4. Teach a client the value clarification process.
5. Teach another nurse or student nurse the following procedures:

   A. behavioral contracting
   B. imagery for problem solving
   C. imagery for performing competently
   D. imagery for healing
   E. imagery for decreasing the influence of negative feelings
   F. affirmation

6. Devise research questions and carry out the research for the following:

   A. relationship of centering to active listening
   B. relationship of level of differentiation to client healing
   C. relationship of value clarification to willingness to change
   D. relationship of behavioral contracting to change
   E. relationship of imagery problem solving to decision making
   F. relationship of Movie of the Mind procedure to future competence
   G. relationship of healing images to healing
   H. relationship of affirmation to lifestyle changes

REFERENCES

Bandler, R., and Grinder, J. (1982). *Reframing.* Moab, UT: Real People Press, pp. 1-37.

Berni, R., and Fordyce, W. (1973). *Behavior Modification and the Nursing Process.* St. Louis: Mosby.

Bowen, M. (1978). *Family Theory in Clinical Practice.* New York: Jason Aronson.

Brown, N., et al. (1983). The relationship among health beliefs, health values, and health promotion activity. *Western Journal of Nursing Research,* 5(2):155–163.

Clark, C. C. (1981). *Enhancing Wellness: A Guide for Self-Care.* New York: Springer.

Collar, C. F. (1977). The effective personal integration model and its impact on locus of control. Unpublished doctoral dissertation, Denton, TX: North Texas State University.

Conference on Future Directions in Health Care: The Dimensions of Medicine. (1975). New York: Blue Cross, p. ii.

Davis, M., Eshelman, E., and McKay, M. (1982). *The Relaxation and Stress Reduction Workbook.* Oakland, CA: New Harbinger.

Hover, D. (1983). Enhancing family communication using neuro-linguistic programming. In *Family Health A Theoretical Approach to Nursing Care*, Ed. by I. Clements and F. Roberts. New York: Wiley, pp. 83–91.

Kern, D., and Stejskal, J. (1983). Relaxation in the classroom: reduce your students' anxiety while improving their learning and recall. *Journal of Holistic Nursing*, 1(1):17–20.

Kirschenbaum, H., and Simon, S. (1974). Values and the future movement in education. In *Learning for Tomorrow: The Role of the Future in Education*, Ed. by A. Toffler. New York: Vintage Books, pp. 257–271.

Kirschenbaum, H. (1976). Clarifying values clarification: some theoretical issues and a review of research. *Group and Organization Studies*, 1(1):99–115.

Krieger, D. (1979). *The Therapeutic Touch*. Englewood Cliffs, NJ: Prentice-Hall.

McKay, M., Davis, M., and Fanning, P. (1983). *Messages, the Communication Book*. Oakland: New Harbinger.

Miller, S. R., and Winstead-Frey, P. (1982). *Family Systems Theory in Nursing Practice*. Reston, VA: Reston Publishing Co.

Ornstein, R. (1972). *The Psychology of Consciousness*. San Francisco: W. H. Freeman and Co., p. 52.

Pender, N. (1982). *Health Promotion in Nursing Practice*. Norwalk, CT: Appleton-Century-Crofts.

Peplau, H. E. (1952). *Interpersonal Relations in Nursing*. New York: G. P. Putnam, pp. 119–157.

Raths, L., Harmin, M., and Simon, S. B. (1966). *Values and Teaching*. Columbus, OH: Charles E. Merrill Books.

Ray, S. (1976). *I Deserve Love*. Millbrae, CA: Les Femmes.

Rotter, J. (1966). Generalized expectations for internal vs. external control of reinforcement. *Psychological Monographs*, 80(1):1–28

Samaroff, A. J. (1980). Issues in early reproductive and care-taking risk: review and current status. In *Psychosocial Risks in Infant Environment Transactions*, Ed. by P. B. Savin et al. New York: Brunner/Mazel, pp. 343–359.

Samuels, M., and Samuels, N. (1975). *Seeing with the Mind's Eye*. New York: Random House.

Scalese, V. (1978). Effects of electromyographic feedback training on the perception of locus of control and accuracy of person perception. Unpublished doctoral dissertation, Kalamazoo, MI: Western Michigan University.

Selye, H. (1956). *The Stress of Life*. New York: McGraw-Hill.

Selye, H. (1974). *Stress Without Distress*. Philadelphia and New York: J.P. Lippincott.

Sheehy, G. (1974). *Passages: Predictable Crises of Adult Life*. New York: E. P. Dutton, p. 251.

Simmons, L. W. (1950). The relation between decline of anxiety reducing and anxiety resolving factors in a deteriorating culture and its relevance to bodily disease. *Proceedings of the Association of Research Neurological and Mental Diseases*, 29:127.

Wagner, E., et al. (1982). An assessment of health hazard/health risk appraisal. *American Journal of Public Health*, 72(4):347–352.

3

POSITIVE RELATIONSHIP BUILDING

This chapter explores two important aspects of relationship building:

- Empathy
- Assertiveness

Humans are social beings who require interaction with one another to grow. Two important skills for nurses and clients are empathy and assertiveness: one allows understanding of others, and the other allows individuals to stand up for their own thoughts, feelings, and desires. At the beginning level, the nurse struggles to be empathic and assertive; at the advanced level, the nurse is ready to begin modeling and teaching clients these skills. The Integrative Learning Experiences at the end of this chapter, Case Studies, and Clinical Examples mirror this differentiation of beginning and advanced skills. The nurse models and teaches clients to use these critical skills for positive relationship building.

EMPATHY

Empathy is the ability to accurately perceive the feelings and meanings of others. When working with others, empathy forms the basis for a helping relationship. Empathy is the opposite of telling others, "I know what your health problems are" or "I know why you're having a hard time attaining wellness." When being empathic, the nurse does not lose separateness from others and take on their feelings or views (sympathy), but does try to *understand* what their feelings and views are. Empathy can be rated from low to high (Carkhuff, 1969; Kalish, 1973).

Assessing Empathy

Table 14 gives examples of different levels of empathy and the kind of comments the nurse may make to convey these different levels of empathy.

Table 14. Levels of Empathy

Low Empathy: The other's feelings are ignored or their full meaning is not grasped. Example 1:

NURSE: You should exercise more.

CLIENT: Why? I'm as healthy as you are.

NURSE: You'll be sorry when you're older!

CLIENT: I can't see running around getting a heart attack.

NURSE: Well, if you're not going to exercise, let's talk about something else.

Example 2:

CLIENT: I'd like more information on nutrition.

NURSE: You'd like more information so you can lose weight? *(assumption)*

CLIENT: Yes, but I wonder why I get tired and my skin feels crawly after I eat certain foods. It kept me up all night—I was at my wit's end and . . .

NURSE: *(interrupting)* As I told you before, this book will help you with that small matter *(plays down client's perception of the importance of his feelings)*

Beginning Empathy: The nurse conveys an accurate awareness of the conspicuous current feelings and their meaning to the client.

Example:

CLIENT: I've noticed I feel very tired and groggy lately, and I get depressed a lot.

NURSE: What's your reaction to this? (*gets more information*)

CLIENT: Well, I wonder if I should go get a prescription from my doctor for an antidepressant.

NURSE: You're wondering if medicine will help? *(reflects client's ideas)*

CLIENT: Yes, but I tried them once before and they didn't help. Maybe there's something wrong with my attitude or the way I eat. I've been dieting to lose weight so I cut out bread and cereal and live pretty much on cottage cheese. Yesterday, I really got scared. I got very dizzy and saw black spots before my eyes.

NURSE: You were really scared yesterday when you got dizzy. *(reflects feeling verbally conveyed by client)*

CLIENT: Yes, I suppose I better plan a better reducing diet. Maybe I can find one that allows me to feel good while I lose weight.

NURSE: You want to find a reducing diet that allows you to feel good. I think I can help you with that.

Table 14 *(continued)*

High Empathy: The nurse communicates accurately and confidently the current conspicuous and deeper feeling of the client.

CLIENT: You're so high and mighty, always telling us what to eat and what to do! *(angrily)*

NURSE: You really feel angry when I tell you what to do. *(reflects feeling tone of client through own tone .of voice)*

CLIENT: Yes! Since I was little someone has always been telling me what to do! I can take responsibility for myself—that's why I'm in this class.

NURSE: You're feeling angry because you want to take more responsibility for yourself.

CLIENT: Yes, you got it.

When the nurse *assumes* the client's meaning, low empathy occurs. Judging others' current feelings based on past experiences or the expectation of how others always act, feel, or think is invalid in an empathic relationship. Empathy allows the nurse to understand another's feelings while still maintaining differentiation of self. For example, the nurse can be empathic with a crying child without resorting to sympathetic tears and helplessness. Empathy provides a balance between emotional acceptance and intellectual objectivity.

Empathy provides an emotional mirror for the reflection of others' feelings. Empathic people learn to use the words and language of those they care about and reflect feelings and ideas back (Kalisch, 1973) to check whether this is how the client feels. Advice is not given unless it has been asked for, and then only if there has been an attempt to solve the problem together. Behavior is not labeled as "childish" or "crazy." Instead, the nurse uses the tone of voice or mood conveyed by the client. Reflection does not take on the tone, "Here is what you are saying"; it is made in a tentative manner, such as, "It sounds as if you're really angry," unless there is no doubt about the matter.

Sometimes it is difficult to understand the other's point of view. Using a relaxation and imagery exercise may help in these cases. The nurse finds a quiet spot and focuses on relaxing. Picturing oneself as the client may provide help in learning how clients view situations; to do this effectively, it is necessary to totally immerse oneself in the thoughts, feelings, and actions of clients—to walk in their shoes, so to speak.

Empathy requires the ability to listen actively and to reflect the essence of the client's communication. Although listening seems simple and passive, it is difficult to stop trying to solve other people's problems for them, telling them what the nurse would do under similar circumstances, or pooh-poohing the problem by discounting its importance

("What are you worrying about, look at Mr. Jones over there."). In most conversations, the person who is not speaking is often not listening very carefully to what is being said, but instead is getting ready to interrupt, preach, moralize, boast, discount what the other has just said, convince, reassure, or give advice. Many conversations sound like double mono-logues, with both wanting to be listened to, but neither listening to the other person.

When the nurse is an active listener, there is a conscious desire to listen attentively without preconceived notions, trying to understand not only the words but also the emotions and body movement of what the other person is communicating. Active listening is necessary to produce reflective communication. Reflective communication helps the client clarify what is really being experienced in the depth of the gut. To be effective, reflective communication combines a statement of the words and emotional content just conveyed by the other person. Although it sounds simple, it is not easy to do without sounding like a parrot.

Reflective communication acknowledges that clients may often ask for advice but seldom take it, or if they do, there is no permanent change or growth unless they have come to alter their way of thinking by increasing their ability to see their options. Reflective communication provides a sounding board against which clients learn to be more independent while experiencing a sense of caring, closeness, and help in clarifying their thoughts and feelings, expanding their consciousness and wholeness as people, and working out their own solutions.

Helping Clients Develop Empathy

There are a number of measures nurses can use to help clients develop empathy, including:

1. Paraphrasing. Ask clients to "say back to me what you heard me say." The paraphrased information can then be discussed in terms of what was not heard or recalled. Nurses or clients can tape record the initial words and the paraphrase and compare them for accuracy. Once clients understand that they are not listening actively, they may be ready to work on their empathy skills.

2. Providing reading material on empathy and its use. After clients have read the material, the nurse and client can discuss what was read and identify examples of empathy (or its lack) in future conversations.

3. Analyzing nurse empathy. (This is a more difficult skill and requires the nurse's willingness to take criticism.) The client can be asked to tell the nurse whenever client meaning is overlooked or not acknowl-

edged. A signal system can be used to encourage client participation. For example, the nurse can provide a card the client can hold up whenever the nurse misses the client's meaning, overlooks a feeling, changes the subject, etc. Once the nurse demonstrates willingness to examine self-empathy, the client will probably be more willing to do so also.

ASSERTIVENESS

Assertiveness is the ability to stand up for thoughts, feelings, or desires. It means being able to define and stand up for reasonable rights, while being respectful of others' rights, setting goals for wellness, acting on these goals by following through consistently, and taking responsibility for the consequences of actions.

"I"-Messages vs. "You"-Messages

Being assertive requires taking a risk by clearly stating what is expected from others and what they can expect from the nurse. "I" messages are used, e.g., "I would like to . . .," "I suggest we settle it by . . .," "I feel angry when I'm called lazy."

Contrarily, aggressiveness has an element of control or manipulation. "You"-messages, such as "Why didn't you . . .?," "You should have . . .," "I think you are crazy" prevail when agressiveness occurs. A common pattern that develops when assertiveness is missing is the avoidance of a confrontation or wellness issue, build-up of resentment, blow-up or angry outburst, feelings of guilt and recrimination, and a return to avoidance. Thus, aggressiveness/avoidance are intimately connected, and assertive behavior is in a different realm in which issues are addressed, thoughts and feelings are expressed when they occur, and action is taken to enhance wellness.

Sometimes "You"-aggressive messages masquerade as assertive ones, e.g., "I think *you're* wrong!," "I feel *you* ought to change," "I want *you* to do as I say." In these messages, the speaker tries to control the listener by judging behavior, or attempting to force change or action; *these messages are aggressive and avoid the responsibility each person has for his or her behavior* (Clark, 1978).

Some "We"-messages can also be assertive, especially if they imply collaboration, such as "We can meet and work this out." (Undifferentiated messages, such as, "Let's take our bath now," are *not* assertive *or* collaborative.)

"You"-blaming messages are apt to put others on the defensive; for this reason alone they ought to be deleted. In addition, they absolve the speaker of his or her responsibility in the issue at hand. Examples of this type of aggressive statement are: "Why didn't you take care of that?," "Why can't you do it right?," "I think this is your fault," "Why are you going around upsetting everyone?"

Some assertive messages do use the word *you*, but there is neither blame nor coercion attached to assertive "you" messages. ("Would you like to tell me your point of view?," "I want to thank you," "I thought I heard you say. . . .")

Assertiveness is a useful nursing skill for several reasons: nurses can role model for clients and assist them to be more assertive; assertive communication also lets both parties know where they stand and frees energy to deal with the situation as it really is instead of being used to decipher what the other person *really* means.

Assertiveness and Stress

Assertiveness is also useful as a stress reduction measure. People who are unable to express their thoughts and feelings directly or who feel unappreciated or exploited often report having psychosomatic complaints such as headaches or stomach problems. Assertive people often report increased feelings of self-confidence, reduced anxiety, decreased bodily complaints, and improved communication and response from others. There are a number of strategies to use to become more assertive.

Controlling Anxiety, Fear, and Anger with Relaxation Procedures

One way to reduce anxiety and fear about being assertive is to regularly practice relaxation exercises (see Chapter 2). Assertiveness requires presenting oneself in a confident, self-assured manner. When body musculature is tense and constricted, a self-confident presentation is difficult. A relaxed body increases the probability that others will be approached in a direct, open manner.

Techniques for Enhancing Assertiveness

Nurses may not be aware of how they come across to others. There are a number of strategies that can be used to provide feedback about presentation of self. Mirror practice gives feedback about facial expression, posture, and whether words fit with gestures and body position. It can also be helpful in rehearsing assertive statements prior to trying them with the real-life person. This kind of rehearsal can build confidence so that assertiveness in the real-life situation is more likely.

Audio- and videotape recorders also provide excellent practice in assertion. Audiotape provides clues about whether there are sufficient pauses, whether tone of voice is assertive, whether statements are made too quickly, if words are said with sufficient firmness and authority, and whether the issue is stated clearly and adhered to. Tape recorders are also useful for recording (and providing instant replay about) ability to limit interruptions, express feelings appropriately, take a stand on an issue, disagree, admit a mistake, reward or thank another person, give positive criticism, say no, express distress about the way a relationship is moving, and ask for collaboration. Some statements to record on a tape recorder and evaluate for effectiveness are:

- I cannot talk to you now. I'll talk to you at 1 o'clock.
- I feel really angry about this!
- I have made up my mind on this.
- I see your point, but I disagree.
- I *did* make an error.
- Let's sit down and work this out together.
- No, I will *not* reconsider this; this item is not negotiable.
- I'm upset about our relationship and I'd like to talk with you about it.
- I appreciate your help.
- We agreed your report would be on my desk yesterday. What happened?

Another use of audiotape is to record relaxing or reward messages that can be played back at a later time. Relaxation exercises can be found in Chapter 2; some rewarding messages to consider recording are:

- You are working toward wellness in a useful, helpful way. Congratulations on your effort. Keep up the good work.
- Congratulations on not smoking. Give yourself a hug or find someone to hug. Be proud of yourself. Allow yourself to feel good about your accomplishment.
- Congratulations on meeting your fitness goal. Treat yourself to a reward and be sure to allow yourself to feel good about your accomplishment!

Videotape feedback adds the extra information of eye contact, body posture and positioning, gestures, facial expressions, verbal responses that are too quick or hesitant, conciseness of statements, and confidence of presentation. Probably the best use of videotape is to record upcoming or past situations. Scripts can be written for two people and then recorded and evaluated according to each of the information components. Table 15 provides a completed guide for assessing an assertive presentation of self that has been videotaped. (The "Goals for Next Role Play" can be used if working with a partner.)

Another way to use videotape is for *role playing*. In this approach, one person tells the other about an upcoming or past situation. (It is best to choose two-person situations, avoiding those with a long history of emotional overlay; strive for choices that are likely to end in a successful role play, not in frustration because deep-seated issues are involved.) The first person gives the other a description of what is to be said, which

Table 15. Assertiveness Assessments

Nonverbal Presentation of Self	Examples/Comments
Frequent and direct eye contact Speaking loudly enough and firmly enough Open, direct body communication Gestures match words said	"I kept looking at the ceiling when talking. I crossed my arms and looked angry when talking about being pleased."
Verbal Presentation of Self	
Remain on the point of discussion without changing topics Use "I" messages, e.g., "I can't help you now," "I feel angry when . . .," "I'd like to talk with you about . . .," "I don't like to be shouted at . . .," "I realize you're concerned, but please don't make decisions for me," "I did make a mistake." "Thank you." "I'd like to do a joint evaluation with you." "I think we can work this out." Refrain from using "You-blaming" messages, e.g., "You didn't . . .," "You should have . . .," "It's your fault that . . .," "You aren't doing that right."	"I let her lead me away from my goal and we started talking about her sore leg instead of my raise. I used the following blaming messages: I think you should give me a raise. I feel you overlooked me."

Goal(s) for Next Role Play
1. Maintain eye contact
2. Uncross my arms
3. Tell my partner I feel angry instead of giving an inconsistent message
4. Get feedback from partner

role each person will take, how the other should act to approximate the real-life situation, and how the interchange will end and begin. A 3 to 5 minute script is sufficient when extraneous discussions are omitted and the issue is adhered to. The other role player needs to be coached to be helpful and should be told that making it easy for the other person is *not* helpful. Being as aggressive or avoiding as the real life person will provide much better practice and will prepare the other person in a better way. Some directions that might be given are: "Be sure to try to make me feel guilty about saying no," or "Every time I try to stick to the issue, you change the subject," or "Use a really angry tone of voice, but pretend you're not angry."

Using a script and trying it out will help the nurse identify areas that require further practice or more information. For example, if asking for a raise or a decision of some type, it is necessary to "do one's homework," coming up with alternate solutions for problems and providing adequate information for the other person to support a point of view. Merely asserting without having appropriate data to support a stand is less likely to end in a positive resolution. All of the procedures discussed as applicable for the nurse are also appropriate when assisting clients to be more assertive.

What Prevents Nurses From Being Assertive

Nurses often fear being assertive because they fear not being liked, being rejected, being retaliated against, etc. It is important to be aware of which of these fears (or others) may be preventing assertiveness and take action to dispel them (see Chapter 5 for additional stress reduction measures to use to dispel irrational beliefs).

The same fears seem to operate in both sexes; nurses of both sexes seem to be most fearful of rejection and tend to bend over backwards to please. When asked what prevents them from being assertive, they often say, "I don't want to hurt their feelings." Male nurses are less concerned with hurting others' feelings and are more apt to confess, "I don't want them to get the better of me, so I end up being aggressive." Males in the profession report that they feel pressured by female nurses to "be strong and never show our feelings."

Both of these reactions can be traced back to early family experiences in which girls are raised to be nice, not fight, not show anger, and (often) are judged on how they look or socialize, not on their competence in the task. As a result, many girls grow up to be women who underestimate their achievements, attribute their success to luck, and doubt their ability even when highly competent. Men assume they are competent and readily set out to prove it (Rivers, Barnett, & Baruch, 1979, pp. 106–107).

Early school experiences also influence the assertiveness of male and female nurses. Dweck (1975) found that teachers expect boys to be rowdy and inattentive about schoolwork, but girls are expected to be well-behaved, dutiful, and exerting their best effort. When boys fail, they are told to try harder (a motivation problem), but girls are just told they have done something incorrectly (may be interpreted as a lack of ability).

Early life experiences explain why nurses (predominately females) have difficulty being assertive with doctors (predominately male), and why male nurses may not have as great a difficulty being assertive with doctors, but may have more difficulty sharing responsibility and asking for help than their female counterparts. Both male and female nurses have some assertiveness issues with which to deal. And lines may not be as clearly drawn as presented; there may be some female nurses who feel more competent than their male peers. Indeed, assertiveness appears to be situational. Some nurses may feel more comfortable being assertive at work, while others feel more comfortable being assertive at home. Perhaps one of the few generalizations that can be made is that everyone has some assertiveness issue to deal with; no one is totally unassertive nor totally assertive. There is a continuum.

CASE STUDY: *Assertiveness With Peers*

> Bob Smith was working to obtain his B.S.N. When assertiveness was discussed in a seminar, he shared the following comment: "Why is it that everyone expects you to be strong and handle every situation?" As the discussion group helped Bob explore the issue further, it became clear that Bob's (female) nursing peers gave him verbal and nonverbal messages to be strong and not show any of the unsureness he felt about dealing with some nursing situations. It was suggested that Bob set up a time to talk with his female counterparts about how he felt and to share how difficult it was to always be the one who was expected to be strong and competent. The next week in class, Bob shared how he had met with his female peers and seemed surprised that they were surprised about how he felt; they decided to ask each time a stressful situation occurred how each one felt about taking responsibility in that situation. Bob reported feeling greatly relieved that "Things are now out in the open."

Assertive Strategies for Dealing with Criticism

There are three strategies for assertively responding to criticism: acknowledgment, clouding, and probing (McKay, Davis, & Fanning, 1983 pp. 124–128). Constructive criticism can lead to improvement; feedback from others can help you learn not to repeat the error. Extract the growth-promoting aspects of criticisms from others and use them to grow. Dispel irrational beliefs that criticism means failure or wrongness. Sometimes criticism is accurate, but not constructive.

Acknowledging. Whenever criticism is received, an assertive response includes acknowledging the critic's comment. Some examples are: (1) "You're right, I am half an hour late for work," (2) "You're right, I did misspell a lot of words," (3) "Yes, I am late in handing in this report."

Excuses and apologies are not part of an assertive response. Consider them automatic leftovers from childhood when excuses and apologies were demanded; parents and teachers expected an explanation and so one was compiled. As adults, individuals have the right to choose whether to give an explanation or not. Often, it is not advantageous to give an explanation because it provides further ammunition for the other person and does not present a picture of competence. Consider the two situations below; the first presents the nurse as blame-fixing, childlike, and incompetent; the second presents the nurse as assertive and adult. The major difference between the two situations is that the nurse gives an excuse in the first instance and does not acknowledge error; in the second instance, the nurse acknowledges error and does not give an excuse.

Situation 1: Non-Acknowledging

SUPERVISOR: You're late again! How long do you think I'm going to tolerate this?!

NURSE: Oh, I'm so sorry, please forgive me, the car broke down again and my husband wouldn't give me a lift!

SUPERVISOR: You've always got an excuse, but this time I'm not buying it. I'm writing you up and docking you for 15 minutes.

Situation 2: Acknowledging

SUPERVISOR: You're late again! How long do you think I'm going to tolerate this?!

NURSE: You're right, I am 15 minutes late.

SUPERVISOR: I'm docking you for the 15 minutes.

Clouding. Clouding is a useful technique when nonconstructive, manipulative criticism that is disagreed with is received (McKay, Davis, & Fanning, 1983, p. 125). It allows nurses to stand their ground while continuing to communicate with the other person. Clouding requires careful listening to what is being said to find something that can honestly be agreed with, either in part, in probability, or in principle. The idea is to agree with the part of the person's statement that makes some sense, but not agree to change.

Situation 1: Agreeing in Part

SUPERVISOR: You always have an excuse for not working overtime. What's the matter with you anyway?

SUPERVISEE: Yes, I do have many family responsibilities.

SUPERVISOR: You don't seem to care for the patients here at all.

SUPERVISEE: You're right; I guess it seems that way.

Situation 2: Agreeing in Probability

PHYSICIAN: Putting on a little weight, aren't you, sweetie?

NURSE: It may be that I've gained a few pounds.

PHYSICIAN: Time to put you on a reducing diet.

NURSE: You may be right that it is time.

Situation 3: Agreeing in Principle

FACULTY MEMBER: If you don't study more than you do, you're going to fail.

STUDENT: You're right; if I don't study, I will fail.

Probing. Criticism is often used by others to avoid important feelings or wishes. Assertive probing assists in determining whether criticism is constructive or manipulative, and clarifies unclear comments. The first step in assertive probing is to listen carefully and isolate the part of the criticism that seems most bothersome to the critic. The next step is to ask the critic, "What is it that bothers you about . . .?"

Situation 1: Assertive Probing

SUPERVISOR: You're not doing a very good job here. Your work is not up to par.

NURSE: What is it about my work that bothers you?

SUPERVISOR: Well, everyone else is working overtime, but you waltz out of here two out of three nights.

NURSE: What is it about my leaving on time when other people work overtime?

SUPERVISOR: I don't like working overtime either, but the work has to be done. It's not right that you just work by the clock.

NURSE: What is it that bothers you when I work by the clock?

SUPERVISOR: When you leave, someone else has to finish your work. I want you to make sure your work is completed before you leave.

NURSE: I see. Thanks for explaining the situation to me.

Additional Assertive Strategies

Broken Record. This approach is useful when others do not seem to hear or accept what is being said, or when an explanation would provide the other person with an opportunity to continue a pointless discussion. It is especially useful for saying no to others' requests.

The first step in broken record is to clarify exactly what the limits of what will be done are. The second step is to formulate a short, specific statement about what is wanted; avoid giving excuses or explanations since they give the other person ammunition to undermine the original statement. The third step is to use consistent body language that supports the statement, including maintaining eye contact, standing or sitting erect, and keeping hands and arms quietly at the side of the body. The fourth step is to calmly and firmly repeat the chosen statement as many times as necessary until the other person realizes there is no negotiation possible. The first few times a statement is said, the other person may give an excuse or attempt to derive a different answer. The fifth step is an optional one and includes briefly acknowledging the other's ideas, feelings, or wishes before returning to the broken record statement, e.g., "I hear you saying you're upset, but I don't want to work any more overtime."

Situation 1: Broken Record

PERSON 1: I just got an opportunity to fly to Aspen to ski. Won't you help me out and switch vacation schedules with me?

PERSON 2: How great for you. *No, I don't want to switch schedules.*

PERSON 1: You mean you're not going to help me? What kind of a friend are you?

PERSON 2: I understand that you're disappointed, but *I don't want to switch schedules.*

PERSON 1: But I have to go to Aspen and you're the only one who can help me.

PERSON 2: *No, I don't want to switch schedules.*

PERSON 1: Boy, you're really hard-hearted. What happened to you, you used to be so nice, now suddenly, Wanda the Witch.

PERSON 2:   *No, I don't want to switch schedules.*
PERSON 1:   Boy, you're not going to give on this, are you?
PERSON 2:   No.

Content-to-Process Shift. When the focus or point of the conversation drifts away from the original topic, the content-to-process shift can be used to shift from the subject being discussed (the content) to what is occurring between the two speakers (the process), e.g., "We're off the point now, let's get back to what we agreed to discuss."

Content-to-process shift can involve self-disclosure of current thoughts or feelings, e.g., "I'm feeling uncomfortable discussing this now, and I notice we're both tense." This approach is especially useful when voices are raised and anger is present: "We seem to be getting into a battle about this." The trick is to comment neutrally about what is observed so an attack will not be experienced by the other person.

Momentary Delay. In many social situations there is a compelling aspect to situations. There is often the implied command from the other person that a question must be answered right away. Rather than being swayed by the emotion of the moment, the professional nurse can take a deep breath and a momentary (or longer) delay. This procedure allows for further understanding and analysis of the pros and cons of each available response.

Situation 1: Momentary Delay

SUPERVISOR: I'd like you to read the riot act to the aides; they aren't doing their work. You have to do something right now!
NURSE: (takes a deep breath) I'll need more information before I can act.

Situation 2: Momentary Delay

SUPERVISEE: I think I deserve a raise; here is a summary of the things I have brought to this job and the outcomes I have achieved.
SUPERVISOR: There may be something in what you have to say; let me think about this for a few minutes.

Time Out. When the conversation reaches an impasse, but the discussion is an important one, the conversation can be delayed to a later time; time out is only assertive if a specific time in the near future is set to continue the discussion.

Situation 1: Time Out

TEENAGER: I think you're blaming me unfairly.

PARENT: We've been talking about this quite a while now and I don't think we're getting anywhere. Let's sleep on it and I'll see you at 9:00 a.m. tomorrow.

Joining and Circling the Attacker. This approach is derived from the martial art of Aiki, in which the attacked person accepts the attack and turns with it, letting the attacker pass in the direction he or she has chosen. According to Dobson and Miller (1978):

> One of the best ways to survive . . . is to . . . flow with them. Harmonize . . . Be the water not the rock . . . The water has direction and flexibility. Eon by eon the rock is worn down, until halfway through eternity it has become a pebble. If the rock would turn with the force of the water, still retaining its place in the stream bed, the rock would lose nothing; the water would continue past. (pp. 87–88)

As in the martial art, there is a pause the attacker takes just before a change in direction. That brief moment is when the attacker loses balance; it is at that precise moment that the defender takes charge and helps the attacker to a new, firmer, less aggressive balance.

> Most attackers are spoiling for a fight. They are overextended, and they need the victim to fight back and preserve their tenuous balance. So if you yell at a yeller, you help him stay upright. (Dobson & Miller, 1978, p. 102)

The focus of energy is on the resolution of conflict and the restoration of harmony, and problem-solving. In each attacking or conflict situation, there are four alternative ways to respond:

1. *Do nothing.* This is an appropriate response when time is needed, when more information is needed to find out what is behind the attack, when the attacked person does not want to dignify the attack by reacting (it is not necessary to answer charges unless the nurse chooses to do so), or when the attack makes no sense. Doing nothing must be a conscious choice, not a response to fear, in order to be an assertive response.

2. *Use diversion, deflection, or humor.* This is an appropriate response to deflect or redirect an attack. "Most attacks . . . come at you along a fairly straight line. By employing . . . surprise you can break that line and cause the attack to misfire" (Dobson & Miller, 1978, p. 73). Changing the subject ("I see you're wearing a new suit") or absurd explanations can be used to create a diversion or deflection.

Situation 1: Using Deflection/Humor

A: You forgot to get that report in! What do you think you're doing?!

B: You're right; I'm sorry I didn't follow through on our agreement.

A: That's no excuse!

B: I would have finished it, but I was attacked by Martians from outer space.

A: That's absurd!

B: I know. So is continuing to rage at someone after he's apologized.

3. *Join with the attackers,* agree with their right to feel as they do. (This is Aiki, confluence, flowing-with; being the water, not the rock.)

Situation 1: Joining the Attacker

PHYSICIAN: What have you done? You're the worst nurse I've ever seen!!

NURSE: I don't blame you.

PHYSICIAN: What do you mean, I don't blame you?

NURSE: It's not up to me to blame anybody for feeling the way they do. You're not happy, and I can't quibble with that.

PHYSICIAN: (puzzled) But you think your work is up to par?

NURSE: It can't be if you're not happy with it. My job is to work with you.

PHYSICIAN: (confused) I don't understand.

NURSE: If you don't think I should be fired outright, let's see if we can't work together on this thing and make it mutually acceptable. What are some of your complaints?

(The nurse's use of surprise combined with joining the attack led to the physician's losing his balance. The nurse has joined the physician and is helping him; the nurse does not take the attack personally, but objectifies the conflict; this leads to confusion. The nurse then takes the lead and helps the physician to deal with the conflict as an adult instead of a child.)

4. *Withdrawal* is an appropriate choice when all else fails and an escape route is open or when the time and place for discussion is wrong. To use withdrawal well, it must be completed clearly and with a single intention. Being unclear about the right to leave the scene can result in confusion. It is important to withdraw with certainty, knowing that it is each person's right to stay out of destructive involvements.

5. *Parley* is most effective when involved in a no-win situation in which the other person has defined the encounter as a contest; in this case, the nurse can remain centered and turn the conflict around, offering a reasonable way out for both parties. Some parleying comments are:

"Shall we see if we can work out a compromise?"
"Let's see if we can't iron out the problem."
"Maybe we can figure out a way to solve both our problems by working together."

6. *Fighting back* is the response of choice when there is no other option, it is a question of life or death, or it is a question of serious priority. Fighting back could include expressing anger directly or standing up to an insult.

Situation 1: Fighting Back

SURGEON: (who has just cornered the nurse in front of several other surgeons and physicians) Listen, kid, my time is too valuable to spend chasing all over the place to find that room you assigned me to just because you're so inefficient you can't get the simplest things through your pinhead! And another thing, where is that new scalpel I ordered?

NURSE: I won't stand here and be insulted. I resent being blamed for someone else's room assigning. We can argue or try to solve the problem together.

SURGEON: I don't have to take this from you! I can have you fired!

NURSE: If you want to stop this, figure out the room assignment and I'll find out about the scalpel. (exiting)

This response focuses the surgeon on the problem and its solution, yet allows the nurse to stand up for her rights, which she has already decided are a high priority for her with this surgeon who has constantly humiliated her in public. If the nurse loses her job (an unlikely but possible resolution), the nurse has already decided she has no intention of continuing to work under these conditions. Most likely the job will not be lost and conditions could improve as the surgeon realizes he cannot bully the nurse.

When the decision to stand up for one's rights has been made, it is important to make several assessments prior to acting, including:

● Does this person have nothing to lose by being aggressive? (If the answer is yes, the nurse may choose to reconsider this response and choose another, since the other person may be irrational in the interchange.)
● What is the minimum amount of energy needed in this situation to make my point? (use the minimum energy needed to restore harmony)
● What is the best time and place for the confrontation?
● What is the best way to stop an attacker's advance?

- What is the best way to focus the conflict on the problem and not on generalities or personalities?
- What do I want my face to say and how can I ensure it says that?
- What do I want my body to say and how can I ensure it says that?
- What spatial relationship to the other person is most likely to end in harmony?

Multiple Attack. An attack from several other people seems intimidating. Examining the geometry of forces, it can be seen that due to the nature of the force exerted by the attackers, they require one another's presence in order to continue the attack. Their forces create a balance due to focusing energy directly on the attackee. If the nurse keeps an attacker between herself or himself, a shield will develop between the nurse and the rest of the attackers, and the attack will be defused.

Situation 1: Multiple Attack

Sandra is a staff nurse who believes in wellness nursing. She tries to collaborate with her clients and help them to take responsibility for decisions about what happens to them. As a result, she spends more time talking with her clients than some of the other nurses do. Her supervisor has noted her "wasting time" talking with clients a number of times and several physicians have demonstrated impatience waiting for her to make rounds or assist them. Sandra is in a bind. She believes in what she is doing but knows she is being evaluated negatively. She knows this cannot go on indefinitely, so she moves in on a straight line to bring the attacks into direct confrontation. She calls a meeting of physicians and her supervisor to discuss the kinds of nursing plans she's implemented. Sandra centers herself, which helps her to remember the group is not there "to get her." They're anxious about their work and worried about time pressures and being evaluated positively by their supervisors.

Ms. Bart, the nursing supervisor, is the most outspoken and demands that Sandra spend less time talking with patients and more time assisting physicians and completing her paperwork. Sandra pays attention to her breathing and keeps centered so she doesn't scream out, "Look here, I went to nursing school to learn these special skills I have and I know what's the best way to practice nursing!" Sandra realizes that Ms. Bart, in the best tradition of attackers, has attacked with such force that she has almost lost her balance. Sandra decides to slide around Ms. Bart toward the other attackers. She asks for comments from the physicians, thanks them for their concern about patients, and asks if all the physicians agree with Ms. Bart about her spending less time providing care for their patients. The physicians disagree with one another and raise unrelated questions. Sandra refrains from becoming defensive and continues to go back to Ms. Bart's demands, keeping her between herself and the physicians. Sandra eventually offers to speak at the next grand rounds, sharing with the physicians her nursing interventions and outcomes for various "difficult" clients.

Situation 2: Multiple Attack

Sue Anderson, R.N., is working with a client, Emily Weiss, who is constantly complaining her teenage kids seem to be down on her lately. They argue about performing household tasks and complain about her cooking and "nagging." As a result, Emily feels cut off and resentful. Sue suggests a family meeting to bring the attacks into direct confrontation. Emily resists at first, until Sue does some role playing with her to help her decide exactly what she wants to say to her family. Emily practices centering herself prior to the family meeting and resists becoming defensive when the complaints start. Emily pays attention to her breathing, thanks them for being so candid, slides around the children's attacks, and keeps her husband between herself and the kids. Emily offers to stop nagging them in exchange for their agreeing to each cook one meal a week. The next week she reports to Sue that things are better around the house.

Hidden Agendas. Hidden agendas are unstated issues that are played out through interaction with others. Hidden agendas are excellent defensive maneuvers for low self-esteem. They protect against rejection by creating the desired impression at the expense of intimacy and authenticity. Nurses and clients use them to put up a smoke screen of carefully selected stories and calculated remarks. Clues that hidden agendas are operating include making the same point again and again and trying to prove something. The problem with hidden agendas is that they are obstacles to authentic, positive relationships. Therefore, it is important to assess the tendency for operating from a hidden agenda and take steps to devise self-instructions to counteract the pretense.

McKay, Davis, and Fanning (1983, pp. 78–83) list eight major hidden agendas:

1. *I'm Good.* Many of the statements from a person using this agenda demonstrate how caring and sensitive the person is; a fine character is created, but not an authentic self. No one is entrusted with the parts of oneself that are less than wonderful. People who always present them-

selves as good, honest, loyal, generous, successful, powerful, strong, wealthy, self-sacrificing, etc. tend to bore other people, and an intimate relationship becomes difficult.

2. *I'm Good (But You're Not).* In this agenda, the person attempts to raise his or her self-esteem by showing how stupid, incompetent, selfish, unreasonable, lazy, frightened, or insensitive others are. One nurse often complained, "Do you think I can ever get anyone around here to help me? I'm the only one doing the work!" This hidden agenda gives a temporary boost to self-esteem, but others feel threatened and put down and defensive maneuvers on their part soon follow.

3. *You're Good (But I'm Not).* People who constantly flatter others have this agenda. More complex forms involve worship of smart, beautiful, or strong people. This agenda can also be used to ward off anger, rejection, and high expectations; who expects much of someone who is incompetent and self-berating?

4. *I'm Helpless, I Suffer.* This agenda portrays the person as a victim who has suffered misfortune, injustice, and abuse. The implied message is that the person is helpless and not responsible for what happens. Variations include presenting a problem and then proving nothing will help resolve it, and trading "horror stories" with another to form a bond of sympathy.

5. *I'm Blameless.* This is the agenda of people who have innumerable excuses for their failures. The basic position is: "I didn't do it." ("The doctor did it . . . The patient did it . . . The family interferes . . . My boss is the problem . . .")

6. *I'm Fragile.* The basic stance is, "Don't hurt me, I can't take it." The person tells or shows others he needs protection from the truth. ("I don't want to talk about it, it upsets me," "You're giving me another of my headaches," and "This reminds me of my parents fighting, let's not get into it" are typical comments from this stance.) On most hospital units there is one person who does not do his or her work but is not confronted by others because "She's fragile and couldn't take it."

7. *I'm Tough.* A variation is the super nurse whose communication is often a harried listing of things done or to do; the underlying message is "I work harder, longer, and faster than anyone." The purpose of the agenda is to ward off hurt and protect a fragile self-esteem.

8. *I Know It All.* This is the agenda of the perpetual instructor, constantly moralizing as a protection from re-encountering early experiences of shame of being inadequate and not knowing.

McKay, Davis, and Fanning (1983, p. 83) suggest using self-instructions for overcoming hidden agendas (see Table 16); the statements can be said as mantras over and over again, can be taped to a bathroom mirror, the inside of a briefcase or carried on 3 × 5 cards.

Table 16. Self-Instructions for Overcoming Hidden Agendas

Agenda	Self-instructional statement
I'm Good	"I'm a mixture of strengths and weaknesses; I can learn to be balanced."
I'm Good (But You're Not)	"I don't have to put you down to make me feel good; I can feel good on my own."
You're Good (But I'm Not)	"I can get attention for my strengths without making excuses."
I'm Helpless, I Suffer	"I experience joy as well as pain; I can allow myself to experience both."
I'm Blameless	"I'm responsible for what happens to me."
I'm Fragile	"I can learn to deal with upset."
I'm Tough	"I can be safe without being tough."
I Know It All	"I can learn a lot from others if I listen, watch, and ask questions."

INTEGRATIVE LEARNING EXPERIENCES

Beginning Level

1. Make a verbatim recording of a 3 to 5 minute conversation with three clients. Assess your level of empathy. Write higher level empathic responses for each client and demonstrate them with those clients or with three others.

2. Keep a record of your I-Messages and You-Messages for a week. Change the You-Messages into I-Messages and devise a plan for implementation of increasing the percentage of I-messages you use.

3. Choose an assertiveness interchange of high priority for you. Be sure the situation does not have a long history of emotionally-charged behavior and involves only you and one other person (builds in success). Write an assertiveness script for the situation. Practice the situation using a mirror and assess and (based on your assessment) change your verbal and nonverbal behavior during mirror practice to approximate an assertive presentation.

4. Use the assertiveness situation you have perfected through mirror practice and practice the situation with a nursing peer, obtaining feedback from the other person about your tone of voice, facial expression, body position, words chosen, and consistency between words and nonverbal presentation. Be sure to coach your peer to play the other person's role so you obtain helpful practice.

5. Use an audio recorder and practice saying no until your evaluation

identifies assertiveness and you make no excuses and do not apologize for saying no. (NOTE: overplay this past the point you would speak in the real-life situation to give you practice in bluntly saying no; this will allow you to say no in the real-life situation with more ease once you have passed the point of your usual response and encountered no negative effects.)

6. Choose another assertiveness situation and complete the following:

   A. Write a script for a two-person situation of high priority for you.
   B. Find a peer and fill him/her in on the specifics of playing the role as the real-life person would.
   C. Practice the situation on videotape until pleased with your performance. Use Table 15 to assess your behavior.

7. Identify situations in your past life that have contributed to non-assertiveness.

8. Work with a peer and videotape your responses to criticism using the following nurse responses:

   A. acknowledgment
   B. clouding
   C. probing
   D. agreeing in part
   E. agreeing in probability
   F. agreeing in principle
   G. broken record

   H. content-to-process shift
   I. momentary delay
   J. time out
   K. doing nothing
   L. using deflection/humor
   M. joining the attacker
   N. standing up for your rights

9. Identify hidden agendas you use; develop a plan for implementing self-instructional statements.

Advanced Level

1. Complete any of #1–9 that have not been completed previously.

2. Work with a client to help him/her develop empathy using paraphrasing, relevant reading material, and client feedback.

3. Teach a client the difference between assertiveness and aggressiveness/avoidance.

4. Teach a client a relaxation procedure to use prior to attempting assertiveness.

5. Assist a client to audiotape or videotape an assertiveness situation and evaluate the results. Assist the client to devise a plan for practicing the behavior in the real-life situation.

6. Teach a client how to assess his/her level of assertiveness using Table 15.

7. Assist a client to identify what prevents him/her from being assertive.

8. Assist a client to deal with criticism using a different situation each time to exemplify:

A. acknowledging the criticism
B. clouding
C. agreeing in part
D. agreeing in probability
E. agreeing in principle
F. broken record

G. content-to-process shift
H. momentary delay
I. time out
J. joining and circling the attacker
K. deflection/humor
L. standing up for one's rights

9. Assist a client to identify hidden agendas.

10. Assist a client who has identified hidden agendas to develop self-instructions for overcoming the agenda(s).

REFERENCES

Carkhuff, R. and Berenson, B. (1976). *Beyond Counseling and Therapy.* New York: Holt, Rinehart and Winston, Inc.

Clark, C. C. (1978). *Assertive Skills for Nurses.* Rockville, MD: Aspen Systems.

Dobson, T. and Miller, V. (1978). *Giving In to Get Your Way.* New York: Delacorte.

Dweck, C. (1975). Sex differences in the meaning of negative evaluation in achievement situations: Determinants and consequences. Unpublished paper presented at the Society for Research in Child Development, Denver, CO.

Galassi, M. D., and Galassi, J. P. (1977). *Assert Yourself!* New York: Human Sciences Press.

Kalish, B. (1973). What is empathy? *American Journal of Nursing,* 73(9):1548–1552.

McKay, M., Davis, M., and Fanning, P. (1983). *Messages, The Communication Book.* Oakland, CA: New Harbinger.

Rivers, C., Barnett, R., and Baruch, G. (1979). *Beyond Sugar and Spice: How Women Grow, Learn and Thrive.* New York: Ballantine.

4

STRESS MANAGEMENT

This chapter discusses the following topics:

- Assessing stress symptoms and stress management skills
- Stress management approaches for specific symptoms
- Breathing
- Biofeedback
- Use of progressive relaxation as a nursing intervention
- Self-hypnosis
- Autogenics
- Thought stopping
- Refuting irrational ideas
- Coping skills procedures
- Time management
- Hardiness

ASSESSING STRESS SYMPTOMS AND STRESS MANAGEMENT SKILLS

Stress can be experienced as a result of the interactions of one or more of the wellness dimensions. For example, it is possible to experience stress due to under- or overnutrition, negative interpersonal relationships or nagging thoughts about others or situations, insufficient exercise or ineffective body movement, negative environmental factors or conflicting values or beliefs.

In 1914 Cannon described the *fight or flight response* or "emergency reaction" that prepares the individual to fight or run. Physiological changes include: increase in blood pressure, heart rate, respiration, metabolism, epinephrine, blood glucose, peripheral vascular constriction, dilation of the pupils, and decreased testosterone levels (Benson & Klipper, 1976; Cannon, 1914; Selye, 1956). If stress is chronic, the immune system weakens, lowering resistance to disease (Zeagans, 1982). With chronic stress, temporary conditions can become permanent, turning transient high blood pressure into hypertension, stomach upset into colitis or ulcers, and so forth. Stress has been related to many diseases and ailments including headaches, peptic ulcers, arthritis, colitis, diarrhea, asthma, cardiac arrhythmias, sexual problems, circulatory problems, muscle tension, and cancer (Davis, McKay, & Eshelman, 1982, p. 6).

It is not possible or even wise to turn off innate fight or flight responses to threats. It is possible and wise to learn to interpret and label experiences differently, thereby lessening negative stressor impact.

The first step in reducing stress is to assess the major sources of stress. The Holmes *"Schedule of Recent Experience"* was developed by Thomas Holmes at the University of Washington School of Medicine in Seattle, Washington. It gives a value for each life event (such as divorce, change in financial state, sexual difficulties, death of a spouse, vacation, etc.) and allows the respondant to obtain a total score. The assumption is that the more change an individual has to adjust to, the more likely he or she is to get sick. Holmes found that 80% of the persons he studied who had a score over 300 were apt to get sick in the near future.

A major controversy about the Holmes scale concerns the idea that some changes are not stressful and may even be pleasant. For example, although Holmes claims that a job change is stressful, it may be less stressful to take a new job in pleasanter surroundings than it is to stay in a job that is dead-end, draining, and results in ongoing resentment. Table 17 presents information for assessing and reducing stressful life changes.

Symptom relief can be a powerful motivator for nurses and clients to begin stress management procedures. Table 18 offers a Stress Symptom Assessment.

Physical symptoms may have physiological sources, so it is unwise to proceed on the assumption that all symptoms are completely stress-related. Stress management procedures are generally of two types: those that focus on relaxing the body and those that focus on handling stress differently. Often it is useful to use at least one approach from each broad category. For example, breathing exercises and progressive relaxation may be used to calm the body and refuting irrational ideas may be used to reduce perspectives on events that increase stress (Davis, McKay, & Eshelman, 1982, p. 15).

It is useful to keep a *Stress Awareness Diary* to make note of times that a

Table 17. Assessing and Reducing Stressful Life Changes

1. Identify sources of stress by listing changes in the following areas in the past 2 years.
   - school
   - work
   - close relationship with friends, family, and significant other people or pets
   - living arrangements or place of residence
   - life style
   - financial matters
   - sudden challenges
   - amount of worry about the future

2. Identify which changes were negative (–) and which were positive (+) by placing a + in front of positive changes and a – in front of negative ones.
3. For the negative changes, decide on a procedure for limiting the effects of unresolved stress.* (See Table 18)

Source of Continued Stress   Stress Management Procedure

4. List changes anticipated in the next year and identify at least two procedures to use to reduce the effects of the change on the level of stress.

*Read the rest of this chapter for ideas.

Table 18. Stress Symptom Assessment

Rate the stress-related symptom for degree of discomfort on a scale of 1 (slight discomfort) to 10 (extreme discomfort). After ensuring the symptom does not have a purely physiological source, choose the appropriate procedure from list of codes and proceed to use it. After the procedure has been mastered, reevaluate degree of discomfort for each symptom experienced; this will provide a measure of the effectiveness of the procedure.

	Pre-practice degree of discomfort (1 – 10)	Procedure*	Post-practice degree of discomfort (1 – 10)
Anxiety in specific situations			____
Test anxiety	____	PR, B, M, I, SH	
Deadline anxiety	____	TS, RII, CS, TM	
Interview anxiety	____		____
Other performance anxiety	____		____
Anxiety in personal relationships		PR, BR, SH, AS	
with spouse/date	____	AF	
with parents	____		____

83

Table 18 *(continued)*

	Pre-practice degree of discomfort (1–10)	Procedure*	Post-practice degree of discomfort (1–10)
with children	——		——
other	——		——
Generalized anxiety	——	PR, BR, M, I, A, TS, RII, CS, E, B, AF	——
Depression	——		——
Hopelessness	——	PR, BR, M, TS, AF	——
Powerlessness	——	RII, CS, AS, N, E	——
Low self-esteem	——		——
Hostility	——		——
Resentment	——	BR, M, A, RII,	——
Anger	——	I, B, N, E	——
Irritability	——		——
Phobias	——	PR, TS, CS,	——
Fears	——	I, BR, AF	——
Unwanted thoughts	——	BR, M, TS, I, AF	——
High blood pressure	——	PR, M, A, BN, E, I, AF	——
Headaches	——		——
Neckaches	——	PR, ISH, A, B, N, E, AF	——
Backaches	——		——
Indigestion	——		——
Irritable bowel	——	PR, SH, A, B, N, E, AF	——
Ulcers	——		——
Chronic constipation	——		——
Muscle spasms	——		——
Tics	——	PR, I, SH, B, E	——
Tremors	——		——
Fatigue, chronic	——	PR, BR, SH, I, A, TS, N, E	——
Insomnia	——	PR, SH, A, TS, B, N, E, I, AF	——
Obesity	——	N, E	——
Weakness	——	E, N, I, AF	——

CODES

A = Autogenics	CS = Coping skills	PR = Progressive relaxation
AF = Affirmation	E = Exercise	RII = Refuting irrational ideas
AS = Assertiveness	I = Imagery	SH = Self-hypnosis
B = Biofeedback	M = Meditation	TS = Thought stopping
BR = Breathing	N = Nutrition	TM = Time management

stressful event occurs and the time a physical or emotional symptom could be related to stress. In time, it is possible to recognize where the body stores muscular tension. With increased awareness, specific procedures for releasing tension in those areas can be practiced. Keeping a record of progress will assist in the change process because it reinforces success and points out what needs further focus.

STRESS MANAGEMENT INTERVENTIONS

Breathing

Breathing is essential for life, yet many breathe in the upper part of the chest, not allowing sufficient blood to reach the lungs, brain, and other tissues. Under stress, many people restrict their breathing even further, increasing fatigue, muscular tension, irritability, and anxiety (Davis, McKay, & Eshelman, 1982, p. 30).

While breathing exercises can be learned readily, it is important to maintain continued practice of them in a nonstressful, relaxing environment to attain the full benefits. The first step in enhancing breathing is breathing awareness.

Breathing Awareness

Nurses are best able to teach the client the procedure if they practice it first. The first step is to lie on a rug or blanket on the floor with legs straight and slightly apart and toes pointed comfortably out, with arms at sides, not touching the body, and with palms up and eyes closed.

Attention is brought to breathing and one hand is placed on the spot that seems to rise and fall during inhalation and exhalation. The other hand is placed on the abdomen and breathing is very gently brought to the abdominal area.

The Relaxation Sigh

The relaxing sigh can be used by nurses prior to approaching a client or can be taught to clients who want to reduce tension levels. The relaxing sigh can be completed in the standing or sitting position. Upon exhalation, a deep sigh is used to let out a sound of deep relief as the air rushes out of the lungs. Inhalation is allowed to occur automatically. The procedure is repeated as necessary, as many times as necessary.

Breathing and Imagery

Breathing can be combined with imagery to provide a powerful healing stimulus. The breath is accomplished in a comfortable position while sitting or lying. The hands are placed on the abdomen; upon inhalation, energy is pictured rushing into the lungs and moving into the solar plexus for storage. Upon exhalation, energy is pictured flowing to all parts of the body. In the case of an injury or illness, energy can be pictured flowing to the injured or ill part.

Alternate Breath

The alternate breath has been found useful for general relaxation and to alleviate tension or sinus headaches (Davis, McKay, & Eshelman, 1982, p. 36). The procedure is accomplished while sitting in a comfortable position using good posture. The index and second finger of the right hand rest on the forehead, and the right nostril is held closed gently by the thumb. Inhalation occurs through the left nostril. The left nostril is then gently closed with the ring finger and the right thumb is simultaneously removed from the right nostril. Air is exhaled slowly and soundlessly through the right nostril. The cycle is continued in a slow and even manner: inhale through right nostril, close right nostril with thumb and open the left nostril; exhale through the left nostril; inhale through the left nostril. Five cycles are suggested for beginners, slowly working up to 10 or 25 cycles.

Biofeedback

Biofeedback means getting feedback from the body about internal processes. Thus, breathing with awareness, imagery, and any intervention that allows feedback about the body is biofeedback.

More specifically, the term is used to refer to the use of instrumentation to develop the ability to read tension in various body systems. Instruments are especially useful when the client is unable to identify signs of stress, such as decreased hand temperature, increased muscle tension, or increased blood pressure. However, reading the signs of tension is only the first step in reducing stress. Once the clues have been identified, the client will still need assistance in learning to let go of the physical tension.

According to Davis, McKay, and Eshelman (1982, p. 164), biofeedback works as follows:

> Biofeedback instruments monitor selected body systems that can be picked up by electrodes and transformed into visual or auditory signals. Any internal change instantly triggers an external signal, such as a sound, a flickering light, or readings on a meter.

The following symptoms have been treated with biofeedback: tension headache, migraine, hypertension, insomnia, spastic colon, muscle spasm or pain, epilepsy, anxiety, phobic reactions, asthma, stuttering, and teeth grinding (Davis, McKay, & Eshelman, 1982, p. 164.).

Clients may come to a sophisticated biofeedback center for treatment, or they can purchase inexpensive monitoring equipment for home use. Levels of in-home equipment vary. Sometimes measures are broadly calibrated and may not be completely accurate. Treatment will probably be most effective when the client works with a professional who has high quality equipment and who can assist in overcoming roadblocks that might interrupt progress. A directory of certified biofeedback practitioners is available from The Biofeedback Society of America, 4301 Owen Street, Wheat Ridge, CO 80030. The following publications can also provide useful information: *Biofeedback Network*, Dub Rakestraw, Editor, 103 South Grove, Greensburg, KS 67054; *Somatics*, Thomas Hanna, Editor, 1516 Grant Ave., Suite 220, Novato, CA 94947; and *Biofeedback and Self Control*, Aldine Publishing, 1323 W. 18th Pl., Chicago, IL 60608.

Progressive Relaxation as a Nursing Measure

Progressive relaxation was developed by Jacobson in 1938 and involves tightening and relaxing the muscle groups of the body, beginning with the hand and moving to the upper and then the lower arm, the forehead, eyes and nose, mouth, neck, upper back, abdomen, buttocks, thigh, calf, and foot for 5 to 7 seconds. The client is encouraged to check for relaxation prior to moving to the next major muscle group. If the nurse is working directly with the client in a relaxation session, the nurse and client can agree that if the client is tense, the index finger of the right or left hand will be raised when the nurse checks for relaxation.

Scandrett and Uecker (1985, p. 33) suggest that a careful assessment of the client is essential prior to employing relaxation techniques. Symptoms need to be identified and an anxiety scale or anxiety symptom checklist may prove useful. Baseline and posttreatment vital sign measures will validate physiological changes associated with relaxation. Essential components of the pretreatment interview include assessing:

- a report of the client's identification of the most bothersome symptom
- onset, duration, and full description of symptoms
- family history of similar complaints
- client interventions and a description of the results

- an investigation of why the client now seeks help for this symptom
- current and recent medications, including over-the-counter drugs
- physical limitations or illnesses
- previous experience with relaxation training
- use of alcohol or mind-altering drugs
- dietary patterns, especially use of caffeine, sugar, and daily alcohol intake
- sleep patterns
- exercise patterns
- overview of daily routine, including stressors
- psychiatric history, including screening for major depressive or psychotic disorders
- willingness to learn and practice at home

Scandrett and Uecker (1985, p. 34) include self-hypnosis, biofeedback, autogenics, and meditation under the rubric of relaxation therapy and suggest the following nursing diagnoses as appropriate for intervention with it: anxiety, sleep disturbance, activity intolerance, powerlessness, ineffective breathing pattern, comfort alterations in pain, ineffectual coping, impaired physical mobility, and fear.

Progressive relaxation has been used as a nursing measure for over a decade. A review of studies that have used relaxation techniques is pertinent in establishing a scientific basis for practice.

Morris (1979) reported on a study to reduce stress in a medical clinic. The subject was post myocardial infarction and was taught muscle tensing and relaxing via taped instructions. The measurement used was vital signs; measurements were taken 1 year after progressive relaxation was taught. The results included a decrease in blood pressure from 190/100 to 154/84, a decrease in cholesterol from 34.4 to 24 mg, a decrease in triglycerides from 302 to 118 mg, a decrease in uric acid from 10 to 8.4 mg, and reported decrease in angina.

Moore and Altmaier (1981) reported the use of progressive relaxation in decreasing anxiety associated with clinic visits and chemotherapy. Nine clients diagnosed with cancer receiving chemotherapy were given six practice and educative sessions. Adjustment was measured by the Affect Adjective Checklist (Zuckerman & Lubin, 1965) interview, sleep and appetite patterns, participation in decision making, and correlation between client and physician description of prognosis. Two clients dropped out of the program; four adjusted according to the Affect Adjective Checklist; and three did not adjust but reported reduced anxiety.

Greziak (1977) reported the use of progressive relaxation for pain associated with spinal cord injury. The technique included muscle relaxation, letting the mind drift to a pleasant image, and concentration on that image. Four case studies of quadriplegia and paraplegia were reported. Measures included subjective reports and staff observation. Clients reported some relief and altered attitudes toward the experience of pain; staff noted mood elevation.

Aiken and Henrichs (1971) reported the effect of progressive relaxation on postoperative complication for 15 post open heart surgery clients who were matched with a similar group. The treatment group listened to a relaxation tape four times a day. The Minnesota Multiphasic Personality Inventory (MMPI) and postoperative complications were the measures of effectiveness. The expected complication rate was 40%; the treatment group was found to have an 8% complication rate. There were significant differences in anesthesia time, bypass time, units of blood required, and degree of hypothermia in those who practiced progressive relaxation.

Flaherty and Fitzpatrick (1978) reported the study of 42 clients who had undergone general surgery. They looked at the effect on comfort of getting out of bed the first time after surgery. There were significant differences in those who learned the relaxation technique from those who did not in terms of narcotic dose, incisional pain, body distress, blood pressure, and heart rate.

Bohachick (1984) reported the use of progressive relaxation training in cardiac rehabilitation. Eighteen clients received 3 weeks of relaxation training in addition to their exercise therapy; a control group of 19 was not taught the technique. The Spielberger State-Anxiety Scale and selected dimensions of the Symptom Checklist-90-Revised were used as measures. Posttreatment anxiety and depression scores for the treatment group were significantly lower (p=0.05) than the control group. (Earlier investigators have reported that those who have suffered myocardial infarction tend to be more depressed and anxious than the general population.)

Although progressive relaxation has proven effective in most studies, some precautions for its use include the following (Snyder, 1984, p. 57):

- In persons who are depressed, relaxation may precipitate further withdrawal.
- In persons experiencing hallucinations and delusions, loss-of-reality-contact reactions may occur.
- The toxic effects of medications can be increased by the relaxation state.
- Tightly tensing muscles can increase blood pressure; those with cardiac conditions should use nontensing relaxation exercises.

• Some clients may experience heightened pain by focusing their attention on body functions; for these clients, imagery may be the treatment of choice.

Self-Hypnosis

Hypnosis is a wakeful state of deep relaxation; there is an alteration in the conscious level of thinking and remembering, and an increase in the ability to focus in on a particular situation. Hypnosis is a heightened state of awareness during which people are more open to suggestion; most people have experienced a trance state at one time or another, e.g., while daydreaming, or when concentrating intently on a book, movie, television program, or work project. All hypnosis is really self-hypnosis because no one will accept a suggestion unless he or she really wants to; thus, the "self" is always in control.

When using self-hypnosis as an intervention, the client usually begins by listening to a taped relaxation and suggestion session or works with a health care professional skilled in the maneuver. With practice, clients can learn quite quickly to relax and put themselves in a trance state. Table 19 gives basic instructions for self-hypnosis. As with all procedures in the book, the nurse should try it out first to understand what the experience is like and to anticipate any difficulties clients might have with the procedure.

For hypnosis to be effective, positive suggestions must be used. Suggestions are used all the time by lay and professional people, but often they are in a negative form. Both negative and positive suggestions affect the subconscious mind even when asleep or unconscious. Adverse suggestions, such as "She'll never recover from this," or "It's malignant, the patient doesn't have a chance," or "You can't be helped, you will have to learn to live with the condition" are heard and acted upon by the hearer. The last comment seems innocuous, but taken literally it means the client will die if the symptom is lost (LeCron, 1964).

Table 20 gives suggestions for coaching clients in self-hypnosis.

Suggestions are most effective and wellness-enhancing when phrased in a positive form, e.g., "I will feel comfortable and confident during the interview tomorrow" (as opposed to "I will not feel tension tomorrow"). Formulating suggestions in the becoming mode is often most effective, e.g., "My comfort is gradually increasing" (instead of "I am totally comfortable"). The best results are forthcoming when only one or two suggestions are focused on. Bombarding oneself with numerous suggestions dilutes the force of all of them.

Eighty to 90% of people can be hypnotized, but those who are severe-

Table 19. Basic Instructions for Self-Hypnosis

1. Sit or lie in a comfortable position. Remind yourself that whenever you want to come out of hypnosis you can.

2. Use a candle, picture, crack in the ceiling, fire in the fireplace, or some other object to encourage eye fixation.

3. While watching the object, suggest your eyes are getting heavier, are beginning to sting, or are starting to flutter (whichever works best) to induce eyelid heaviness.

4. Preselect a word or phrase to use at the moment your eyes close. The words "relax now," or a color or a place that is beautiful and has special meaning to you, can also be used.

5. With eyes closed, begin relaxing all your muscles, starting with forearms and biceps; first tighten, then relax them. Move to the face, neck, shoulders, chest, stomach, lower back, buttocks, thighs, calves, and toes.

6. Picture the top of an escalator with the steps moving down in front of you. As you step on, count back slowly from 10 to 0. Repeat counting back slowly for two more floors.

7. Begin to notice a feeling of heaviness in your right arm (if right-handed, or left arm if left-handed); then notice your arm getting lighter and lighter as if balloons are tied to it, lifting it higher and higher. Soon your hand will begin to move, imperceptively at first, but then it will float, moving closer and closer to your face. When your hand touches your face, you will be in hypnosis.

8. When ready, return from hypnosis, feeling refreshed and relaxed.

Table 20. Coaching Clients in Self-Hypnosis

Directions to Give Clients

1. If uncomfortable with the word "hypnosis," tell the client the experience will increase comfort and relaxation.

2. Encourage the client to practice self-hypnosis regularly; provide praise for a practice attempt; reinforce practice and success and reduce resistance to self-hypnosis by responding with "Good, you are beginning to learn the technique" to whatever they report as effects of their practice.

3. Tell clients they may feel tingling, warmth, or some other sensations, but whatever they experience will be relaxing; this suggestion will reduce resistance and assist clients to integrate transitory reactions.

4. Word suggestions positively and simply; try stating suggestions in a louder, firmer voice.

5. Use rhythm, repetition, and a monotone voice when coaching.

6. If there is a distracting noise during a practice session, give clients the suggestion, "The sounds you hear will tend to deepen your relaxation."

7. Assist the client in setting up a schedule for self-hypnosis practice and agree on a helpful (not nagging) way the nurse can encourage practice and the client or nurse can reward success or practice attempts.

ly emotionally disturbed, depressed, or suicidal respond more positively to psychotherapy then to hypnosis. Others who may not respond positively to hypnosis include: 1) people with psychosomatic illnesses— who deny any emotional component to their problems—and 2) those who are neurologically impaired or mentally retarded (LeCron, 1964).

Clients expected to respond most favorably to hypnosis include those who are highly motivated to learn the technique, are optimistic, willing to try something new, able to concentrate easily, receptive to rather than afraid of hypnosis, and have a good imagination. Clients who do not possess all the above characteristics can learn self-hypnosis if they are willing to practice the technique more frequently.

Some people respond best to permissive suggestions ("I can feel more relaxed and refreshed") while others respond best to commands ("I will feel more relaxed and refreshed"). Experimentation is the best method of determining whether suggestions should be phrased in the permissive or the command mode.

Self-hypnosis can be used to reduce stress related to smoking, drinking, overeating, taking harmful drugs, destructive anger, timidity, anxiety, allergies, itching, asthma, anger, study problems, and pain. The basic self-hypnosis state is induced (see Table 20), but the suggestions used differ depending on the stressor. Suggestions can be said aloud, played on an audio tape, or written and then read to oneself or the client. Bernhardt and Martin (1977, pp. 19–20) suggest the following suggestions be used:

For my body, not for me, smoking (this harmful drug, destructive anger, anxiety, timidity, head symptom, drinking, overeating) is a poison. I need my body to live, I will protect my body as I would protect (name of loved one).

Suggestions for itching, allergies, and asthma would follow the same format with slight variation (Bernhardt & Martin, 1977, pp. 60–74).

For itching:
Not for me, but for my body, this itch is damaging; it means my body is out of balance. To live comfortably, I need my body in balance. To the point I wish to live in comfort, I will itch when I choose to and at the body location I choose.

For allergies, asthma, or colds, the basic suggestion is used and the following is added:
If I choose to live this day symptom-free, I can, because I have power over my body. I can tell my nose when to get stuffed up and when not to. I can declare myself master of my body.

Self-hypnosis is also useful in slowing the heart or breathing rate, using the suggestion: "My pulse is slowing down a few beats a minute, and I am relaxing" or "I am beginning to breathe more slowly and comfortably." Clients can be instructed to take their pulse after several minutes until it has slowed sufficiently; at this point, the following suggestion can be used: "This is the heart rate (or pulse) I am comfortable with and want to remain at."

When learning self-hypnosis, some people may not respond well to either muscle relaxation *or* visualization. Poems that use rhythm, repetition, and imagery can be used in that case, or children can be held and rocked rhythmically. Older children (age 4–16 years) can draw a clown face on their preferred thumbnail. They then place a quarter between that thumb and their forefinger while looking at the clown face. Children are told to look only at the clown face and as they do, the coin will slowly become heavy and slip down and fall. When the coin slips, the children are told their eyes will close and they will be very relaxed. Next, the children are told to place their hands on their legs and answer questions by raising their "yes" hand or their "no" hand. (Which hand is which is agreed on prior to the induction technique.) Questions are then asked that pertain to the problem at hand. For example, for bedwetters, the question is asked, "Would you like to have dry beds at night?" Before asking questions about the problem area, children are asked questions of a neutral type such as, "Do you like ice cream?" Those who answer "yes" to the bedwetting question are told they can learn a "trick" but they must practice it very hard every day, and then the "trick" will help them urinate only in the toilet. The children are asked to practice saying the following statement every time the quarter falls out of their hand:

> When I need to urinate, I will wake up all by myself, go to the bathroom all by myself, urinate in the toilet, and return to my nice dry bed. (Bricklin, 1976)

Dr. Karen Olness, Assistant Professor of Medicine at George Washington University, tried this with 20 girls and 20 boys. Within the first month, 20 were "cured" (and had no recurrence of bedwetting 6 months after the study), six others improved, one did not practice, one had a urinary tract operation, and one answered "no" when asked if he wanted a dry bed; this client was referred to psychiatric evaluation (Bricklin, 1976).

Self-Hypnosis and Pain

There are many advantages of using relaxation and self-hypnotic techniques with clients, particularly with those who are immobile due to physical or emotional difficulties. Those who are hospitalized may benefit from this approach because it can replace the sense of mastery and control they have lost due to the process of hospitalization. Being taught self-hypnosis techniques also provides a special experience for them when the health practitioner says, "I understand that you are having a lot of pain (discomfort, trouble, etc.) and I'm going to teach you a special way to feel better."

Using relaxation and self-hypnotic techniques in a health care institution also does something for the staff working there. First of all, it gets them involved in something special. Zahourek (1978) suggests nurses on a unit be taught the technique so they can help coach the client in the absence of the primary practitioner. In cases where a client is labeled "difficult" or "demanding" or "noncompliant," self-hypnosis can provide hope for the client and the staff.

Often, merely conveying a firm, clear message of intent to help with pain will provide relief. Some comments to use in this regard are: "I am here to help you relieve your pain," or "I want to work with you to reduce your pain." Other types of statements that are helpful are: "What is the pain?" "Describe the pain to me." "What does this pain mean to you?" "How often do you have the pain?" "What do you do to relieve the pain?" "I would like to suggest other ways you can learn to relieve your pain." This discussion is then followed by a decision by the client (if possible) regarding his or her choice of pain relief measure. Approximately 30 minutes after the choice and implementation, the nurse discusses the measure if necessary. Assuming clients have pain if they say they have pain, having confidence they can help, using measures other than medication, checking to ensure the relief measure works, finding out which warnings of pain people have and helping them intervene in the pain before it becomes intense are helpful nursing measures.

Individuals in chronic, ongoing pain tend to take on the pain as part of their identity. They can be encouraged to question, "What meaning does this pain have for me?" "Can I imagine myself without pain?" "Is it worth it to me to give up this pain?" while deeply relaxed in self-hypnosis. Clients with this kind of pain may require self-hypnosis sessions of 15 minutes or more twice a day. Nurses working with these clients must be willing to spend additional time with them and realize that there may be times when hypnosis does not work.

Clients may experience excruciating pain at meaningful times; for example, one person who had survived a fire that killed her daughter had a great deal of pain (despite hypnosis) at noon, the time the fire had occurred (Zahourek, 1976).

Clients who have ongoing pain begin to ask themselves, "Can I stand this pain indefinitely?" A suggestion to use with these people during self-hypnosis is "No pain lasts forever." Clients who have been through life-threatening situations may come to associate pain with being alive, since the feeling of pain may be the one thing that reassures them they are alive. This idea can remain in their subconscious as a self-given suggestion ("If I did not have this pain, I'd be dead"). These clients will often claim to have pain even while asleep. A suggestion that may be helpful in this case is: "When other signs of life were missing, the pain was reassuring, but now it is preferable to be alive without this ongoing pain than to be alive with it." According to Ewin (1978), this type of psychic pain can be distinguished from the pain of cancer, arthritis, or fracture in that psychic pain is always present whereas pain from other afflictions is intermittent.

When using self-hypnosis, it is important to involve as many of the senses as possible (smelling odors, feeling ocean spray or warm sun, touching cool water, tasting salty spray, hearing waves on the beach, etc.). A relatively quick way to induce relaxation is to ask the client to picture him- or herself in a quiet, relaxing, comforting place and to hear, smell, taste, feel, and see everything associated with that place. The nurse can remain with the client and ask that the index finger of the client's right hand be raised to indicate complete relaxation and the index finger of the left hand to indicate lack of relaxation. The nurse can ask the client to indicate level of relaxation after a few minutes; if relaxation has not been attained, the nurse can try progressive relaxation or some other method. For more information regarding the use of self-hypnosis, the reader can consult: Zahourek, Rothlyn P. *Clinical Hypnosis and Therapeutic Suggestion in Nursing,* Grune and Stratton, 1985.

Autogenics

Autogenics is a form of self-hypnosis that allows the participant to induce the feeling of warmth and heaviness associated with a trance state. Johannes H. Schultz, a Berlin psychiatrist, combined autosuggestion with some Yoga techniques and developed a system of autogenic training. The system has been found effective in the treatment of disorders of the respiratory tract, the gastrointestinal tract, the circulatory system, and the endocrine system, as well as anxiety, irritability, and fatigue. The exercises can be used to increase resistance to stressors, reduce or eliminate sleep disorders, and modify pain reactions.

Autogenic therapy is not recommended for children under 5 years old, or for adults who lack motivation or have severe emotional disorders. Those with diabetes, hypoglycemic conditions, or heart conditions should discuss the use of the method with their physicians. Occasionally, a client may experience a sharp rise or drop in blood pressure when doing the exercises; those with high or low blood pressure should take or have their blood pressure taken to ensure the exercises are useful.

The exercises can be completed in a comfortable sitting or lying position. It may take up to 10 months to master the six exercises. Ninety second sessions five to eight times a day are recommended for mastery. The client assumes an attitude of passive concentration; initially this will be difficult to attain, but a wandering mind can easily be brought back to concentration. Clients often experience some reactions that are normal but distracting, including a sensation of weight or temperature change, tingling, electric currents, involuntary movements, stiffness, some pain, anxiety, a desire to cry, irritability, headaches, nausea, or hallucinations. These discharges are transitory and will pass as the program is continued.

Each session is ended with a statement to oneself such as, "When I open my eyes I will feel refreshed and alert" and a few deep breaths and stretches until normal awakeness is achieved. Early exercises are focused on heaviness; this cues muscles to relax; the client repeats the following statements, working up from 90 seconds to 4 minutes four to seven times a day. "My right (dominant) arm is heavy." "My left (non-dominant) arm is heavy." "Both my arms are heavy." "My right leg is heavy." "My left leg is heavy." "Both my legs are heavy."

Later exercises focus on warmth, which assists in attaining relaxation in blood vessels. The client repeats the following statements working up from 90 seconds to 10 minutes a day: "My right (dominant) arm is warm." "My left (non-dominant) arm is warm." "Both my legs are warm." "My right leg is warm." "Both my legs are warm." "My arms and legs are warm."

Next, the client focuses on heartbeat and repeats the following statement: "My heartbeat is calm and regular." Clients who have difficulty becoming aware of their heartbeat can rest their hand over their heart. Those who experience any discomfort are counseled to move to the next three themes and return to the heartbeat theme following the forehead theme.

When focusing on the breathing theme, the client repeats, "It breathes me" or "My breathing is calm and relaxed." The client can picture him- or herself breathing easily to potentiate the effect of slow, deep respiration.

The solar plexus theme is not used for clients who have ulcers, diabetes, or any condition involving bleeding from the abdominal region. The statement that is focused on for other clients is: "My solar plexus (abdomen, stomach, or belly) is warm."

The forehead theme is best repeated while lying on the back since dizziness can result. The client repeats, "My forehead is cool."

Autogenics can also be used for organ-specific work. For example, for blushing, the client can repeat: "My feet are warm" or "My shoulders are warm." For coughs, the statements, "My throat is cool" and "My chest is warm" are helpful. For asthma, clients use, "It breathes me calm and regular."

Additional statements that can be interspersed with standard themes include: "I feel quiet." "My whole body feels quiet, heavy, comfortable and relaxed." "My mind is quiet." "I withdraw my thoughts from the surroundings and I feel serene and still." "My thoughts are turned inward and I am at peace." "I feel an inward quietness." "Deep within my mind, I can visualize and experience myself as relaxed and comfortable and still" (Davis, McKay, & Eshelman, 1982, pp. 81–88).

Thought Stopping

Thought stopping is an approach that is especially useful when nagging, repetitive thoughts interfere with wellness. Unwanted thoughts are interrupted by the client with the command "stop," an image of the letters of the word stop, a loud noise (such as a buzzer or bell), or a negative stimulus, such as wearing a rubber band around the wrist and snapping it when the unwanted thought occurs.

Thought stopping may work because (a) distraction occurs, (b) the interruption behaviors serve as a punishment and what is punished consistently is apt to be inhibited, (c) it is an assertive response and can be followed by reassuring or self-accepting comments, and (d) it interrupts the chain of negative and frightening thoughts leading to negative and frightening feelings, thus reducing stress level.

For effective mastery, regular practice for 3 to 7 days is needed. The client chooses the problematic thought; if necessary, the client can be assisted to prioritize interfering thoughts and focus on the most bothersome one.

Next, the nagging thought is brought to attention. Clients are asked to close their eyes and imagine a situation during which the stressful thought is likely to occur. The next step is to interrupt the nagging thought with an egg timer, alarm clock, snap of the fingers, or an image or verbalization of the word, "STOP."

When clients are able to conjure up and dispense with the nagging thought at will, positive, assertive statements are used to replace the nonconstructive one, e.g.:

- fear of flying: "This is a beautiful view from up here."
- food obsession: "My body is using the food I have eaten to sustain me."
- fear of attack: "I am safe if I use the approaches I have learned to protect myself."

Choosing the best extinguishing behavior and the best replacement statements involves an open discussion with clients; the nurse enumerates the possible extinguishers and may hint at assertive replacement statements, but clients are encouraged to choose based on their knowledge of what is helpful to them.

Clients who experience failure with the approach can choose a less intrusive thought to begin with; once success is achieved, the more troublesome thought can be attempted. Clients need to know that distressful thoughts may return in the future, especially during times of stress; the procedure discussed above can be repeated in these cases.

Refuting Irrational Ideas

Human beings engage in almost continuous self-talk during their waking hours. *Self-talk* is the internal language we use to describe and interpret the world. When self-talk is accurate and realistic, wellness is enhanced; when irrational and untrue, stress and emotional disturbance occur.

Albert Ellis (*A Guide to Rational Living*, 1961) developed a system to attack irrational ideas or beliefs and replace them with more realistic interpretations and self-talk. At the root of irrational thought is the idea that something is being done *to* the person; rational thought is based on the idea that events occur and people experience these events. Irrational self-talk tends to lead to unpleasant emotions; rational self-talk is more likely to lead to pleasant feelings and a positive interpretation of experiences.

One common form of irrational self-talk is statements that "awfulize" experience by making catastrophic, nightmarish interpretations of events, e.g., interpreting a momentary chest pain as a heart attack, a grumpy word from a supervisor as intent to fire, or silence as negative criticism.

The kinds of statements Ellis considers irrational are:

1. External events cause most human misery—people simply react as events trigger their emotions.

2. Happiness can be achieved by inaction, passivity, and endless leisure.
3. People must be unfailingly competent and perfect in all endeavors.
4. It is easier to avoid than to face life's difficulties and responsibilities.
5. The past determines the present.
6. It is horrible when people and things are not the way they should be.
7. It is a necessity for adults to have love and approval from peers, family, and friends.
8. Unfamiliar or potentially dangerous situations always lead to fear and anxiety.
9. People are helpless and have no control over what they experience or feel.
10. People are fragile and cannot be told the truth.
11. Good relationships are built on sacrifice and giving.
12. Rejection and abandonment are the result if one does not always try to please others.
13. There is a perfect love and a perfect relationship.
14. A person's worth is dependent on achievement and production.
15. Anger is bad and destructive.
16. It is bad and wrong to go after what you want and need.

Goodman (1974) developed several guidelines for turning irrational thinking into rational thought, including:

1. The situation does not do anything to me; I say things to myself that produce anxiety and fear.
2. To say things should be other than they are is to believe in magic.
3. All humans are fallible and make mistakes.
4. It takes two to argue.
5. The original cause of a problem is often lost in antiquity; the best place to focus attention is on the present: what to do about the problem *now*.
6. People feel the way they think; the interpretation of events leads to emotions, not the events themselves.

Refuting irrational ideas is a skill and requires practice in the following five steps:

1. Write down the facts of the event, including only the observable behaviors.

2. Write down self-talk about the event, including all subjective value judgments, assumptions, beliefs, predictions, and worries.
3. Note which statements are classified by Ellis as irrational; a star or some other symbol can be used.
4. Focus on the emotional response to the event using one or two words, e.g., angry, hopeless, felt worthless, afraid.
5. Select *one* irrational idea to refute.
6. Write down all evidence that the idea is false.
7. Write down the worst thing that could happen if what is feared happens or what is desired is not attained.
8. Write down positive effects that might occur if what is feared happens or if what is desired is not attained.
9. Substitute alternative self-talk.

Table 21 provides an example of the use of Ellis's format for refuting irrational ideas.

Table 21. Refuting Irrational Ideas

1. *Activating event:* An L.P.N. complained about my nursing care to a client's family.

2. *Rational ideas:* I know she's under a lot of pressure because she's new to the unit.

3. *Irrational ideas:* I can't stand being humiliated in public. Feelings of rage and wanting to kill her are taking over. I'm falling apart.

4. *Main feeling(s):* Rage, anger, humiliation.

5. *Refuting the irrational idea(s):* I'm falling apart.
    a. Being put down in public is not pleasant, but I can handle it.
    b. I'm mislabeling rage and anger as falling apart.
    c. I usually get along O.K. with that L.P.N. and once I calm down, I will again.

6. *The worst thing that could happen:* The worst thing that could happen is that I could put down the L.P.N. in the future to get back at her.

7. *Good things that could occur as a result of this incident:* I can learn to handle put downs without feeling out of control.

8. *Alternate thoughts:* I'm O.K. It's O.K. to feel anger and rage and know I can still function. I can learn to handle this situation and feel good about myself for doing so.

9. *Alternate emotions:* I'm angry, but feel less out of control. The anger is starting to fade and I am feeling calmer.

Coping Skills Procedures

Coping skills training grew out of relaxation and systematic desensitization procedures that were expanded and refined by Meichenbaum and Cameron (1974). The procedures include a combination of progressive relaxation and stress coping self-statements that are used to replace the defeatist self-talk called forth in stressful situations.

Coping skills procedures can be used to rehearse via the imagination for real life events deemed stressful. First, a stressful situation is called forth. Next, progressive relaxation is practiced. Finally, coping skills statements are repeated until the situation can be thoroughly completed in rehearsal without feeling stressed.

The procedures have been shown effective in the reduction of general anxiety and interview, speech, and test anxiety and appear to be effective in the treatment of phobias, especially the fear of heights. Davis, McKay, and Eshelman (1982, p. 120) report the effects of 2-year follow-ups of hypertense, postcardiac clients showing that 89 percent were still able to achieve general relaxation using coping skills training, 79 percent could still generally control tension, and 79 percent were able to fall asleep sooner and sleep more deeply. According to Davis, McKay, and Eshelman (1982, p. 120), coping skills procedures can be mastered in approximately 1 week, once progressive relaxation has been learned (1–2 weeks for mastery).

Coping thoughts can be divided into statements useful for different stages of the stressful situation: preparatory, the situation, and reinforcing success. Examples of statements found effective for each stage follow; clients and nurses can develop their own list and memorize them and/or carry a copy with them for use in stressful situations.

Preparatory Stage:

- I can handle this.
- There's nothing to worry about.
- I'll jump in and be all right.
- It will be easier once I get started.
- Soon this will be over.

The Situation:

- I will not allow this situation to upset me.
- Take a deep breath and relax.
- I can take it step by step.
- I can do this; I'm handling it now.
- I can keep my mind on the task at hand.
- It doesn't matter what others think; I will do it.
- Deep breathing really works.

Reinforcing Success:

- Situations don't have to overwhelm me anymore.
- I did it!
- I did well.
- I'm going to tell ___ about my success.
- By stopping thinking about being afraid, I wasn't afraid.

Time Management

According to Davis, McKay, and Eshelman (1982, p. 151), symptoms of inappropriate time management include: rushing, fatigue, or listlessness with many slack hours of nonproductive activity, chronic vacillation between unpleasant alternatives, chronic missing of deadlines, insufficient time for rest or personal relationships, and the sense of being overwhelmed by demands and details.

Most methods of time management include three steps:

- establishing priorities
- eliminating low priority tasks
- learning to make decisions

Effective time management has been found effective in minimizing deadline anxiety, avoidance anxiety, and job fatigue (McKay, Davis, & Eshelman, 1982, p. 152).

The first step in time management is exploring how time is currently being spent. An easy way to do this is to divide the day into three segments: waking through lunch, end of lunch through dinner, and end of dinner until bedtime. A small notebook is carried and the number of minutes for each activity engaged in in each time segment is logged. The inventory is kept for 3 days. At the end of the time, the total amount of time spent in each of the following categories is noted: Table 22 provides a time management assessment for Eloise Strates, R.N. Based on a review of the inventory, she made the following decisions:

1. Put out clothes for the next day prior to going to bed.
2. Get up at the alarm and limit shower to 5 minutes.
3. Make breakfasts that don't require cooking, cut dinner preparation to 30 minutes, and enlist family to do food preparation 3 days/ week.
4. Ask for a late lunch to take advantage of most productive work hours (11 a.m. to 2 p.m.).

Table 22. Time Management Assessment

Activity	Time (minutes)	Activity	Time (minutes)
Waking through Lunch		After Lunch through Dinner	
Lying in bed and think-	20	Working with clients	90
ing about getting up		Daydreaming while	20
Shower	20	staring at paper-	
Decide what to wear	25	work	
and dress		Shift report	20
Cook breakfast	15	Socializing	30
Read paper/eat	30	Commute	30
Phone friend	15	Shopping	45
Commute to work	30	Phone calls	30
Routine paperwork	30	Cooking	90
Daydream	10	Eating	30
Nonmandatory meet-	60	After Dinner Until Retiring	
ing		Phone calls	60
Working with clients	120	Television	90
Lunch	45	Study	90
		Prepare for bed/read	30

5. Use thought stopping to limit daydreaming.
6. Stop attending nonmandatory, nonproductive meetings.

Eloise's next step was to set priorities. She began by making a list of things she most wanted to accomplish in the near future and comparing it to how she spent her time. She visualized herself being told she only had 6 months to live and began to imagine how she could best spend the time. She made the list without stopping to evaluate or judge what she wrote and suggested others might also find this the most helpful way to proceed.

Eloise's next step was to make a list of 1-month and 1-year goals she believed she could reasonably accomplish in terms of work, improvement, and recreation. Then she sat back and reflected that she now had long, medium, and short range goals. Next, Eloise prioritized each list by deciding which were the top drawer items (most essential or desired), middle drawer items (can be put off for a while, but still important), and bottom drawer (can easily be put off indefinitely with no harm done).

Eloise then chose two top drawer goals for her lifetime goals, 1-year goals, and 1-month goals to begin working toward.

T-1: Buy a new car (1-year goal).
T-2: Write an article for a nursing journal (lifetime goal to contribute to the profession).
T-3: Have dinner out with husband once a week (1-month goal).
T-4: Investigate ways of becoming a nursing consultant (lifetime goal to communicate nursing knowledge).
T-5: Dance lessons with husband (1-year goal).
T-6: Complete old records pile at work (1-month goal).

Since Eloise was overwhelmed by the six goals, she decided to break each one down into manageable steps. For example, her goal of investigating ways of becoming a nursing consultant was divided into the following steps:

1. Borrow a friend's book on consultation and read a chapter a week.
2. Talk with other nurses who are currently consultants; ask one or more to be my mentor.
3. Make a list of my nursing knowledge and trends in nursing, and combine them to make a list of saleable consulting skills.
4. Purchase stationery, business cards, and brochures detailing my consulting skills.

Eloise found it so difficult to get started even after breaking down her priorities into manageable steps that she developed a daily "To-Do" list including everything she wanted to accomplish that day. She rated each item top, middle, or bottom priority and worked only on the top priority items for the day.

This approach helped somewhat, but Eloise still had difficulty until she discovered the rules for making time (McKay, Davis, & Eshelman, 1982, pp. 158–159):

1. Learn to say "no"; remind yourself this is your life and your time to spend as best befits you. Only when your boss asks should you spend time on bottom priority items. Be prepared to say, "I don't have the time." If necessary, take an assertiveness training course.
2. Build time into your schedule for unscheduled events, interruptions, and unforeseen occurrences.
3. Set aside several time periods during the day for structured relaxation; being relaxed will allow you to use the time you have more efficiently.
4. Keep a list of short, 5-minute tasks that can be done any time you are waiting or are between other tasks.

5. Learn to do two things at once; plan dinner while driving home or organize an important letter or list while waiting in line at the bank.
6. Delegate bottom drawer tasks to sons, daughters, secretaries, or in-laws.
7. Get up 15 to 30 minutes earlier every day.
8. Allow no more than 1 hour of television-watching for yourself daily. Use it as a reward for working on your top drawer items.

Part of time management is the ability to make decisions. Procrastination is the great time robber. Procrastination can often be overcome by (Davis, McKay, & Eshelman, 1982, pp. 159–161):

1. Recognizing the unpleasantness of making some decisions versus the unpleasantness of putting it off; analyze the cost and risks of delay.
2. Examine the payoffs you receive for procrastinating, e.g., you won't have to face the possibility of failure, you can be taken care of by others, you can gain attention by being chronically unhappy.
3. Join the resistance you have created by exaggerating and intensifying whatever you are doing to put off the decision. Keep it up until you are bored and making the decision seems more attractive than whatever you are doing to procrastinate.
4. Take responsibility for your delaying tactics by writing down how long each delay took.
5. When making unimportant decisions, choose south or east over north or west; pick left over right; smooth over rough; pick the shortest; choose the closest; pick the one that comes first alphabetically.
6. Take small steps toward the decision: if you want to decide to sew on a button, take out the thread and materials and place them by you as a lead-in to the decision to begin.
7. Avoid beginning a new task until you have completed a predecided segment of the current one; allow yourself to fully experience the reward of finishing something, one of the great payoffs of decision making.

Hardiness

Dr. Suzanne Ouellette Kobasa has researched the ability of people to survive stress. She found that *psychological "hardiness"* or the ability to survive is composed of three ingredients: 1) Commitment to self, work, family, and other important values; 2) a sense of personal control over one's life; and 3) the ability to see change in one's life as a challenge to master.

Dr. Kobasa tested executives, lawyers, women in gynecologists' offices, telephone foremen, operator supervisors, U.S. Army officers, and college students; the results were the same: biology is not destiny. A hardy personality is more important than a strong constitution. It is possible to come from a family with chronic illness and do better under stress if one is hardy than to come from a "healthy" family but have few inner resources (Kobasa, 1984).

Exercise is a good antidote to stress but may be short-term. Jogging after an argument can help that evening, but the next morning stress levels can rise if the stress-provoking situation is re-encountered. Hardiness skills may be long-term innoculations against stressors.

Three techniques Dr. Kobasa found helpful for increasing hardiness skills are: focusing, restructuring stressful situations, and compensating through self-improvement. Focusing is a technique developed by Eugen Gendlin that can assist in recognizing signals from the body that stress is interfering with comfort. Dr. Kobasa found that executives are so used to pressure in their temples, tightened necks, or stomach knots that they have stopped noticing these signals that something is wrong. A beginning question might be: "Where is my tension located in my body?" Those who have learned to tune out body signals can begin with a progressive relaxation tape; this will assist in identifying body locations of stress and tension. Another step is to make a list of "Things That Are Bothering Me Today." The list is then reviewed and the question, "What is keeping me from feeling terrific today?" can assist in the process. Using an affirmation such as, "This day is getting better and better" may help also.

The second technique (reconstruction of stressful situations) is accomplished by thinking about a recent episode of distress, writing down three ways it could have gone better, and three ways it could have gone worse. This exercise increases the ability to put the situation in perspective, a useful procedure for reducing stress.

The third technique (compensating through self-improvement) works most effectively with stressors that cannot be avoided: an illness, impending divorce, unexpected death or loss of a loved one, etc. The feeling of loss of control that results due to this kind of unexpected event can be balanced by taking on a new challenge. Learning to sew, knit, or scuba dive or teaching someone a skill can reassure that life can still be coped with adequately.

INTEGRATIVE LEARNING EXPERIENCES

Use Table 23 for Beginning and Advanced Experiences when called for in this and other chapters. You will note that the "Evaluations" column is divided into "Client Behaviors" and "Nurse Behaviors." The following guidelines will help you in evaluating the effectiveness of your interventions in each category:

Client Behaviors

- Elicit client evaluative comments, such as:
  "I'm sleeping better."
  "I'm less fatigued."
  "I can listen to criticism without getting mad."
  "You've been very helpful to me with . . . but I expected you to do more. . . ."
  "That feels good."
  "I feel whole, peaceful." (Centering)
  "It's getting easier to do my morning workout."

- Note or record body changes (in bodywork, centering, therapeutic touch, hypnosis, and relaxation procedures—breathing becomes deeper and lower, swallowing may indicate relaxation of throat, skin color changes as circulation improves).

Nurse Behaviors

Did you (or another nurse):

- Use effective communication skills (initiating, timing, validating, open body posture, consistency of words with gestures/facial expressions/tone of voice, listening, sharing, using "I" or "We" collaborative messages, using clear/concise messages, providing constructive feedback, staying on agreed-upon goal, sharing)?
- Collaborate with client?
- Involve client in decisions?
- Teach client to prioritize wellness needs?
- Assist client to choose wellness goal based on client priorities?
- Assist client to identify blocks to goal attainment?

- Assist client to plan specific measures to overcome blocks to goal attainment?
- Assist client to learn/choose wellness interventions?
- Teach client to evaluate progress toward wellness goal?
- Practice ethically and legally?
- Take steps to ensure client safety?
- Demonstrate interventions correctly without omitting steps?
- Complete interventions within time frame?
- Identify strengths?
- Identify need for further learning/practice?

Table 23. Nursing Process in Promoting Wellness

Assessments	Interventions	Evaluations
(Include teaching or communication problems and nursing diagnoses)	(Include any steps taken by nurse or client to deal with assessments; include nurse–client contracts and reinforcement of positive behaviors)	(Evaluate the effectiveness of interventions based on specific observed behaviors; give specific examples for each item; obtain videotape, peer, or faculty feedback regarding effectiveness)

Client Behaviors

Nurse (own) Behaviors

Beginning Level

1. Complete the information requested in Table 17 with you as client.
2. Complete the information requested in Table 18 with you as client.
3. Keep a Stress Awareness Diary for 1 week; summarize your findings.
4. Practice the breathing exercises in this chapter and write a summary using Table 23 to organize the information.
5. Practice progressive relaxation to mastery.
6. Practice self-hypnosis (using Table 20) to mastery.
7. Practice autogenics to mastery.
8. Practice thought stopping to mastery.
9. Practice refuting one of your irrational ideas using approaches provided in this chapter.
10. Develop coping skills statements for an upcoming situation of your choice.
11. Assess your time management skills, following Eloise's examples.
12. Assess your hardiness and practice skills suggested by Kobasa.
13. Devise interventions for the following clients:
   (Give the intervention(s) of choice, *specific* comments you would use to introduce the intervention to a client, and *specific* observations or measurements you would use to evaluate intervention effects.)

   A. a student complaining of test anxiety
   B. a new graduate complaining of interview anxiety
   C. a new R.N. on the unit who fears working with I.V.s
   D. a first time parent anxious about bonding with the infant
   E. a nursing home resident who feels hopeless
   F. a nursing student with low self-esteem
   G. a nurse resentful that she must return to school for a B.S.N. in order to advance in her career
   H. a 19-year-old college sophomore who is afraid to leave the dormitory to attend class
   I. a 34-year-old secretary who is obsessed with thoughts that she will be raped
   J. a 50-year-old executive with hypertension
   K. a student with recurring headaches without organic etiology
   L. a young executive jogger with backache (no organic etiology)
   M. a mother with irritable bowel
   N. a student with insomnia

O. an overweight R.N.
P. a victim of an automobile accident who complains of pain despite pain medication
Q. an 84-year-old-man diagnosed with terminal cancer
R. a client 2 days postoperative open heart surgery
S. a postoperative client who is scheduled to get out of bed for the first time
T. a cardiac rehabilitation client
U. a client who wishes to quit smoking
V. a client suffering from chronic itching
W. an 8-year-old boy who wets his bed
X. a 28-year-old woman who believes she has no control over what happens to her
Y. a 40-year-old teacher who is always missing deadlines, unable to make decisions, and complains of fatigue and insufficient rest

14. Imagine you are about to teach a client self-hypnosis. What questions or resistances might you anticipate? How would you intervene with each?
(Be *specific;* include exact words or actions.)
15. Role play teaching the following to a client; use Table 23 to summarize the experiences. Discuss the information in *each* column with a nurse peer and get *written* feedback concerning what is omitted, what is well-presented, and hints for further study/practice.

A. Breathing	F. Thought stopping
B. Progressive relaxation	G. Refuting irrational ideas
C. Stress awareness diary	H. Coping skills
D. Self-hypnosis	I. Time management
E. Autogenics	J. Hardiness

Advanced Level

1. Complete any exercises in the beginning level not already completed.
2. Use Table 17 with three clients; compare your findings among clients with the findings of a nurse peer with her clients (sample = 6).
3. Use Table 18 with three clients; compare your findings among clients with findings of a nurse peer with her clients (sample = 6).
4. Teach a client how to keep a Stress Awareness Diary, including how to set up the diary, length of recordkeeping, how often

progress will be checked and by whom, reinforcement(s), and evaluation procedures. Use Table 23 format. Compare your findings with a nurse peer teaching the same procedure.

5. Teach three clients progressive relaxation; be sure to complete a pretreatment interview. Use Table 23 format to organize your assessment, interventions, and evaluation. Obtain written feedback from a nurse peer.

6. Teach three clients breathing exercises. Use Table 23 format. Obtain written feedback from a nurse peer.

7. Teach three clients self-hypnosis. Use Table 20 and Table 23 format. Obtain written feedback from a nurse peer.

8. Teach three clients autogenics. Use Table 23 format. Obtain written feedback from a nurse peer.

9. Teach three clients thought stopping. Use Table 23 format. Obtain written feedback from a nurse peer.

10. Teach three clients how to refute an irrational idea they hold. Use Table 23 format. Obtain written feedback from a nurse peer.

11. Teach three clients coping skills. Use Table 23 format. Obtain written feedback from a nurse peer.

12. Teach three clients time management skills. Use Table 23 format. Obtain written feedback from a nurse peer.

13. Teach three clients hardiness skills. Use Table 23 format. Obtain written feedback from a nurse peer.

REFERENCES

Aikin, L., and Hendrichs, T. (1971). Systematic relaxation as a nursing intervention technique with open heart surgery patients. *Nursing Research*, 20(2):212–217.

Benson, H., and Klipper, M. (1976). *The Relaxation Response*. New York: Avon.

Bernhardt, R., and Martin, D. (1977). *Self-Mastery Through Self-Hypnosis*. New York: Signet.

Bohachick, P. (1984). Progressive relaxation in cardiac rehabilitation: Effect of psychological variables. *Nursing Research*, 33(5):283–287.

Bricklin, M. (1976). *The Practical Encyclopedia of Natural Healing*. Emmaus, PA: Rodale, pp. 289–290.

Cannon, W. (1914). The emergency function of the medulla in pain and the major emotions. *American Journal of Physiology*, 33:356–372.

Davis, M., McKay, M., and Eshelman, E. (1982). *The Relaxation and Stress Reduction Workbook*, 2nd ed. Oakland, CA: New Harbinger.

Ellis, A., and Harper, R. (1961). *A Guide to Rational Living*. North Hollywood, CA: Wilshire Books.

Ewin, D. (1978). Relieving suffering and pain with hypnosis. *Geriatrics*, 33(6):87–89.

Flaherty, G., and Fitzpatrick, J. (1978). Relaxation technique to increase comfort level of postoperative patients: a preliminary study. *Nursing Research*, 27(6):352–355.

Goodman, D. (1974). *Emotional Well-Being Through Rational Behavior Training*. Springfield, IL: Charles C Thomas.

Greziak, R. (1977). Relaxation techniques in treatment of chronic pain. *Archives of Physical Medicine Rehabilitation*, 58(6):270–272.

Jacobson, E. (1938). *Progressive Relaxation*. Chicago: University of Chicago Press.

Kobasa, S. (1984). How much stress can you survive? *American Health*, 3(7):64–77.

LeCron, L. (1964). *Self-Hypnosis*. New York: Signet, pp. 78–92.

Meichenbaum, D., and Cameron, R. (1974). Modifying what clients say to themselves. In *Self-Control: Power to the Person*, M. Mahoney and R. Cameron, Eds. Monterey, CA: Brooks/Cole.

Morris, C. (1979). Relaxation therapy in a clinic. *American Journal of Nursing*, 79:1958–1959.

Scandrett, S., and Uecker, S. (1985). Relaxation training. In *Nursing Interventions: Treatments for Nursing Diagnoses*, G. Bulecheck and J. McCloskey, Eds. Philadelphia: W. B. Saunders, pp. 22–48.

Selye, H. (1956). *The Stress of Life*. New York: McGraw-Hill.

Snyder, M. (1984). Progressive relaxation as a nursing intervention: an analysis. *Advances in Nursing Science*, 6(3):47–58.

Zahourek, R. (1978). Use of relaxation and hypnotic techniques in the care of the difficult patient. Workshop for nurses at Downstate Medical Center, Brooklyn, NY, November 1, 1978.

Zeagans, L. (1982). Stress and the development of somatic disorders. In *Handbook of Stress: Theoretical and Clinical Aspects*, L. Goldberger and S. Brezwitz, Eds. New York: Free Press.

Zuckerman, M., and Lubin, B. (1965). *Manual for the Multiple Affect Adjective Checklist*. San Diego: Educational and Industrial Testing Service.

5

NUTRITIONAL WELLNESS

This chapter discusses the following topics:

- Food and wellness
- Guidelines for reading nutritional information
- Food myths
- Suggested dietary goals
- Vitamins, minerals, and supplements
- Nutrients for prevention
- Drug–nutrient interactions
- Weight maintenance

FOOD AND WELLNESS

Until recently, the focus of most funded research has been the study of microbes as the cause of disease. Knowledge is just beginning to accumulate regarding the preventive and healing aspects of food and the detrimental effects of poor nutrition. Information gathered by the Senate Select Committee on Nutrition and Human Needs (1977) associated poor nutrition with six of the 10 leading causes of death, "including heart disease, some cancers, stroke and hypertension, arteriosclerosis, diabetes, and cirrhosis of the liver." Table 24 identifies signs of balanced eating. Table 25 provides one way for assessing what the body needs to be well.

One of the greatest gifts the nurse can give the client for developing nutritional wellness is the ability to find and analyze the conflicting

Table 24. Signs of Balanced Eating

One way to ensure your body gets what it needs is to check for signs of balanced eating. Some signs to look for are:

- good endurance and high energy level
- alertness and responsiveness with good attention span
- shiny, lustrous hair
- healthy scalp
- thyroid gland of normal size
- clear, bright eyes
- lack of circles or puffiness around eyes
- moist lips of good color
- pink tongue with papillae present
- pink, firm gums
- clean, straight teeth
- smooth, slightly moist skin
- flat abdomen
- well-developed legs and feet
- lack of tenderness, weakness, or swelling in legs or feet
- normal weight for height, age, and body build
- erect posture with straight back, arms, legs, abdomen in and chest slightly out
- well-developed, firm muscles
- feelings of calm
- good appetite and digestion
- easy and regular elimination
- sleeping well

Table 25. What Does Your Body Need?

Because of conflicting opinions and views on nutrition, a useful approach to take at this time is to assume that your body knows what it needs and will begin to tell you when it is not adequately nourished. Some clues your body might give are: ability to sleep after ingesting a particular food, stool the day following eating that food, breath and body odor, and energy level. You might want to begin to chart your body's reactions to one or more foods by asking the following questions:

1. How well does this food seem to go through my digestive system? Does this food seem to be soothing or cleansing or health-promoting?
2. How do I sleep after ingesting this food?
3. What sort of stool is produced the day after I eat this food?
4. How are my breath and body odor the day after I eat this food?
5. How is my energy level the day of and the day after I eat this food?
6. How does what I am eating affect my skin, hair, and fingernails?
7. How does what I am eating affect my body shape and weight?
8. How does what I am eating affect my ability to concentrate?
9. How does what I am eating affect my relationships with others?
10. How does what I am eating affect how I feel about me and my life?

sources of nutritional information. To do this, the nurse must first be knowledgeable about nutrition resources.

GUIDELINES FOR READING NUTRITIONAL INFORMATION

Some guidelines to keep in mind when reading nutritional information include:

1. Determine the author's background, specificity, and comprehensiveness of references. All authors have biases; be sure you know which ones the author you are reading has. Many authors do not use complete references, up-to-date references, or only include references supporting their point of view; determine as much as possible which variables are operating.
2. Go back to the original reference whenever possible to determine unreliable reporting.
3. Determine the source of funding of the periodical or book; e.g., if food producers are funders, question whether the results or types of research being reported may be biased.
4. Read as many different kinds of nutritional information as possible in order to get a balanced view of the issues.
5. When a relatively nonbiased source is found, keep returning to it for information in the future and tell clients about it.

An example of a source of information that appears to be relatively nonbiased is: Center for Science in the Public Interest, 1755 S Street, N.W., Washington, D.C. 20009.

FOOD MYTHS

Nurses need to be aware of food myths they hold or that are held by clients. Some of the most frequently used ones are:

1. *Meat contains more protein than other foods.* Actually, meat contains only about 25% protein and is about in the middle of the protein quantity scale, ranking below soybeans, fish, milk, soybean flour, and eggs.
2. *Large quantities of meat must be eaten to provide sufficient protein to grow and replace body tissues.* Most Americans eat twice the amount of protein

their bodies can use; the recommended daily allowance of protein, 58–60 grams, can be reached even when all meat, fish, and poultry are eliminated from the diet. For example, by combining wheat and beans, milk and rice, milk and peanuts, or beans and rice, dishes containing all the amino acids necessary for the body can be obtained.

3. *Meat offers the highest quality protein available.* Quality of protein refers to amount of protein available that is usable by the body; eggs and milk are more usable by the body than meat is, and soybeans and whole rice are as usable (Lappe, 1975).

4. *Sugar is sugar.* Sugar occurs naturally in milk, fruits, and vegetables; although sugar is being eaten in the food, it is being ingested with fiber, minerals, vitamins, and protein, thus providing a superior combination of nutrients as compared to processed sugars in candy, sodas, and other sweets.

5. *Sugar is a good source of energy.* Refined sugar leads to less energy because the food is digested quickly, and the blood level of sugar (glucose) rises very rapidly. As a result, insulin is released in excess into the blood, and liver reserves of glycogen (stored glucose) are used, leading to fatigue, shakiness, irritability, faintness, and (in some people) violent behavior. Eating refined sugar results in highs and lows and more coffee (with sugar) or another soda or piece of candy to get a "lift." For high energy, frequent, high-protein meals or complex carbohydrates such as grains or vegetables are recommended.

6. *Starchy foods put on weight.* Complex carbohydrates such as whole grain pasta, baked potatoes, unrefined rice, and whole grain breads and cereals contain a great deal of fiber that is filling; it is only when butter, margarine, sour cream, or other fillings or toppings are used that calories accrue.

SUGGESTED DIETARY GOALS

The Senate Select Committee on Nutrition of the United States Senate adopted seven dietary goals in 1977 as follows:

Goal 1. To avoid overweight, consume only as much energy (calories) as expended. Decrease energy intake and increase exercise if overweight. One in three Americans is overweight. The Dietary Goals recommends reducing foods high in fat, refined and processed foods, sugars, and alcohol, and increasing high-fiber foods such as fruits, vegetables, whole grains, and legumes.

Goal 2. Increase consumption of fresh fruits and vegetables and whole grains to 48% of food intake. Complex carbohydrates are satisfying and protect against cardiovascular disease, constipation, cancer, and overweight (American Cancer Society, 1984; Hirayama, 1979; Painter, 1972). To consume 55–60% of total calories as carbohydrate, meat becomes a condiment, as in Oriental cooking and rice, pasta, potatoes and other starches the main dish. Guidelines for increasing complex carbohydrates and fiber in the diet:

- Choose whole and fresh foods over processed and refined ones; if fresh, local foods are not available, choose fresh-frozen ones, avoiding heavy sauces.
- Choose whole wheat products over white, refined flour. The average white flour retains only 76% of the original wheat grain. When refined to white flour, 10–100% of the trace minerals, vitamins, and fiber are lost; only a small minority is replaced in "enriched" products.
- Select whole grain products for breakfast; leftovers from brown rice, bulgar, kasha, or whole grain noodles can be used as cereal. If no leftovers are available, choose hot cereals (avoiding "instant" or "quick cooking" varieties, which imply greater processing) over cold, ready-to-eat cereals made from refined grain products.
- Become creative in increasing complex carbohydrate meals, e.g., chili without beef, salads, soups, sandwich spreads from one or more types of beans and other vegetables, pocket bread sandwiches, vegetable and pasta or rice casseroles.

Goal 3. Reduce consumption of refined and processed sugars to 10% of daily intake. Refined sugars add empty calories that increase weight, rob the body's stores of vitamins and minerals during metabolism, and replace nutritious foods or lead to weight gain. According to Garrison and Somer (1985, p. 195), sugar has been linked with tooth decay, heart disease, cancer, and diabetes. Although the research is not conclusive, data indicate that an intake of sugar of more than 30% of total calories may lead to a wide range of biochemical abnormalities similar to the ones present in cardiovascular disease (Reiser et al., 1979; Yudkin, 1980). Guidelines for reducing sugar in meal planning are (Garrison & Somer, 1985, pp. 195–196):

- Read labels and avoid foods containing sucrose, raw sugar, glucose, brown sugar, turbinado honey, dextrose, fructose, corn syrup, corn sweetener, and natural sweetener; the closer the sugar is to the beginning of the list of ingredients, the greater the amount of sugar present.
- Substitute fruit juices, nonfat milk, unsweetened tea, mineral water with a slice of lemon, vegetable juice, and water for sugared, fruit-flavored drinks and soft drinks. Although commercial diet soft

drinks are low in sugar, they may be high in additives, dyes, phosphates (calcium-robbing), and caffeine.
- Choose fresh fruits or fruits canned in unsweetened juice.
- Choose ready-to-eat cereals with sugar listed as the fourth or lower item on the ingredients list; sweeten cereal with fruit.
- Begin reducing sugar in recipes gradually; use a juice concentrate instead of sugar in recipes.

Goal 4. Reduce fat consumption to 30% of daily intake.

Goal 5. Reduce intake of saturated fat to 10%, and take in 10% of calories in polyunsaturated fats and another 10% in monounsaturated fats.

Goal 6. Reduce cholesterol consumption to 300 grams/day. Saturated fats and cholesterol are strongly associated with increased risk of cardiovascular disease, hypertension, obesity, atherosclerosis, and other degenerative diseases. Polyunsaturated fat is associated with increased risk of cancer. Some guidelines for meeting goals related to dietary fat include:

- Reduce intake of high fat foods: french fries, hamburgers, whole milk, whole milk cheeses, ice cream, bacon, prepared salad dressings, cream, non-dairy creamers, hydrogenated oils (available on the grocery shelf and in many prepared foods; read ingredients list on all foods purchased), and whipped cream substitutes.
- Obtain needed essential fatty acids from vegetable oils that are relatively nonprocessed (virgin olive oil; dark, unprocessed oils), unprocessed nuts and seeds, fish, and unprocessed whole grains.
- Reduce dietary cholesterol by lowering intake of eggs, liver, and organ meats, red meats, animal fats (lard and chicken fat or skin), and high-fat dairy products.
- Use yogurt or cottage cheese as a garnish for baked potatoes.
- Prepare salad dressing from yogurt, nonfat cottage cheese, garlic, onion, spices, vinegar, and lemon juice.
- Select broiled or baked meat, fowl, and fish; remove fat and skin prior to eating.
- Avoid foods implying that fat is used in the preparation, including descriptions such as: refried, creamed, cream sauce, au gratin, parmesan, escalloped, au lait, à la mode, marinated, prime, pot pie, au fromage, stewed, basted, casserole, hollandaise, or crispy.
- Choose foods that are steamed, in broth, in its own juice, poached, roasted, or in tomato or marinara sauce; these imply low-fat preparation.
- Read nutrition information panels prior to purchasing processed foods. Avoid purchasing foods containing: animal fat, egg and egg yolk solids, butter, bacon fat, lard, palm oil, shortening, vegetable

fat, hydrogenated or partially hydrogenated oils, whole milk solids, cream and cream sauces, coconut oil, coconut, milk chocolate.
- Elevate meat, fowl, or fish when roasting or broiling; do not baste with drippings; use wine, fruit juice, or broth instead.
- Roast at a low temperature (325–350° F) to enhance flavor and fat removal. High temperatures seal fats into the meat.
- Chill meat or fowl drippings and remove fat prior to preparing sauces or gravies.
- Sauté vegetables in defatted chicken stock.

Goal 7. Limit intake of table salt to 5 grams/day. The usefulness of restricting sodium intake is still being debated and tested. See Table 26 for information concerning the low sodium debate. Until the debate is settled, use the following guidelines to reduce sodium:

- Read food and medication labels to identify and eliminate foods processed with salt or containing sodium additives, including baking soda, monosodium glutamate (MSG), cough medicines, laxatives, aspirin, sedatives, sodium phosphate, sodium alginate, sodium nitrate, etc.
- Reduce consumption of food processed in brine—olives, sauerkraut, pickles—or soak in water prior to eating.
- Avoid commercial snacks including potato and corn chips, salted peanuts, pretzels, and crackers.
- Avoid salted or smoked meats, sandwich meats, bacon, hot dogs, corned or chipped beef, sausage, and salt pork.
- Reduce or eliminate salted condiments: catsup, mustard, Worcestershire sauce, bouillon cubes, soy sauce, barbeque sauce.
- Limit processed and high salt cheeses; choose the low salt varieties.

VITAMINS AND MINERALS

There are arguments for and against the need for vitamin and mineral supplementation. Some of the reasons cited in favor of vitamin supplementation due to changes in the available food sources are:

Justification for Supplementation

- Some soils are depleted and produce crops that are nutritionally inferior.
- Toxic insecticides leave harmful residues on food and kill important soil microorganisms and earthworms.

- The increasing use of chemicals in the processing of food has depleted them nutritionally.
- Increasing numbers of people eat vitamin-free sugar as 25% of their daily food intake.
- Chemical additives replace other essential food elements and may also be toxic.
- Numerous life experiences require additional vitamin and mineral stores to reduce stress, including: any difficulty with the digestive tract (diarrhea, colitis, liver or gall bladder disorders); pregnancy; breastfeeding; increased physical activity; infections; the use of antibiotics, aspirin, estrogen, steroids, sulfa drugs, or anticoagulants; inhaling polluted air; drinking polluted water; prolonged emotional stress; smoking or being in a smoke-filled room; fractures; alcohol intake.
- A change in life style in America to a more hectic pace has decreased effective meal planning and led to more "fast-food" meals.

Table 26. The Low Salt Controversy

Until recently, low salt foods were thought to be beneficial for lowering blood pressure. Current research suggests low salt diets may be harmful. One reason may be that salt retains water and keeps the blood from getting too thick; when salt intake is low, water is flushed out of the bloodstream and the blood thickens. This effect may not be dangerous to those with normal blood pressure, but it can cause undue work for the heart muscles of those who do, according to Drs. Drayer of the University of California and Devereux of New York Hospital. The researchers found that those with high blood pressure had thick or viscous blood; their antidote? Drink more water and follow a food plan that's neither high nor low in salt. Losing weight helps, too. Diuretics, which used to be prescribed to increase the flow of urine and reduce fluid, may be an outdated idea (*American Health*, Nov. 1984).

Another group of researchers have been studying the effect of moderate sodium restriction; they found that it resulted in a significant lowering of blood pressure in about 40% of the men in their study. The researchers called these men, "salt sensitive" and found they had significantly higher blood pressure and lower salivary sodium levels with their usual salt intake than did the others, and also more had family histories of high blood pressure. The researchers propose that about 40% of young adults with normal blood pressure may have a susceptibility to sodium-induced intake which may be genetically determined; for these people, reducing sodium intake may prevent the development of high blood pressure. Measurement of the saliva for sodium level may be a simple screening test for salt sensitivity (Skrabal et al., *Hypertension*, Mar./Apr. 1984).

Epidemiological (examining which people develop which diseases) and animal studies have shown that decreased calcium intake is associated with high blood pressure. Recent studies have also shown that sodium intake is inversely related to incidence of hypertension and that the anti-high blood pressure effect of calcium may depend on eating foods that contain adequate sodium. When an attempt is made to restrict sodium, dairy foods (high in calcium) are often eliminated. Calcium supplementation is suggested as a prevention and treatment measure in these cases (Parrott-Garcia & McCarron, *Nutrition Review,* June 1984).

McCarron et al. (*Science,* June 29, 1984) collected dietary intake information from 10,372 adults not taking any drugs to lower blood pressure nor adhering to special diets. They found that the nutrient most consistently associated with blood pressure was calcium, a mineral known to both contract and relax smooth muscles such as the heart. People with high blood pressure (greater than 160 mm Hg) had an average calcium intake nearly 20% less than those with lower systolic pressure and only 74% of the recommended daily allowance for the mineral. People with high blood pressure also had lower intakes of potassium, sodium, and vitamins A and C than those with lower blood pressure; cholesterol intake was not consistently different. Lower intake of dairy products was the one food group characteristic of those with high blood pressure. Eating to lower the intake of calories, sodium, or cholesterol may at the same time reduce the intake of calcium and other protective nutrients.

Diet-conscious Americans, especially women, may consume fewer than 500 mg of calcium a day, even though the recommended allowance is 800 mg or higher. Some sources of calcium are low-fat dairy foods; sardines; canned salmon (eaten with the bones); green, leafy vegetables; molasses; whole wheat bread; fish; tomatoes; and lean beef. Calcium carbonate tablets are another possibility; calcium gluconate tablets contain less calcium and calcium lactate tablets may be more difficult for most adults to absorb. Bone meal and dolomite provide calcium but may also contain toxic metals, so they may not be a good choice (*American Health,* Jul./Aug. 1984.)

A study showing seemingly contrary evidence was completed by Lindahl et al. (*British Journal of Nutrition,* Jul./Aug. 1984). They found that when a strict vegetarian diet (no milk or eggs) was given to 26 hypertensive people, aged 25–70 years, their blood pressure decreased, they rated their condition as better, and the number of symptoms such as headache, dizziness, and tiredness was reduced from an average of 3.7 to 0.2 per person. A number of previous studies of vegetarians have demonstrated that such a meal plan is associated with lower blood pressure. One explanation for the seeming contradiction is that the calcium was obtained from sources other than dairy and egg products. (Adapted with permission, Copyright 1985, *The Wellness Newsletter,* 6(2):2.)

(Author's note: One group for whom calcium supplementation may not be a good idea is pregnant women. Research at the U.S. Department of Health and Human Services has shown that maternal calcium absorption in the gastrointestinal tract increases during pregnancy. Pregnant women who took calcium supplements tended to secrete urinary calcium and their vitamin D levels were markedly elevated. This condition is like the kidney stone forming state and is probably dangerous. Source: *NIH Program Highlights,* 1981.)

For these reasons, even if it were possible to eat a wide variety of foods, vitamin and mineral supplementation may be necessary. As early as 1943 the Food and Drug Administration (FDA) recognized that food processing was destroying important nutrients. Regulations were passed requiring "enrichment" of processed foods; at that time, the FDA noted that enriched foods were second best to unprocessed ones.

The argument against vitamin and mineral supplementation is that if everyone eats a wide variety of foods, all essential nutrients are available. This argument may be most relevant for the ambulatory, well-informed consumer who is able and willing to eat the wide variety of foods necessary.

Additional information that may be useful as a reference source for nurse and client appears in the following tables: Vitamin Functions, Deficiency Signs, and Food Sources (Table 27), RDAs and Reasons for Supplementation (Table 28), Reference to Minerals (Table 29), and Wellness-Enhancing Foods (Table 30).

NUTRIENTS FOR PREVENTION

Although nutrients may be effective preventive agents for numerous diseases, the best researched in this regard are cancer and cardiovascular disease. The benefits of a vegetarian food plan for life appear in Table 29. Other conditions that are currently being investigated are aggressiveness and osteoporosis. Each category will be considered below.

Cancer and Preventive Nutrients

Beta-Carotene and Cancer. As early as 1926, the connection between vitamin A and cancer was made. Laboratory animals deficient in dietary vitamin A developed gastric carcinoma. The two-step model of cancer included an initiation stage and a promotion stage. Plant derived provitamin A (the carotenes) can affect both phases (Garrison & Somer, 1985).

Major dietary studies have found a correlation between the incidence of various types of cancer (lung, colon, stomach, prostate, and cervical) and beta-carotene intake (Hirayama, 1979; Kummet & Meyskens, 1983; Kvale, Bjelke, & Gart, 1982). Foods rich in beta-carotene include carrots, tomatoes, spinach, apricots, peaches, and cantaloupes. Cruciferous vegetables also seem to exert a cancer-protective effect for gastrointestinal and respiratory tract tumors. Examples of cruciferous vegetables include cabbage, broccoli, Brussels sprouts, kohlrabi, and cauliflower (Garrison & Somer, 1985, p. 143).

Vitamin C and Cancer. Nitrosamines are compounds that have been demonstrated to cause cancer in animals. A variety of foods, cigarette smoke, and food preservatives (nitrates and nitrites) have been linked in animal studies to cancer. Vitamin C has been found useful in inhibiting nitrosamine formation from nitrates and nitrites (Bharucha, Cross, & Rubin, 1980).

Table 27. Vitamin Functions, Deficiency Symptoms, and Food Sources

Vitamin	Functions	Deficiency symptoms or signs	Sources
A	helps fight infection, maintains cell wall strength, and prevents viruses from penetrating and reproducing; blocks production of cancerous tumors	night blindness, itching and burning of eyes, redness of eyelids, drying of mucous membranes, colds or respiratory troubles, dry rough skin, pimples or acne, susceptibility to eye infections, difficulty urinating or performing sexually	carrots, brocoli, kale, spinach, eggs, milk fat, fish liver oils, apricots, cantaloupes, organ meats*
B₁ (thiamine)	promotes appetite and good digestion, plays an important role in oxidation, blood and protein metabolism, and growth	tiredness with inability to sleep, swelling legs, loss of appetite, lack of enthusiasm, forgetting things regularly, aching or tender calf muscles, rapid heartbeat, overreacting to normal stress, constipation, feeling of going crazy	sunflower seeds, brewer's yeast, beef kidney,* whole-wheat flour, rolled oats, green peas, soybeans, beef heart, lima beans, crabmeat, brown rice, asparagus, raisins, desiccated liver, wheat germ
B₂ (riboflavin)	contributes to protein and carbohydrate metabolism, tissue repair and formation, growth in infants, proper nitrogen balance in adults, light adaption	feeling trembly, dizzy, or sluggish, burning feet, chapping lips, tiring easily, being overly nervous, having digestive disturbances, scaling of skin, having bloodshot eyes	beef, liver, kidney, or heart,* ham, chicken, hazelnuts, peanuts, hickory nuts, soybeans, soy flour, wheat germ and whole-wheat products, spinach, kale, peas, lima beans, brewer's yeast, sunflower seeds, eggs

Table 27 *(continued)*

Vitamin	Functions	Deficiency symptoms or signs	Sources
B₃ (niacin)	dilates blood vessels, aids in carbohydrate metabolism and the use of Vitamins B₁ and B₂	having cold feet or body numbness, having a swollen bright red tongue or gums, feeling overly anxious, weak, or tired, having memory loss, developing prickly heat rash	wheat germ, wheat bran, brewer's yeast, salmon, prunes, lentils, chicken, peanuts, sunflower seeds, tuna, turkey, rabbit
B₆ (pyridoxine)	activates enzymes, aids in metabolism of fats, carbohydrates, potassium, iron, protein, and formation of hormones, nucleic acids, antibodies, hemoglobin, and lecithin, dissolves cholesterol and regulates water imbalance, may be useful in fighting off cancer, one form of anemia, and tooth decay	feeling tense, irritable or nervous, not being able to concentrate or sleep, having tics, tremors, twitches, bad breath, seborrheic dermatitis or eczema, bloating, puffiness, soreness, or cramping in menstruating or menopausal women	brewer's yeast, sunflower seeds, toasted wheat germ, brown rice, soybeans, white beans, liver, chicken, mackerel, salmon, tuna, bananas, walnuts, peanuts, sweet potatoes, cooked cabbage
B₁₂	maintains normal red blood cell formation and nervous system, aids in RNA and DNA manufacture, conversion of folic acid to folinic acid, carbohydrate, fat, and protein metabolism, fertility, and growth and resistance to germs	feeling apathetic, moody, forgetful, suspicious, soreness in arms or legs or having difficulty walking or talking, jerking of arms or legs	organ meats,* raw beef, clams, oysters, sardines, crab, crayfish, mackerel, trout, herring, eggs, some cheeses, nutritional yeast, sea vegetables (kombu, dulse, kelp, wakame), fermented soyfoods (tempeh, natto, and miso)

124

	Function	Deficiency symptoms	Food sources
Folic acid	vital to blood formation, cell growth, synthesis of RNA and DNA, resistance to infections and to proper mental functioning	looking pale and wan, feeling "pooped," getting brownish spots on face and hands, panting with slight exertion	asparagus, desiccated or fresh liver,* fresh dark green uncooked vegetables, wheat bran, turnips, potatoes, orange juice, black-eyed peas, lima beans, watermelon, oysters, cantaloupe
Pantothenic acid	protects against environmental stress and infection, works with pyridoxine and folic acid to create antibodies, assists in production of body energy, protects against side effects of some antibiotics, aids in expelling trapped intestinal gas	having balky bowels, chronic gas or distention, feeling fatigued or not hungry, having constant respiratory infections, strange itching or burning sensations	soy flour, sunflower seeds, dark buckwheat, sesame seeds, brewer's yeast, peanuts, lobster, wheat bran, broccoli, mushrooms, eggs, oysters, sweet potatoes, cauliflower, organ meats*
Biotin	aids in metabolism of carbohydrates, proteins, and fats, assists in growth, maintenance of skin, hair, nerves, sebaceous glands, bone marrow, and sex glands	having poor appetite, sore mouth and lips, dermatitis, nausea and vomiting, depression, pallor, muscle pains, pains around the heart, tickling sensation in hands and feet	nutritional yeast, liver,* eggs, mushrooms, lima beans, yogurt, and a variety of nuts, fish, and grains

Table 27 *(continued)*

Vitamin	Functions	Deficiency symptoms or signs	Sources
Inositol	not clear, but seems to be useful in controlling cholesterol level	not known	wheat germ, oranges, grapefruit, watermelon, peas, cantaloupes, whole-grain breads, and cereals, molasses, nuts, brewer's yeast, bulgar wheat, lima beans, oysters, peaches, lettuce, brown rice
Choline	essential to nerve fluid, liver functioning, keeping blood pressure down, increasing body resistance to infection	not known	egg yolks, soybeans, liver,* brewer's yeast, fish, peanuts, wheat germ, lecithin
C (ascorbic acid)	contributes to health of blood vessels, gums, teeth, and bones, essential to assimilation of iron, aids body in fighting off infection and cancer-producing substances and in normalizing blood cholesterol level, detoxifies some of the poisons due to smoking, aids in healing process, process, essential to collagen (body "glue"), slows down aging, and protects against stress	frequent bruises, poor healing, bleeding gums when toothbrushing, frequent infections, feeling run down, having an aching back due to disc lesions	green peppers, honeydew melon, cooked broccoli or brussel sprouts or kale, cantaloupes, strawberries, papaya, cooked cauliflower, oranges, watercress, raspberries, parsley, raw cabbage, grapefruit, blackberries, lemons, onions, sprouts, spinach, tomatoes, rose hip tea or powder

D	vital for maintaining health and growth of bones, for using calcium, and for metabolic functions affecting eyes, heart, and nervous system	weakness and generalized bone aches, localized back pain on arising or bending over, pain in areas where spinal vertebrae may have collapsed, brittle bones that break easily, pain in mid- to lower back	fish liver oil, Vitamin-D-enriched milk, eggs, salmon, tuna
E	seems to be useful in any condition where there is actual or threatened clotting, decrease in blood supply, increased oxygen need, externally when there are burns, or sores to heal, or to protect against exposure to radiation	not known	nutritional yeast, wheat germ, peanuts, outer leaf of cabbage, leafy portions of broccoli and cauliflower, raw spinach, asparagus, whole-grain rice or wheat or oats, cold pressed wheat germ, cottonseed, or safflower oil
K	essential to blood clotting	some types of bleeding without clotting	spinach, cabbage, cauliflower, tomatoes, pork liver,* lean meat, peas, carrots, soybeans, potatoes, wheat germ, egg yolks

*Remember: Any chemicals ingested by animals concentrate in their organs and especially their livers; if you decide to eat organ meats to ensure adequate intake of vitamins, you might consider taking extra amounts of the vitamins that detoxify your body, such as Vitamin C and pantothenic acid.

Source: C. C. Clark, *Enhancing Wellness: A Guide for Self-Care,* pp. 48–52. New York: Springer Publishing Co.

Table 28. RDAs of Vitamins; Reasons Supplementation May Be Needed

Vitamin	RDA	Reasons supplementation may be needed
A*	Adults: 5,000 I.U. daily Nursing mothers: 4,000 I.U. daily Pregnant women: 6,000 I.U. daily Children over 12: 4,500–6,000 I.U. daily Children under 12: 1,500–3,500 I.U. daily	Americans are eating 30 pounds less fresh fruit and 20 pounds less vegetables per capita per year than in 1950; cooking dramatically decreases the value of the vitamin; widespread use of fertilizers and pesticides interferes with body's ability to convert carotene into Vitamin A; high-protein diets require more Vitamin A to process; cold temperatures, air pollution require additional amounts of the vitamin.
B₁	1.2–1.5 mg daily	Cereal and rice producers remove thiamine when germ and outer coating is removed; large quantities are lost in cooking water; people who eat little or no organ meats, fresh vegetables, oatmeal, potatoes, and beans may receive little thiamine, as do people who have diarrhea, who eat excess sugars or carbohydrates, drink coffee or alcohol, take antibiotics, or smoke, and those exposed to stress or aging processes.
B₂	1.6–1.8 mg daily	Supplements are needed by people who eat snack foods, processed desserts, or commercial baked goods; the vitamin is destroyed by cooking or when antibiotics or oral contraceptives are taken; it is destroyed when milk bottles or meat containers are left exposed to light.

Nutrient	Dosage	Notes
B₃	18–20 mg daily	Heavy intake of highly refined and/or carbohydrate foods requires more B₃ to metabolize; it is lost during cooking; its metabolism is interfered with when taking oral antibiotics; illness and taking alcoholic beverages decreases its absorption.
B₆	Adults: 2 mg daily Nursing and pregnant women: 2.5 mg daily	Losses of B₆ are due to refining, cooking, processing, storing, and to eating a high-protein diet; there is an increased need when taking steroids (such as cortisone and estrogen), oral contraceptives, or when pregnant or menstruating.
B₁₂	2 micrograms (mcg) daily	When eating only vegetarian meals.
Folic acid	400 mcg daily	Needed during pregnancy, when taking oral contraceptives, when growing or aging, when faced with trauma, infection, or chronic daily stress, or when drinking alcoholic beverages.
Pantothenic acid	10 mg daily	Needed to supplement processed food; greater need when subjected to infection, environmental stress, x-rays, surgery, or antibiotics.
Biotin	300 mcg daily	Needed when eating raw eggs or taking antibiotics or sulfa drugs or when eating beef (cattle are routinely given antibiotics and hormones).
Choline	non established yet	Infants need it if not breastfed (cow's milk does not contain this vitamin, but breast milk does).

Table 28 (continued)

Vitamin	RDA	Reasons supplementation may be needed
C	30–45 mg daily	Needed to slow down aging processes, increase healing of infection, disease, or injury; decreases effects of toxic chemicals in the environment; if taking aspirin, more of this vitamin is needed; when smoking or drinking, more is required; soaking vegetables and fresh fruits in water or exposing fruit or juices to air destroys this vitamin.
D*	400 I.U. daily	Calcium is not absorbed without sufficient Vitamin D; needed at times of insufficient sun exposure in winter, when soot and air pollution filter out sun rays, when spending long hours in offices or indoors; when taking steroids, or when smoking.
E	30 I.U. daily	When outer leaves of vegetables are not eaten; when vegetables are placed in vigorously boiling water to cook (rather than bringing the water to a boil); when eating processed foods, exposed to smog, drinking chlorinated water, undertaking strenuous exercise, when exposed to air purifiers, static electricity, sun, x-rays; by those who take oxygen as a therapeutic measure, have had a heart attack or burn.
K	no requirement	People who are elderly, women with prolonged menstruation, people with liver disease, diarrhea, colitis, or who take antibiotics or anti-coagulants (blood-thinners) .

*Note: Vitamins A and D are the only two vitamins that can be toxic if taken in excess; extra amounts of other vitamins are excreted by the body. If you note symptoms of overdosage in Vitamins A or D, discontinue taking it until symptoms disappear, then take a smaller dose.
Symptoms of Vitamin A overdosage: bone or joint pain that comes and goes, fatigue, insomnia, loss of hair, dryness and fissuring of lips, loss of appetite, peeling and flaking of skin, dizziness.
Symptoms of Vitamin D overdosage: nausea, weight loss, loss of appetite, head pain, calcification of bones, and in children a reduction in growth rate [35].

Table 29. Reference to Minerals, RDAs, Functions, Sources, Factors Leading to Insufficient Intake

Mineral	Functions	Sources	Factors leading to insufficient intake
Calcium RDA: 1000 mg/day; 1.4 g for menopausal women	Keeps body framework rigid and teeth strong; creates tranquility in nervous system and calms nervousness; necessary for transmission of nerve impulses and for muscle contraction, clotting, some enzymes, "glue" (collagen) that holds body together and cells in place, and to regulate transport of substances in and out of cells	milk, cheese, eggs, green leafy vegetables, fish, butter, tomatoes, lean beef, whole wheat bread, yogurt, canned sardines, molasses, dolomite, soy milk, buttermilk	dieting to restrict calories or cholesterol; eating snack foods; drinking soft drinks; having a high protein intake
Chromium RDA: none established; no estimate available	Helps to keep blood sugar levels in check	brewer's yeast, wheat germ, calf's liver, black pepper, and animal proteins except fish	refinement of cereal and grain products remove chromium; the elderly and those who are pregnant or protein-calorie malnourished are at risk for deficiency

Table 29 *(continued)*

Mineral	Functions	Sources	Factors leading to insufficient intake
Iron RDA: 10 mg/day	Works with copper to produce hemoglobin, an essential substance that carries oxygen to and from the body	organ meats, red meats, kidney beans, molasses, egg yolk, whole-grain breads and cereals	infants remaining on milk for long periods of time or those who are born of women who have low stores of iron; women who are menstruating, pregnant, breastfeeding or postmenopausal
Iodine RDA: 130–150 mcg/day	Necessary for normal functioning of thyroid gland; may protect against breast cancer	seafood, brown rice, beans, bananas, green leafy vegetables, kelp	living in areas where soil is low in this mineral (Great Lakes and Rocky Mountain regions)
Magnesium RDA: 350 mg/day	Works with calcium to ensure good muscle movement and a strong heart beat; seems to prevent blood vessel and heart disease	whole-grain bread and cereals, fresh peas, brown rice, soy flour, wheat germ, nuts, swiss chard, figs, green leafy vegetables, citrus fruits, dolomite	having diarrhea, vomiting, taking diuretics, drinking soft water, eating processed foods
Manganese RDA: none established; estimate 2.5–7 mg/day needed	Important to fat metabolism, bone formation, brain function, reproduction, and may protect against cancer of the pancreas	nuts, seeds, whole grains, fruits and vegetables, dry beans and peas, oatmeal	high levels of calcium and phosphorus diminish absorption of manganese

	Helps form / Protects	Food Sources	Depletion Factors
Phosphorus RDA: 800 mg/day	Helps form nucleic acids; a component of cell membranes; aids in metabolism and storage and release of energy; a component of B vitamin coenzymes	liver, yogurt, milk, brown rice, wheat germ, sunflower seeds, brewer's yeast, meat, seafood, nuts, eggs, peas, beans, lentils	people with kidney disease; taking high doses of antacids
Potassium RDA: none, estimated need: 2.5 g/day for adults; .98 to 3.9 g/day for children	Works in concert with sodium to move materials through cells walls (osmosis) and maintains acid-base balance; helps muscles contract, heart to beat regularly, nerves to carry impulses properly, and food to be turned into energy	shredded raw cabbage, bananas, turkey, apples, fresh apricots, cooked broccoli, baked potato, wheat germ, molasses, spinach, dried fruit, fresh fruits and vegetables of all kinds	using convenience foods and highly processed foods; profuse sweating; taking certain diuretics (water pills) to lose fluid; taking cardiovascular drugs, steroids, laxatives, enemas; eating licorice candy; breastfeeding, having depression or ulcerative colitis
Selenium RDA: 50–200 mcg/day	Protects against heart disease and cancer; detoxifies the body from effects of pollutants and radiation; important for healthy skin and hair and for production of sperm cells	high protein foods such as meats, seafoods; whole-grain breads and cereals; brewer's yeast; asparagus, garlic, mushrooms	eating beef fed on corn or eating grains grown in selenium-poor soil (northeast, Florida, parts of Washington and Oregon, parts of the midwest); exposure to industrial pollutants

Table 29 *(continued)*

Mineral	Functions	Sources	Factors leading to insufficient intake
Sodium RDA: not established	Maintains osmotic pressure in the fluid outside the cells	celery, carrots, beets, cucumbers, string beans, asparagus, turnips, strawberries, oatmeal, cheese, eggs, coconut, black figs	some kidney and adrenal diseases; diarrhea; vomiting
Sulfur RDA: not established	Part of the structure of amino acids, such as keratin, the protein of the hair; component of thiamine and biotin (vitamins); required for many oxidation-reduction reactions and coenzymes; contained in blood and other tissues; detoxifying agent; part of material found in skin, bones, tendons, and cartilage	cabbage, peas, beans, cauliflower, brussel sprouts, eggs, horse-radish, shrimp, chestnuts, mustard greens, onions, asparagus	no information available

| Zinc
RDA: 10–15 mg/day | Necessary for adequate breathing and digestion; important to taste, hearing, smell, appetite, normal growth and sexual functioning and reproduction, wound healing, healthy hair, good complexion; decreases lead toxicity | oysters, herring, liver, eggs, nuts, wheat germ and red meats | exposure to lead in gasoline, paints, joints in food cans, lead dust, drinking water that comes through lead pipes; eating canned tomatoes in quantity; foods containing phytate (beans, whole grains, and peanut butter) or calcium interfere with zinc absorption; being a vegetarian; regularly eating imitation meats, fast foods, white bread, fried potatoes, and rich desserts; drinking alcohol; being pregnant; having a cold or chest infection, kidney disease, heart problems, cancer, or taking birth control pills |

Source: C. C. Clark, *Enhancing Wellness: A Guide for Self-Care*, pp. 61–63. New York: Springer Publishing Co.

Table 30. Wellness Enhancing Foods

Eat these often	Vitamins provided	Minerals provided	Other advantages
Raw spinach*	A_1, B_2, C, folic acid, E, K	calcium, magnesium, potassium, copper, iodine, manganese	provides fiber and complex carbohydrate
Wheat germ (toasted)	B_1, B_2, B_3, B_6, inositol, choline, E	magnesium, potassium, chromium	high protein
Brewer's yeast	B_1, B_2, B_3, B_6, B_{12}, pantothenic acid, biotin, inositol, choline, E	selenium, chromium copper, zinc, magnesium, calcium, potassium	can be sprinkled on foods or in drinks
Kale	A, B_2, C	calcium, magnesium, copper, iodine, manganese	provides fiber and complex carbohydrate
Cantaloupe	A, folic acid, inositol, C	manganese	provides fiber and is a good dessert substitute for "sweets"
Sunflower seeds	B_1, B_2, B_3, B_6, pantothenic acid	manganese	easy to carry for a quick snack

*Spinach contains oxalic acid that can decrease the amount of available calcium, so be sure to eat enough calcium from other sources to make up for this.

Food	Vitamins	Minerals	Benefits
Brown rice	B_1, B_6, inositol	magnesium, iodine	inexpensive, good source of protein when combined with beans, eggs, or milk products
Broccoli	A, folic acid, pantothenic acid, C, E	calcium, magnesium, potassium, copper, iodine, manganese	provides fiber and complex carbohydrate
Eggs	A, B_2, B_{12}, biotin, choline, D, K	calcium, iron, potassium	best source of all essential amino acids; low fat
Chicken (no skin)	B_2, B_3, B_6	copper, chromium	low fat; very usable protein
Whole grains	B_1, B_2, B_{12}, biotin, inositol, E	calcium, magnesium, iron, selenium, manganese, chromium	provides fiber
Wheat bran	B_3, folic acid, pantothenic acid		excellent laxative
Peanuts (unsalted, no oil)	B_2, B_3, B_6, pantothenic acid, choline, E	copper, manganese, magnesium	complete protein when combined with a milk product
Cauliflower	pantothenic acid, C, E, K	manganese	provides fiber and complex carbohydrate
Peas	B_2, inositol, K	magnesium, manganese	low calorie, complex carbohydrate

Table 30 *(continued)*

Eat these often	Vitamins provided	Minerals provided	Other advantages
Lima beans	folic acid, biotin, inositol, B_2	manganese	complex carbohydrate
Grapefruit	inositol, C	magnesium, manganese	low calorie, complex carbohydrate, corrects acid imbalance
Soybeans	B_1, B_2, B_3, choline, K	manganese	inexpensive source of protein
Asparagus	B_1, folic acid, E	manganese	low calorie, complex carbohydrate
Cabbage	B_6, C, E, K	potassium	low calorie, complex carbohydrate
Carrots	A, K	potassium, manganese	low calorie, complex carbohydrate
Fish	B_3, B_6, B_{12}, biotin, choline	calcium, zinc, copper, selenium	low fat, highly usable protein
Yogurt (plain)	D	calcium	high protein, low fat, provides helpful bacteria
Sprouts	A, B_2, B_3, folic acid, pyridoxine, pantothenic acid, E, K	calcium, iron, phosphorus, potassium	low calorie, inexpensive, high protein

Source: C. C. Clark, *Enhancing Wellness: A Guide for Self-Care*, pp. 61–63. New York: Springer Publishing Co.

When dietary habits of large populations are reviewed, foods rich in vitamin C appear to have a cancer-protective effect (Grahm, Schotz, & Martino, 1972), but these foods are also rich in vitamin A and folic acid; all of these and dietary fiber have been shown to offer some cancer protection (National Academy of Science Committee on Diet, Nutrition, and Cancer, 1982).

Vitamin C has been found useful in blocking the formation of N-nitrosos compounds (which are converted to carcinogens), thus decreasing the risk of bladder cancer (Schlegel, 1975), and may be useful in preventing stomach and colon cancer (Bartholomew, Hill, & Hudson, 1980; Dion, 1982).

Selenium and Cancer. The cancer-protective nature of selenium is supported primarily by epidemiological studies. In the United States and other countries where the soil and forage crops in certain regions are deficient in selenium, the incidence of death from cancer of the digestive organs, lung, breast, and lymph cancer is greater than in those areas that have a high-selenium content in forage crops (Shamberger & Willis, 1971). A comparison of evidence collected from 27 countries revealed that the incidence of cancer was significantly lower in populations with high dietary selenium intake (Schrauzer, White, & Schneider, 1977).

When case-control studies have been conducted on those with cancer, their selenium status was significantly lower than that of a control group for cancer of the breast, gastrointestinal tract, Hodgkin's disease, lymphocytic leukemia, pulmonary carcinoma, otolaryngeal carcinoma, genitourinary carcinoma, and colon and skin cancer (Allaway, Kubota, & Losee, 1968; Brogramhamer, McConnell, & Blocky, 1976; Calautti et al., 1980; McConnell et al., 1980; Robinson et al., 1979; Shamberg et al., 1973; Willet et al., 1983.)

It is believed that selenium prevents cancer by protecting cells from peroxide-induced oxidation (Griffin, 1979). When selenium is given as a supplement, it acts as an immune stimulant. Organic forms of selenium (methylated and selenoamino acids) and the selenium found naturally in yeast and whole grains are suggested; inorganic forms of selenium supplements and artificially selenized yeasts have potential for mutagenicity (Noda, 1979). The recommended daily allowance for adults is 50–200 µg (Helzsouer, 1983).

Vitamin E and Cancer. Vitamin E works as an antioxidant, protecting the unsaturated fatty membranes in the body from the formation of the carcinogens, lipoperoxides. Preliminary studies of tumor growth in animals suggests a potential role for vitamin E in inhibiting the carcinogenic process (Prasad & Edwards-Prasad, 1983). Although addi-

Table 31. Does Vegetarianism Protect Against Chronic Disease?

Vegetarianism seems to have a lot of advantages and some disadvantages. Let's look at the research and see why a plant-based meal plan may enhance wellness.

Cancer. Vegetarians eat more beans, whole grains, vegetables, and fruits than meat eaters so they take in more fiber, vitamins A and C, and protease inhibitors (anticancer agents). Vegans, who eat no meat, eggs, or dairy products, get a lower percentage of their calories from fat than do nonvegetarians. A low fat diet is clearly related to protection from cancers of the breast, colon, and prostate (R. L. Phillips et al., Cancer in vegetarians, unpublished research reported in *Nutr Act* 10 (5):9, 1983; *N Engl J Med* 307:1542, 1982)

Osteoporosis (brittle bone syndrome). It is not clear why vegetarians have less osteoporosis, but they do. One explanation is that meat meals cause the body to excrete excess calcium (*J Am Diet Assoc* 76:148, 1980)

Heart Disease. Both types of vegetarians have lower blood cholesterol levels than do nonvegetarians (*J Hum Nutr* 35:437, 1981; *Am J Clin Nutr* 23:249, 1970). A new study (unpublished research reported in *Nutr Act* 19(5):9, 1983) shows they also have lower heart attack rates. Twenty-five thousand Seventh Day Adventists (SDA) were monitored for 20 years. Males who ate meat six or more times a week were twice as likely to die of heart disease as vegetarian SDAs if they were 55 or older and ran four times the risk of a fatal heart attack than vegetarian SDAs if they were aged 40–54

Obesity. Studies show the average lacto-ovo (eats milk products and eggs) vegetarian is slightly leaner than meat eaters and vegans are between 8 and 20 pounds lighter. (*J Hum Nutr* 35:437, 1981; *Am J Med* 36:269, 1964; *N Engl J Med* 292:1148, 1975; *J Am Diet Assoc* 77:655, 1980)

High Blood Pressure. Vegetarianism lowers blood pressure, probably because it helps people lose weight, especially if they omit meat, eggs, and dairy products (*Am J Epidem* 100:390, 1974)

Diabetes. The vegan diet can assist in weight loss and is very similar to the high-complex carbohydrate, high-fiber plan now being used to treat adult onset diabetes. This raises the question of whether the meal plan may also be preventive*

Vegetarianism offers all these potential benefits, but there are a few disadvantages. Although lacto-ovo vegetarians have no more nutritional deficiencies than meat eaters (*J Am Diet Assoc* 77:61, 1980), vegans, particularly children, may have difficulty obtaining sufficient vitamins D and B-12, calcium, zinc, iron, riboflavin, or calories (*Nutr Act* 10 (5):11, 1983).

It appears that the advantages of moving toward a vegetarian meal plan outweigh the disadvantages, especially if you're an adult. And even if you are a child or concerned for a child's welfare, adding fermented soy products, wheat germ, brewers yeast, cooking with iron cookware, and ensuring adequate sunshine should take care of the disadvantages.

---

*Addendum: A vegetarian diet may reduce the risk of *developing* diabetes (D. Snowdon & R. Phillips, "Does a Vegetarian Diet Reduce the Occurrence of Diabetes?" *American Journal of Public Health,* 75(5):507–512, May 1985.

Reprinted with permission of *The Wellness Newsletter,* 5 (2):4–5, 1984.

tional research is necessary before any definitive statement can be made regarding the chemopreventive qualities of vitamin E, animal studies have shown that the vitamin in concert with selenium can inhibit the development of artificially induced breast cancer in rats (Horvath & Clement, 1983). Tables 27 and 29 provide information regarding dietary sources of vitamin E and selenium.

Dietary Guidelines for Reducing Cancer Risks

Dietary guidelines for decreasing the risk of cancer were suggested by the American Cancer Society's Medical and Scientific Committee (Nutrition and Cancer, 1984). The recommendations and elaborations of them as suggested by Garrison and Somer (1985, pp. 142–144) follow.

1. *Avoid obesity.* Obese people (20% or more above ideal weight) have an increased risk for cancers of the uterus, gallbladder, kidney, stomach, colon, and breast.

2. *Cut down on total fat intake.* Excessive use of *either* saturated or unsaturated fat increases the risk of developing cancers of the breast, colon, and prostate.

3. *Eat more high fiber foods (whole grains, fruits, and vegetables.)* There is sufficient evidence to warranty the increase of fiber intake and variety of fiber foods eaten. Simply adding bran to a meal plan is not thought to be sufficient.

4. *Include foods rich in vitamin A and/or carotene and vitamin C daily.* (See explanations above regarding these vitamins.)

5. *Include cruciferous vegetables daily.* A component in these vegetables seems to reduce risk of cancer of the gastrointestinal and respiratory tract.

6. *Be moderate in consumption of alcoholic beverages.* Alcohol increases the risk of cirrhosis, liver cancer, cancer of the oral cavity, larynx, and esophagus. The risk is potentiated in smokers who also abuse alcohol.

7. *Be moderate in consumption of salt-cured, smoked, and nitrite-cured foods.* As mentioned earlier, nitrosamines are cancer precursors. Smoking or barbecuing meats results in the production of procarcinogenic substances.

Cardiovascular Disease and Preventive Nutrients

The likelihood of developing CVD is dependent on the individual's personal decision to avoid or embrace specific risk factors. "Risk factors are any characteristics associated with an above average incidence of a disease" (Garrison & Somer, 1985, p. 149). Risk factors are signals warning that a habit, age, or dietary pattern is associated with disease. If heeded, warning signals can enhance wellness.

Primary Habits Associated with Cardiovascular Disease. The most well-known cardiovascular disease (CVD) risk factor study is the Framingham study (1948) that identified primary habits associated with CVD (hypertension, cigarette smoking, and elevated cholesterol). Since then, elevated low density lipoprotein-cholesterol has been recognized as the fourth primary risk factor. Secondary risk factors include obesity, diabetes, lack of aerobic exercise, stress, male sex, high serum trigly-cerides, increasing age, a family history of heart or blood vessel disease, and stress-prone personality type (Garrison & Somer, 1985, p. 149).

Serum Cholesterol. It is well established that serum cholesterol levels are directly related to CVD (Gordon & Verter, 1969; Scott et al., 1972). In countries where serum cholesterol levels are below 160 mg/dl, CVD is nonexistent (Wissler, 1979). Over half of the American people exceed the level suggested by the American Heart Association; when other risk factors such as smoking or obesity are added, a lower serum cholesterol level would be needed to counteract them.

High Density Lipoproteins. High-density lipoproteins (HDL) are heavy and contain the most protein. They collect cholesterol and trans-port it to the liver; they clean up excess cholesterol lingering in the arteries. (Low-density lipoproteins, or LDL, transport cholesterol from the liver and to the tissues; elevated LDL is the primary source of cholesterol and cholesterol esters in plaque; when LDL is high, deposits of cholesterol line the arterial walls.)

HDL can be raised by reducing dietary fat and cholesterol, not smok-ing, maintaining ideal body weight, and increasing cardiovascular or aerobic exercise. Reduced HDL is primarily caused by obesity and a sedentary lifestyle.

Canadian studies have shown that postmyocardial infarction clients were able to rise their HDL as a result of aerobic exercise. At least 20 km/week of running was required to increase HDL (Kavanaugh, 1983).

Total Fat More Important Than Cholesterol Intake. Total fat in the diet appears to be more important than cholesterol intake. Even in vegetarians, a high fat diet promotes elevated serum lipids, but less so than nonvegetarians; this is to be expected because vegetarians eat high fiber, fatty acid, and polyunsaturated foods. There is no correlation between egg consumption (high cholesterol) and plasma lipids (Lieb-man & Bazzarre, 1983).

The Ratio of Polyunsaturated to Saturated Fat. The ratio of poly-unsaturated to saturated fat must be increased to lower serum choles-terol. Polyunsaturated acids have a strong antilipogenic ability; they lower liver lipoprotein synthesis and increase lipoprotein removal. Polyunsaturated fatty acids (PUFA) lower cholesterol in another way. Linoleic acid, an essential fatty acid, is available only through diet. Increased intake of oils (e.g., safflower) high in linoleic acid decreases platelet aggregation and decreases serum cholesterol (Bazan et al., 1981; Oliver, 1982; Sacks et al., 1983).

Essential Fatty Acids. "Essential fatty acids may also influence other activities of prostaglandins, including smooth muscle contraction, renal functions and numerous cardiopulmonary functions" (Garrison & Somer, 1985, p. 166).

Although PUFA are beneficient in preventing CVD, increased intakes have been correlated with increased risk of cancer; *therefore* it is impor-tant to reduce the intake of saturated fats and keep the intake of PUFA constant. Oils tend to be high in polyunsaturates and low in saturates. Olive oil has a polyunsaturated to saturated ratio of 0.9 (the closest to a 1 : 1 ratio.) Olive oil is used daily in the Mediterranean countries, where coronary artery disease is low compared to the American diet (Garrison & Somer, 1985, p. 168).

Dangers of Hydrogenated Fats. Hydrogenated fats hold special dangers. They supply less PUFA than meats and dairy products. Amer-icans consume 600 million pounds of these frying fats each year in fried and processed foods. A glance at many canned or boxed food items reveals that hydrogenated or partially hydrogenated fats are contained therein.

There are several dangers lurking in hydrogenated fats. For example, they:

1. increase the need for essential fatty acids such as linoleic acid (Beare-Rogers, Gray, & Hollywood, 1979);
2. reduce prostaglandin production and interfere with the conversion of linoleic acid to arachidonic acid in the formation of pros-taglandins (Rutenberg et al., 1983);
3. may elevate serum cholesterol and liver glycerides (Rutenberg et al., 1983);

4. are absorbed, but do not seem to be used readily in cellular energy metabolism, acting more like saturated than unsaturated fats, thereby impairing the cellular function; in heart and smooth muscle this may lead to CVD (McGill, Geer, & Strong, 1965).

It is suggested that food labels be scrutinized and the benefits of a fried or fast food meal be weighed against the disadvantages listed above.

EPA Reduces Risk of Heart Disease. The fatty acid omega-3-eicosapentaenoic acid (EPA), found in cold-water fish, lowers levels of serum cholesterol. Given in supplement form, EPA has produced changes associated with reduced risk of heart disease (Fish oil for prevention of atherosclerosis, 1982). However, EPA supplements do have adverse effects, including thrombocytopenia and hepatotoxicity. Therefore, it is best to obtain EPA naturally in mackerel, salmon, and sardines (Garrison & Somer, 1985, pp. 167–168).

Phospholipids (Lecithin). The generic term for a phospholipid is lecithin. Lecithin is composed of two phosphatides, phosphatydlcholine (PC) and phosphatylethanolamine (PE). Clinical studies have shown that lecithin can favorably affect the risk of CVD by reducing serum cholesterol (Vroulis et al., 1982).

Both phospholipids increase excretion of neutral sterols resulting in reduction of the entry of dietary cholesterol and "the reentry of endogenous cholesterol into the body" (Garrison & Somer, 1985, p. 169). One study concluded that the ability of PC to emulsify cholesterol may make fat more soluble, thereby less likely to form gallstones (ter Well, van Gent, & Dekker, 1974).

Many cholesterol-rich foods *also* contain their own lecithin; for example, eggs contain eight times as much lecithin as cholesterol. In one study, there was no decrease in serum lipoproteins and liver lipids when rats were fed PC in the form of soybeans, but when they were fed egg yolks (PC and PE), serum cholesterol and apoprotein A-I declined (Murata, Imaizum, & Sugano, 1982). Major sources of lecithin include egg yolks, soybeans and soybean products, and lecithin (available in granular form as a supplement).

Dietary Fiber. Dietary fiber includes nondigestible plant materials free of calories. In addition to preventing CVD, dietary fiber protects against constipation, diarrhea, hemorrhoids, gallstones, hiatus hernia, varicose veins, and appendicitis; in populations in which dietary fiber composes a large percentage of the diet, these diseases are unknown. Fiber normalizes bowel activity, reducing the transit time of food through the intestines (thereby eliminating toxic substances more quickly), influences intestinal flora, and may reduce the formation of intestinal carcinogens (Garrison & Somer, 1985, p. 169). Some types of fiber (excluding wheat bran) appear to lower blood cholesterol and lower the mortality rate from CVD (Allbrink, Davidson, & Newman, 1976).

Pectin is another form of dietary fiber that has LDL-cholesterol lowering effects (Baig & Cerda, 1981). It is found in apples and some other fruits, including not completely ripe berries.

Other dietary fibers shown to lower cholesterol include: oat fiber (Anderson et al., 1983), guar and locust bean gums (Zavoral et al., 1983) found in soybean ice-cream substitutes in health food stores, soybeans, chickpeas and peanuts (Malinow et al., 1981), and alfalfa (Malinow et al., 1978).

Although some fiber is beneficial, excessive intake of the substance can bind trace minerals, interfere with their absorption, and irritate the intestinal lining. Thirty-seven g/day of dietary fiber provide the protective effect without producing the negative effects (Garrison & Somer, 1985, p. 170). This amount can be obtained from the following *daily* intake: six servings of *wholegrains* (rice, corn, pasta, bread, kasha, etc.); four servings of fresh fruits and vegetables; and one serving of dried beans. It is worthy of note that this reaffirms the wisdom of a primarily vegetarian meal plan for life. Additionally, when planning servings of wholegrains, it is imperative to ensure whole grains are used; the best way to do this is to read labels and/or purchase the whole grains and cook them rather than purchasing quick cooking or white enriched products with or without some wholewheat or other flour added.

Unraveling the Complex Interrelationships of CVD. Focusing on one food factor is not a wellness approach to CVD. Since 70–80% of blood cholesterol is manufactured in the body, the building blocks of cholesterol require study. Some of the factors that interact to influence the manufacture and excretion of cholesterol include amino acids, vitamins, minerals, garlic, inositol, aging, and fasting.

Amino Acids in Soybeans Lower Cholesterol. Vegetable-based protein products appear to reduce serum cholesterol levels (Sirtori, Gatti, & Manter, 1979; Kritichevsky et al., 1982) regardless of egg consumption. Soybeans are relatively high in the amino acid arginine and low in lysine—a combination that seems to lower cholesterol (Check, 1982). Taking supplements rather than eating soybeans and soybean products may *not* produce the desired effect; lysine alone may stimulate cholesterol synthesis (Schmeisser et al., 1983). Although it is important to be cautious in extrapolating findings from chicks to human beings, it is wise to remember the principle found here: it is generally safer to obtain nutrients from whole foods rather than supplements whenever possible.

B-Vitamins Important in Lipid Metabolism and CVD. The following B-vitamins are important in lipid metabolism: pantothenic acid, B_2, B_6, and niacin. Substantial amounts of vitamin B_6 are lost in the production of grains and other foods; this is not one of the four nutrients added back when refined foods are "enriched."

Vitamin B_6 needs are dependent on protein intake. The American diet, already too high in protein, could aggravate a possible borderline deficiency and lead to CVD.

Vitamin C, Cholesterol, and CVD. Vitamin C is found primarily in fruits and vegetables. An absence of these in the daily food plan has been correlated with increased incidence of CVD (Acheson & Williams, 1983). One explanation for this correlation is that vitamin C is important in the synthesis of collagen, the "glue" that strengthens and supports body tissue. Vitamin C (along with pyridoxine, essential fatty acids, zinc, and possibly niacin) also appears to encourage prostacyclin synthesis, encouraging collateral circulation to ischemic areas of the heart (Garrison & Somer, 1985, pp. 173–174). Studies have demonstrated a direct correlation between vitamin C intake and a reduction in cardiovascular death rates (Knox, 1973).

Low ascorbic acid (vitamin C) levels were found in clients with coronary atherosclerosis in one study (Ramirez & Flowers, 1980). Vitamin C affects the cholesterol content of the blood and positively influences triglyceride and lipoprotein levels. Giving vitamin C supplements to men and women with CVD resulted in a reduction in total serum cholesterol for both groups and a reduction in LDL in men (Horsey, Livesley, & Dickerson, 1981; Ginter, 1979).

Vitamin C is most available when food is kept from exposure to air, minimally cooked, not reheated, and when cooking water and juices are eaten. Additionally, vitamin C is destroyed when foods are stored; it is best to purchase small amounts of local, fresh produce. Some factors that deplete the body of vitamin C include: cigarette smoke, stress, birth control pills, alcohol, and the consumption of fast foods; the latter tend to be high in fat, salt, and sugar, with little, if any, vitamin C. "Although the potato is a reasonable source of the vitamin, once it has been sliced, stored, fried in hot oil and held under warming lights, little, if any, of the original vitamin C remains" (Garrison & Somer, 1985, p. 174).

The Fat Soluble Vitamins and CVD. Vitamins A and E play a protective role in CVD because they function as antiperoxidants, antiaggregants, affect oxygen transport and utilization, increase HDL, and enhance hypolipidemic action of niacin (Garrison & Somer, 1985, p. 174). On the other hand, vitamin D in excess promotes atherosclerotic lesions, especially when combined with cholesterol (Seelig, 1983).

Vitamin E is a mild antiaggregatory agent, relieves intermittent claudication, and is a powerful antioxidant. Research suggests a possible advantage to vitamin E supplementation for prevention of blood clotting and other complications of atherosclerosis; questions remain unanswered in some respects. People with vitamin K deficiencies could worsen a poor blood-clotting mechanism if they ingest large quantities of vitamin E. Since the issue remains unsettled, it is probably wise to obtain vitamin E from food sources.

Studies in humans and animals have shown optimal intakes of sodium, magnesium, zinc, calcium, iodine, and chromium reduce the risk of CVD (Garrison & Somer, 1985, p. 175). Garlic is another food substance shown to reduce cholesterol levels, increase HDL, and lower LDL; 15 mg of garlic oil or eight to nine cloves of garlic produced this effect in one study (Bordia, 1981).

Inositol functions to prevent fatty liver infiltration. It works in concert with folic acid, vitamin B_6, choline, vitamin B_{12}, betaine, and the amino acid methionine to stimulate normal liver management of fats (Gavin, 1941). Dietary sources of inositol include grapefruit juice, cantaloupe, oranges, stone-ground whole wheat bread, cooked beans, grapefruit, limes, and green beans (Garrison & Somer, 1985, p. 177).

Aging affects the body's regulation of cholesterol synthesis; an enzyme crucial to this regulation (hydroxymethylglutaryl CoA) declines with age. Fasting may temporarily lower serum cholesterol levels (Garrison & Somer, 1985, p. 177).

Aggressiveness and Nutrition

The studies correlating nutrition and aggressiveness have been completed with institutionalized subjects; this presents some problems in extrapolating to the noninstitutionalized population; however, it is probably true that metabolism remains fairly constant whether the person is in a prison or hospital or not.

Fishbein (1981) found that incarcerated male offenders in Florida were more apt to display maladaptive, aggressive behaviors when eating refined carbohydrates. Prinz (1980) reported using a double-blind study to examine the effects of diet on hyperkinetic behavior; sugar and artificial food dyes together produced significant behavior changes that were not found when examining the effects of either alone.

Beginning in 1980 and for the next 4 years, Stephen J. Schoenthaler, Ph.D., a criminologist, completed a series of rigorous, large sample sized studies involving over 6,000 inmates in 10 penal institutions in three states. In one study, he found that property offenders benefited most from dietary revision; there was a 53% reduction in antisocial behavior—$n = 124$, $p = 0.002$ (Schoenthaler, 1983a).

To determine whether the lowering of sugar consumption or the increased consumption of other foods led to behavioral changes, Schoenthaler covertly increased the quantity of orange juice served to incarcerated juveniles and then compared their behavior with institutionalized juveniles who had been institutionalized prior to the dietary revision. Juveniles who experienced the "increased orange juice" period had a 41% lower rate of antisocial behavior than the baseline population at the 0.01 level of probability (Schoenthaler, 1983b).

Lonsdale and Shamberger studied a population of 20 clients diagnosed as functionally neurotic by a Cleveland, Ohio clinic; the population ranged in age from 3 to 45 years of age (Lonsdale & Shamberg, 1980). They found all subjects had a subclinical thiamine (beriberi) deficiency. The adolescents studied showed poor impulse control, irritability, and occasional periods of hyperaggressiveness; they angered easily and were sensitive to criticism. After a period of thiamine supplementation, these characteristics changed.

Other studies show iron may play a role in aggressiveness, cognitive functioning, and reasoning. Webb and Oski (1974) found that junior high school boys found to be anemic were restless, irritable, and disruptive; in the most anemic, impaired ability to learn was noted. Pollitt and Leibel (1982) confirmed this finding.

Tucker and his associates (1984) found that iron is involved in left hemisphere activity cognition and also in dopaminergic neurotransmission. Schauss, Bland, and Simonsen (1979) found that delinquents' diets were significantly low in folic acid.

Using the findings of these studies, it is possible to conclude that Schoenthaler's orange juice provided delinquents with the building blocks for less aggressive behavior: vitamin C, which increases non-heme iron absorption, thiamine, and folic acid. Additional controlled studies are needed to examine consumption of orange juice and its relationship to an increase in intracellular nutrient levels.

Osteoporosis and Calcium

Osteoporosis is a degenerative bone disease drastically increasing the probability of bone fracture. It results from dietary imbalances, years of low physical activity, and, for women, hormonal changes of menopause.

In approximately 25–30% of postmenopausal women, osteoporosis is a contributor to major orthopedic problems (Avioli, 1981).

If an insufficient amount of calcium is eaten, it will be mobilized from the bones into the bloodstream, leading to bone fragility. Bone loss proceeds gradually; the first sign may be a loss of height, persistent pain in the lower spine area, "dowager's hump," or loss of weight. In some cases, a small trip and subsequent fracture may be the first sign that osteoporosis has occurred. Once bones suffer extensive calcium loss, it is difficult to regain bone strength. The best prevention is to ensure adequate calcium intake (Garrison & Somer, 1985, p. 106).

See Table 29 (pp. 131–135) for RDAs for calcium; although calcium is abundant in many foods, the average woman's diet is low in the mineral. Women over 45 typically consume little more than half the amount recommended; at this level, a loss of 1.5% of total bone mass could occur within a year's time (Avioli, 1981).

Milk is frequently replaced with soft drinks that are usually buffered with phosphoric acid, which can stimulate the release of calcium from the bones. Additional sources of phosphorous include beef and preservatives.

An intake of 1500 mg of calcium daily will inhibit the age-related bone loss in postmenopausal women (Recker, Saville, & Heaney, 1977). Table 29 provides food sources of the mineral.

Alzheimer's Disease and the Calcium–Aluminum Relationship

Processed foods, aluminum-containing medications (e.g., antacids), and the use of aluminum cookware has led to an excessive body burden of aluminum. Toxicity due to aluminum is associated with Alzheimer's and other neuromuscular disorders, hyperparathyroidism, and bone loss (Garrison & Somer, 1985, p. 106).

When serum calcium levels are high, aluminum accumulation is reduced (Konging, 1981; Marquis, 1983). Therefore, it is suggested that sufficient calcium intake be guaranteed and that cooking be done in nonaluminum cookware. Perhaps the best cookware is iron because cooking in such containers insures adequate iron intake, protecting against anemia; glass or stainless steel are alternatives. The difficulty with aluminum and the potential protectiveness of iron cookware underline the relevance of wellness theory; environment and nutrition can interact to lead to disease or higher levels of wellness.

Calcium May Protect against Eclampsia

Fetal losses from eclampsia range from 30 to 35%; about 10% of maternal mortality is due to this complication. A study of Guatemalan women revealed they have a very low incidence of eclampsia despite the presence of other factors (poor prenatal care, poor nutrition, and geography) that are considered high risk for the condition to occur. When the Guatemalan women were compared with Columbian women of a similar socioeconomic level with very high rates of eclampsia, the only difference between the two groups was a high rate of dietary calcium in Guatemala. This finding supports the contention that sufficient calcium intake could be an important preventive measure for eclampsia (Villar, Belizah, & Fischer, 1983).

Premenstrual Tension Reduced with Magnesium, Zinc, Niacin, and Vitamins C, E, and B₆ Supplements

A study of serum and red cells of women with premenstrual syndrome found magnesium levels were low. The classical symptoms (headache, dizziness, and craving for sweets) responded well to magnesium, zinc, niacin, and vitamin C supplementation. Breast tenderness responded to vitamin E supplementation. Tension anxiety associated with premenstrual syndrome improved with increased doses of vitamin B₆ (Abraham, 1983; Abraham & Lubran, 1981).

Amyotrophic Lateral Sclerosis (ALS) and Aluminum

Young men in Guam have a high rate of amyotrophic lateral sclerosis (ALS or Lou Gehrig's disease) which has been traced to a high level of aluminum and manganese exposure. Following up on this finding, researchers at the Departments of Agronomy and Animal Science at the Louisiana Agricultural Experiment Station administered aluminum sulfate and manganese sulfate to animals in varying doses; manganese had no effect on magnesium, but administration of aluminum resulted in symptoms of magnesium deficiency. When the aluminum was removed, the cramping, gastrointestinal complications, and nervous system disorders decreased (Allen, Robinson, & Hembry, 1984). The researchers concluded that aluminum administration can result in magnesium deficiency. This work confirms other studies' findings that a calcium- and magnesium-rich diet offers some protections against aluminum-induced toxicity.

Chromium and Diabetes

The major role of chromium is that of improved carbohydrate metabolism through facilitation of insulin activity. Long-term ingestion of sugar and other refined carbohydrates is considered a primary factor in chromium deficiency leading to disturbances in the ability to handle sugar. These abnormalities resemble those of maturity-onset diabetes, including high levels of sugar in the blood and urine and an excessive amount of insulin in the bloodstream (Garrison & Somer, 1985, p. 111).

Several studies have shown that supplemental chromium can benefit elderly diabetics. Brewer's yeast was given to older maturity-onset diabetics; they showed improvement in blood cholesterol levels (Boyle, 1970; Offenbacher, 1980).

Chromium supplementation from brewer's yeast has also been shown to be an effective treatment for abnormal glucose tolerance as well as a protective factor in atherosclerotic disease (Rabinowitz et al., 1983; Saner et al., 1983).

Copper, Zinc, and Immunity

Patients with depressed cell-mediated immunity have been found to have a low serum zinc and elevated serum copper level. When given zinc supplements, they improved. This supports the hypothesis that alterations in zinc and copper metabolism due to dietary imbalance contribute to immunodeficiency (Oleske et al., 1983).

Lead and Behavior

Although lead has been removed from gasoline for a number of years, toxicity still remains a factor due to ingestion of lead from dust and pollution and use of lead sealed canned foods. Decreased IQ, increased fatigue, and loss of concentration have been reported from chronic lead impairment (Marlowe & Errera, 1982).

Lead and Sudden Infant Death Syndrome

Lead levels are significantly higher in infants who die of Sudden Infant Death Syndrome (SIDS) than infants who die of other causes. These findings do not prove a cause and effect relationship but do explain reports linking SIDS to environmental toxins (Erickson et al., 1983).

DRUG–NUTRIENT INTERACTIONS

Research suggests that nutrient losses induced by many over-the-counter and prescription drugs may actually encourage the disease for which the medication was taken (Garrison & Somer, 1985, p. 209). As nonmedication approaches to disease are recognized, it behooves nurses to consider their role in the medicating process.

Some drugs increase appetite and others decrease it; it is the appetite depressants that are of most concern for populations that are already at risk nutritionally, including the elderly, those with a chronic disease, dieters, those who abuse alcohol, cigarette smokers, new mothers, adolescents, and certain ethnic minorities. Table 32 displays drug effects on nutrient absorption.

WEIGHT MAINTENANCE

Susan Toth, R.N., M.S.N., Carolyn Montgomery, R.N., A.N.P.-C., and Judith Bunn, R.D. (1984) summarized studies reporting what helps people manage their weight.

Stanford University Heart Disease Prevention Program Study

Because personal preferences and learning styles may differentiate who loses and maintains weight, a survey conducted by Stanford tapped these prefences. They found that most people disliked losing weight in a group. Therefore, they developed a mail order extension course that proved successful.

Indiana University School of Medicine Study

At the Indiana University School of Medicine, M. Peri found that buddies are more helpful when it comes to weight loss, unless spouses are overweight and participate in the weight loss program. (This supports the peer facilitation/role model factors found in Clark's study; see pages 326–328.) In the New York study, 70 obese men and women volunteered for training in self-monitoring of foods eaten, nutritional education, and exercise. They were assigned to one of five groups: training only, training supported by a buddy, training supported by a spouse, training supported by both, and a waiting list that received no treatment or training.

After 10 weeks, those who had received training lost an average of 10.5 lb.; those supported by a buddy lost substantially more (14.5 lb.). Those whose spouses had been enlisted for support lost 8.8 lb., less than those who received behavioral training only. The positive effect of a buddy was counteracted by the support of a spouse; those in the buddy/spouse group did less well (9.6 lb. weight loss) than those in the

Table 32. Drug-Induced Nutrient Malabsorption

Drug	Malabsorption	Drug	Malabsorption
acetaminophen	sodium	dyrenium	folic acid
achromycin	B_{12} or folic acid	gluthethimide	calcium
agoral	vitamins A and D	indocin	iron
alcohol	folic acid; thiamin; riboflavin; niacin; vitamin C, B_6, B_{12}; magnesium; zinc	INH	B_6
		klotrix	B_{12} or folic acid
		k-lyte	B_{12} or folic acid
		k-tab	B_{12} or folic acid
aldomet	B_{12} or folic acid	macrodantin	B_{12} or folic acid
aldoril	B_{12} or folic acid	medrol	B_6 and B_{12}
aluminum hydroxide	aluminum toxicity	mellaril	riboflavin
		micro-k	B_{12}
aluminum magnesium	phosphate depletion	mysoline	vitamin K
apresoline	B_6	neomycin	fat, nitrogen, sodium, potassium, calcium, iron, lactose, sucrose, B_{12}
aspirin	iron; folic acid; vitamin C		
aureomycin	riboflavin; vitamin C, calcium	oral contraceptives	B_6, B_{12}
azulfidine	folic acid	panmycin	B_2, vitamin C, calcium
bactrim	B_{12} or folic acid		
biguanides: metformin and phenformin	B_{12}	para-amino salicylic acid	fat, folate, B_{12}
		percodan	B_{12}
biscodyl	potassium deficiency	phenobarbital	calcium
		phenolphthalein	vitamin D, calcium
butazolidin	B_{12} or folic acid	premarin	B_6, B_{12}
cholestyramine	fat; vitamins A, K, B_{12}, D, and iron	primidone	calcium
		potassium chloride	B_{12}
colchicine	fat, carotene, sodium potassium, B_{12}, D, iron	questran	vitamin A, D, K, folic acid
		rifamate	B_6, niacin, Vitamin D
colestid	vitamins D, K, and folic acid	septra	B_{12}
deltasone	B_6, B_{12}, or folic acid	serapes	B_6
		slow k	B_{12}
depen	B_6	soda mint	folic acid
dilantin	vitamin D, folic acid	sodium bicarbonate	sodium overload
		stelazine	B_{12}
diphosphonates	calcium	sumycin	B_{12}
donnatal	B_{12} or folic acid, B_6	tagamet	B_{12}
dyazide	folic acid	thorazine	riboflavin

Source: Drug-Nutrient Interactions, Robert Garrison, 1984–85 Yearbook of Nutritional Medicine, New Canaan, CT: Keats Publishing, 1985, pp. 93–112.

buddy group. Those on the waiting list gained an average of half a pound.

The Georgia Mental Health Institute Study

In a related study in Atlanta, Loveland and Schonitzer found that participation of the spouse in a weight loss program was insignificant unless the spouse was overweight and participated in the weight loss program, too.

The Health Care Plan Medical Center Study

A weight management program at the Health Care Plan Medical Center in West Seneca, NY helps participants identify situations that promote eating, adjust their eating environment, and make appropriate responses to internal and external cues. Participants receive an 8-week course covering nutrition, body image, assertiveness, appetite control, and stress management. Those who change their behavior are rewarded by receiving up to $30 of their $50 deposit; points are awarded for attending meetings, following the diet, eating breakfast daily, keeping a food diary, exercising three times a week, limiting intake of caffeine, sodium, or cholesterol, submitting tested diet recipes, or reaching the 12-week weight goal. The following activities have also been found successful:

- Each group member cooks a low-calorie dish which is sampled by the others
- A yearly reunion is held in December during the holiday season

Participants lose an average of 12 lb. in the 12 week program; a 6–12 month follow-up indicated that 35% maintained a weight loss of more than 10 lb. More than two thirds of the participants earn refunds, and participants reported increased feelings of well-being, fewer symptoms of arthritis, and decreased use of medication for diabetes and high blood pressure.

Recommendations for Weight Loss

In a review of factors that help people lose weight, Glanz (1984) found that knowledge about how and what to eat is not sufficient for change; what is needed includes:

- an emphasis on changing behavior through keeping food diaries of types and amount of food eaten, time of eating, location, position, mood, and companions
- a review of the diary with a helping person
- setting specific behavior change goals
- rewards for changing are designated: tokens, money, prizes, participant-identified rewards
- a combination of mass media approaches and one-on-one counseling
- a design for creating ways of keeping participants in the program; less than half of the participants remain in a program long enough to achieve their weight loss goals
- emphasis on the immediate benefits of good nutritional practices such as attractiveness and self-confidence

The National Center for Health Education in San Francisco (1982) released a report identifying various approaches that have worked with individuals:

- Identify why weight loss is important, listing the reasons in as specific a way as possible.
- Write down the advantages and disadvantages of becoming thinner.
- Record each incident of eating and the circumstances surrounding it for a week.
- Set goals for becoming thinner and formalize them in a contract; have a trusted other person sign it.
- Set up a reward system: praise or other pleasant happening if weight is lost; forfeit money (or another reward) if pledged weight is not lost.
- Find a buddy or a small group of weight losers with whom to discuss the weight loss process and from whom to garner support; keep the support going after desired weight has been reached to avoid slippage.
- Use imagery to picture oneself as fat as currently or as thin as desired.
- Role play with a buddy how to handle pressure from others to eat.
- Learn relaxation techniques and diversionary tactics (drink a glass of water, take a walk, deep breathe) when eating urges overwhelm.
- Get at least one family member involved in the process to offer support and to help change family eating patterns.

Other common weight loss recommendations found helpful by the author in her work with clients include:

- Analyze eating in detail in an individual or group setting, including:
  —Why do I want to change?
  —What are the advantages and disadvantages of changing?
  —Exactly how do I sabotage my eating plan now?
  —What skills do I need to learn to resist pressure from others to
   maintain old eating patterns? (saying no, refraining from getting
   defensive)
  —What kind of support do I need from others to attain my goals?
   (phone calls or written reminders when I feel I'm slipping)
- Eat only at specified meal times and only while sitting down in the
  one household spot identified for eating; eating while cooking and
  eating while watching television increase chances of inappropriate
  eating.
- Slow down eating pace by putting down the fork after each bite,
  taking a break during the meal, and concentrating on the taste and
  texture of food; when food is eaten quickly there is insufficient time
  for body/mind to identify satiation.
- Never do anything else while eating.
- Set goals guaranteed to bring success; start small and gradually increase expectations as success is achieved.
- Develop an exercise program to increase lean body mass, tone the
  body, increase fitness, and moderate hunger urges.
- Eat whole foods (e.g., a baked potato rather than french fries) to
  increase satiety.
- Cut down on appetite stimulants such as coffee, spices, chocolate,
  sugar, colas, and salt.
- Say or write the following affirmation 25 times each day until it is
  believed: It is getting easier and easier to eat food that is healthy and
  that enhances my wellness.
- Stay away from fad diets, monodiets, and other quick loss ideas
  that end in quick loss and quick weight regain; such a syndrome can
  result in hypertension, frustration, and reduced wellness.

Dr. Roland Weinsier (1985) of the University of Alabama has been
investigating another method of weight management called the *"Time
Calorie Displacement" (TCD) method*. It features high-bulk, low-calorie
foods such as fruits, vegetables, and unrefined starches. These foods
take longer to consume than high calorie, less bulky foods such as
meats, fats and oil, and sugar products. The longer the dieter spends in
eating, the greater the satisfaction and the fewer calories consumed.
Some of the recommended foods are rice pudding made with small
amounts of honey and fiber-rich brown rice and mock pizza sandwiches
made with whole wheat English muffins, part skim milk cheese, and
tomatoes.

Clinical studies with obese participants at the University of Alabama show that the TCD food plan keeps people satisfied on about 1,500 calories a day, is nutritionally balanced, and is effective in loss of fatty tissue. Thirty-five percent of the participants lost more than 20 lb. and 7% lost more than 40 lb. over an average of 26 weeks. Steady but small weight loss allows participants to establish new eating patterns so that excess weight does not reappear.

Weinsier tested 20 people; 10 were obese and 10 were of normal weight. Given as much food as they wanted, all reached the same degree of fullness while eating half the number of calories from the high-bulk, low-calorie meals than from the high-calorie meals and rated both meal plans as equally enjoyable. A separate study showed that skinfold thickness (a measure of body fat) fell significantly while muscle mass was maintained. Blood levels of all essential vitamins and minerals were also maintained without vitamin supplementation.

Theories concerning weight maintenance have changed radically over the years. Earlier theorists claimed overweight people consumed more food than lean ones; some nutritionists still hold onto this theory, despite research to the contrary (Coll, Meyer, & Stunkard, 1979; Garrow, 1974; Wooley, Wooley, & Dyrenforth, 1979).

The lazy-body hypothesis holds that some become overweight because they are physically less active than others. The sluggish-metabolism theory holds that some people need less energy to keep their bodily processes going and store the excess as fat. All three theories are based on the assumption that overweight is an accident.

A newer explanation, *setpoint theory*, holds that fatness is not an accident of fat. "Each body wants a characteristic quantity of fat and proceeds to balance food intake, physical activity, and metabolic efficiency to maintain that amount" (Bennett & Gurin, 1982, p. 62). It is theorized that fat storage is managed by part of the unconscious brain; cells are believed to release chemical signals telling the brain how much fat they contain and, when necessary, asking for more. According to the theory, the brain synthesizes sensory impressions (taste and smell of rich foods raise the setpoint), amphetamines and nicotine may lower the setting, and physical activity may lower the setpoint, perhaps through hormonal signals.

According to the theory, the body does not know the difference between dieting and starvation. In an effort to protect the individual, the body goes into starvation practices, requiring fewer calories to do the work of the metabolic processes. Thus, when individuals attempt to diet, their setpoint rises and fat is held on to, making weight loss difficult when rich foods, inactivity, and short-term fad diets reign.

Rare individuals manage to continue dieting and remain relatively thin, despite permanent hunger. But even dedicated dieters may find, to their dismay, that they cannot lose as much weight as they would like. After an initial loss of 10 or 20 pounds, dieters often reach a plateau where they lose weight at a far slower rate, although they remain as hungry as ever. (Bennett & Gurin, 1982, p. 79)

Studies of animals under starvation conditions and forcefed humans support setpoint theory (Bennett & Gurin, 1982, pp. 64–84).

The Wooleys (1979) have suggested that recurrent dieting may be an important variable affecting weight gain. Dieting leads to a lower metabolic rate; when "normal" eating is resumed, weight is regained. Repeated dieting may be leading many to weight gain after dieting. Bennett and Gurin (1982) suggest alternatives to dieting: change food plan to reduce intake of fat, sugar, and artificial sweeteners; and increase physical activity.

A number of studies have demonstrated that the setpoint can be countered by physical activity. Working at the University of California at Davis, Judith Stern, a nutritionist, collaborated with two exercise physiologists to study six people placed on a low-calorie food plan. As expected, metabolic rates fell after 2 weeks (starvation reaction). The subjects then began an exercise program and metabolic rates returned to normal in half the dieters; one dieter lost 30 lb. that month.

Findings are considered preliminary, but the researcher points out that because basal metabolism decreases at a rate of 2 to 5% with every decade past the age of 30, activity may be the only safe way to diminish the accumulation of fat that is normal with aging (Bennett & Gurin, 1982, p. 252).

Studies of populations who are vigorously active also lend credence to the argument that exercise lowers setpoint. For example, Norwegian woodcutters do not grow fat with age; they maintain about 15% body fat for 40 years (Skrobak-Kaczynski & Andersen, 1975).

If the theory is correct, people should lose weight spontaneously when undertaking an exercise program without dieting. Gwinup worked with a group of obese men and women to test the theory. All participants had been discouraged by repeated failures at dieting. The researcher told the group to forget about what they ate and begin a program of physical activity. Most began with brisk walking for 10 or 15 minutes daily. Although most subjects dropped out, all who reached the point of walking briskly for at least 30 min. 5 days/week lost weight.

The 11 women who stayed with the program chose to increase their activity and within 1½ years each lost 22 lb. on the average and continued a steady, slow loss (Gwinup, 1975). The benefits of losing weight in this manner are that there are no negative effects of dieting, including: weakness, increased nervousness, feelings of deprivation, loss of muscle, or quick release of fat-stored toxins into the bloodstream. More than a third of the weight lost during dieting and two thirds lost during a fast reflect loss of muscle, not fat (DeVries, 1974; Oscai, 1973).

Other investigators have demonstrated the same effect, including Moody (1969) and Leon et al. (1979). Exercise alone is a slow route to weight loss; about one third of a pound is lost per week for the overweight or obese and one tenth of a pound per week for people with ideal weight (Epstein & Wing, 1980).

Frequency of exercise is important in weight loss. People who exercise four or five times a week lose weight three times faster than those who exercise 3 days a week; exercising once or twice a week has *no* effect on weight loss (Epstein & Wing, 1980). So much for the weekend athlete syndrome.

The type of food eaten, though not important to weight loss, is important to wellness. Combining an exercise program with a very low carbohydrate diet is not wise; carbohydrates are needed to replenish the body's store of glycogen. Short-term, low-carbohydrate diets are incompatible with strenuous exercise; listlessness, dehydration, and acetone-breath are correlates of this kind of regime (Phinney et al., 1980). Figure 3 gives information useful for attaining ideal weight.

The idea that your mind controls you body is not new, but how many of us tap our considerable mind power to enhance our wellness? Positive affirmation and visualization can be combined to obtain your ideal weight. Before each meal, try the following exercise:

Step One: Find a quiet, peaceful spot and spend 5 minutes relaxing your body. Keep your eyes closed throughout the exercise.

Step Two: Say, "I see and feel my body as I want it to look and feel." Repeat this sentence 10 times very slowly while picturing your body at your ideal weight.

Step Three: Say, "I am able to move toward my ideal weight with increasing comfort." Repeat this statement 10 times while picturing yourself looking and feeling more comfortable.

Step Four: Say, "I *am* able to move toward higher levels of wellness and positive energy." Repeat this statement slowly five times while visualizing yourself moving to increased states of wellness and becoming filled with positive energy.

Step Five: Slowly open your eyes and prepare to eat, carrying with you the image of yourself at your ideal weight.

Figure 3. Getting to your ideal weight.

Diabetes and Weight Loss

Although the reason is not completely understood, lowering the body's stores of fat leads to an increased sensitivity to insulin. Therefore, diabetic clients need to reduce their weight. The traditional low carbohydrate diet has been called into question. As long as the overall intake of calories is low enough to produce weight loss and large amounts of refined sugar are excluded, complex carbohydrates, especially whole grain foods, are desirable foods for weight loss plans (Simpson et al., 1981).

INTEGRATIVE LEARNING EXPERIENCES

Beginning Level

1. Scan several books and articles in professional journals and consumer magazines. Use "Guidelines for Reading Nutritional Information" (p. 115) to evaluate what you read; write down your findings.
2. Role play a response to a client or peer who tells you, "I need a candy bar for energy."
3. Write down a response to a client who says, "I don't eat potatoes or starches anymore; I'm watching my weight."
4. From the guidelines to meet Goal 2 of the Dietary Goals, select one way you plan to meet this goal in the future. (Optional: draw up a contract to do so.)
5. From the guidelines to meet Goal 3 of the Dietary Goals, select one way you can meet this goal in the future. (Optional: draw up a contract to do so.)
6. From the guidelines to reduce dietary fat, select one way you plan to meet this goal in the future. (Optional: draw up a contract to do so.)
7. Make a list of the pros and cons of vitamin and mineral supplementation.
8. Discuss the pros and cons of eating low sodium foods to lower blood pressure.
9. List the nutrients associated with cancer prevention.
10. From the "Dietary Guidelines for Reducing Cancer Risks," devise a plan to lower your cancer risks.
11. Assess which primary habits associated with cardiovascular disease apply to you. (Optional: devise a plan to reduce your risks.)
12. List the preventive nutrients related to cardiovascular disease; assess which apply to you. (Optional: devise a plan to increase the preventive nutrients in your food plans.)

13. Plot your aggressiveness in relation to sugar intake; write down your conclusions. (Optional: devise a contract based on your findings.)
14. Discuss the relationship between calcium, phosphorus, and osteoporosis.
15. Discuss the relationship between calcium, aluminum, and neuromuscular disorders. (Optional: devise a contract based on these relationships.)
16. FOR WOMEN ONLY: Evaluate yourself for premenstrual tension. Devise a plan based on information presented in this chapter.
17. Discuss the setpoint theory and its application to weight maintenance.
18. Write down nutrients for the following client issues based on information presented in this chapter:

    A. hypertension
    B. constipation
    C. infection
    D. cold feet
    E. surgery
    F. pregnancy
    G. diabetes
    H. high serum lipids
    I. heart disease
    J. varicose veins
    K. gallstones
    L. elevated serum cholesterol
    M. aggressiveness
    N. premenstrual tension
    O. diabetes
    P. overweight

Advanced Level

1. Discuss with at least three clients (individually or in a small group) the following issues; record your findings, using Table 23, p. 108 Nursing Process, as a guide.

    A. Guidelines for reading nutritional information
    B. Food myths
    C. Dietary goals
    D. Pros and cons of supplementation
    E. The low salt controversy

F. Wellness-enhancing foods (Table 30)
G. Nutrients for prevention of cancer
H. Dietary guidelines for reducing cancer risks
I. Cardiovascular disease and preventive nutrients
J. Primary habits associated with cardiovascular disease
K. Refined sugar and behavior
L. Osteoporosis and calcium
M. Alzheimer's disease and the calcium–aluminum relationship
N. Nutrients and premenstrual tension
O. Weight maintenance

2. Use Table 31 to examine 10 client charts; devise a written plan to reduce the harmful effects of drug-induced nutrient malabsorption.

REFERENCES

Abraham, G., and Lubran, M. (1981). Serum and red cell magnesium levels in patients with premenstrual tension. *Am. J. Clin. Nutr.* 34:2364–2366.

Abraham, G. (1983). Nutritional factors in the etiology of the premenstrual tension syndromes. *J. Repr. Med.* 28:446–461.

Acheson, R., and Williams, D. (1983). Does consumption of fruits and vegetables protect against stroke? *Lancet* 1:1191–1193.

Albrink, M., Davidson, P., and Newman, T. (1976). Lipid-lowering effect of a very high carbohydrate, high fiber diet. *Diabetes* 25:324.

Allaway, W., et al. (1968). Selenium, molybdenum and vanadium in human blood. *Arch. Environ. Hlth.* 16:342–348.

Allen, V., Robinson, D., and Hembry, F. (1984). Effects of ingested aluminum sulfate on serum magnesium and the possible relationship to hypomagnesemic tetany. *Nutr. Rep. Int.* 29:107.

American Cancer Society. (1984). Nutrition and cancer: cause and prevention. *Cancer J. Clin.* 34(2):121.

Anderson, J., Chen, W., Story, L., and Sieling, B. (1983). Hypocholesterolemic effects of soluble fiber-rich foods for hypercholesteralemic men. *Am. J. Clin. Nutr.* 37:699.

Avioli, L. (1981). Postmenopausal osteoporosis: prevention versus cure. *Fed. Proc.* 40:2418–2422.

Baig, M., and Cerda, J. (1981). Pectin: its interaction with serum proteins. *Am. J. Clin. Nutr.* 34:50–53.

Bartholomew, B., Hill, M., and Hudson, M. (1980). Gastric bacteria, nitrate, nitrite and nitrosamines in patients treated with pernicious anemia and in patients treated with cimetidine. In *N-Nitroso compounds*, E. A. Walker et al., Eds., IARC Publ. 31:595–600.

Bazan, N., Paoletti, R., and Iaconeo, J., Eds. (19XX). *New Trends in Nutrition, Lipid Research, and Cardiovascular Disease.* New York: Alan R. Liss, Inc.

Beare-Rogers, J., Gray, L., and Hollywood, R. (1979). The linoleic acid and trans fatty acids of margarines. *Am. J. Clin. Nutr.* 32:1805–1809.

Bennett, W., and Gurin, J. (1982). *The Dieter's Dilemma: Eating Less and Weighing More.* New York: Basic Books.

Bharuccha, K., Cross, C., and Rubin, M. (1980). Long-chain acetals of ascorbid and erthorbic acids as antinitrosamine agents for bacon. *J. Agric. and Food Chem.* 28:1274–1281.

Bjelke, I. (1974). Epidemiological studies of cancer of the stomach, colon and rectum: with special emphasis on the role of the diet. *Scand. J. Gastr.* 9:1–53.

Bordia, A. (1981). Effect of garlic on blood lipids in patients with congestive heart disease. *Am. J. Clin. Nutr.* 34:2100–2103.

Boyle, E., Mondschein, B., and Dash, H. (1970). Chromium depletion in the pathogenesis of diabetes and atherosclerosis. *S. Med. J.* 70:1449.

Broganhamer, W., McConnell, K., and Blocky, W. (1976). Relationship among serum selenium levels and patients with carcinoma cancer. *Cancer* 37:1384–1388.

Burrows, M., and Farr, W. (1927). The action of mineral oil per os on the organism. *Proc. Soc. Exp. Biol. Med.* 24:719.

Calautti, P., et al. (1980). Serum selenium levels in malignant lymphoprolifera-tion diseases. *Scand. J. Haematol.* 24:63–66.

Check, W. Switch to soy protein for boring but healthful diet. *JAMA* 247:3045–3046.

Coll, M., Meyer, A., and Stunkard, A. (1979). Obesity and food choices in public places. *Arch. Gen. Psychiat.* 36:795–797.

DeVries, H. (1974). *Physiology of Exercise for Physical Education and Athletics,* 2nd ed. Dubuque, IA: Wm. C. Brown Co., Publishers, pp. 257–258.

Epstein, L., and Wing, R. (1980). Aerobic exercise and weight. *Addictive Behaviors* 5:371–388.

Erickson, M., et al. (1983). Tissue mineral levels in victims of sudden infant death syndrome: toxic metals—lead and cadmium. *Ped. Res.* 17:779.

Federal Food and Drug Administration. Fed. Register, July 1, 1943a.

Fish oil for prevention of atherosclerosis. (1982). *The Med. Letter* 24(622):99–100.

Fishbein, D. (1981). Refined carbohydrate consumption and maladaptive be-haviors. *Int. J. Biosoc. Res.* 2:11–14.

Garrison, R., and Somer, E. (1985). *The Nutrition Desk Reference.* New Canaan, CT: Keats Publishing, Inc.

Garrow, J. (1974). *Energy Balance and Obesity in Man.* New York: American Elsevier, pp. 84–85.

Gavin, G., and McHenry, E. (1941). Inositol: a lipotropic factor. *J. Bio. Chem.* 139:485.

Ginter, E. (1979). Pretreatment serum-cholesterol and response to ascorbic acid. *Lancet* 2:9958–9959.

Glanz, R. (1984). Nutrition education for risk factor reduction. *Pt. Educ. Nsletter* 7(6):3–4.

Grahm, S., Schotz, W., and Martino, P. (1972). Alimentary factors in the epidemiology of cancer. *Cancer* 30:927–938.

Griffin, A. (1979). Role of selenium in the chemoprevention of cancer. *Adv. Cancer Res.* 29:419–442.

Gordon, R., and Verter, J. (1969). *The Framingham Study: An Epidemiological Investigation of Cardiovascular Disease.* Bethesda, MD: NIH.

Gwinup, G. (1975). Effect of exercise alone on the weight of obese females. *Arch. Int. Med.* 135:676–680.

Helzesouer, K. (1983). Selenium and cancer patients. *Seminars in Oncol.* 10:308.

Hirayama, T. (1979). Diet and cancer. *Nutr. Cancer* 1:67–181.

Horsey, J., Livesley, B., and Dickerson, J. (1981). Ischemic heart disease and aged patients: effects of ascorbic acid on lipoproteins. *J. Hum. Nutr.* 35:53–58.

Kavanaugh, T., et al. (1983). Influences of exercise and lifestyle variables upon high density lipoprotein cholesterol after myocardial infarction. *Arteriosclerosis* 3:249–259.

Knox, E. (1973). Ischemic heart disease, mortality and dietary intake of vitamin C. *Lancet* 1:1465–1467.

Konig, J. (1981). Aluminum pots as a source of dietary aluminum. *NE J. Med.* 304:172.

Kritichevsky, D., et al. (1982). Atherogenicity of animal and vegetable protein. *Atherosclerosis* 41:429–431.

Kummet, T., and Meyskens, L. (1983). Vitamin A: a potential inhibitor of human cancer. *Seminars in Oncol.* 10:281.

Kvale, G., Bjelke, E., and Gart, J. (1982). Dietary habits and lung cancer risk. In *Proceedings of the Thirteenth International Cancer Congress.* Seattle, WA: International Union Against Cancer, p. 175.

Lappe, F. (1975). *Diet for a Small Planet.* New York: Ballantine, pp. 62–117.

Leon, A., et al. (1979). Effects of a vigorous walking program on body composition and carbohydrate and lipid metabolism of obese young men. *Am. J. Clin. Nutr.* 32:1776–1787.

Liebman, M., and Bazzarre, T. (1983). Plasma lipids of vegetarian and nonvegetarian males; effects of egg consumption. *Am. J. Clin. Nutr.* 38:612–619.

Lonsdale, D., and Shamberger, R. (1980). Red cell transketase as an indicator of nutritional deficiency. *Am. J. Clin. Nutr.* 33(2):205–221.

Malinow, M., et al. (1978). Effect of alfalfa meal on shrinkage (regression) of atherosclerotic plaques during cholesterol feeding in monkeys. *Atherosclerosis* 30:27–43.

Malinow, M., et al. (1981). Cholesterol and bile balance in Macaco fascicularis. *J. Clin. Invest.* 67:156–162.

Marlowe, M., and Errera, J. (1982). Low lead levels and behavior problems in children. *Behav. Dis.* 7:163.

McConnell, K., et al. (1980). The relationship of dietary selenium and breast cancer. *J. Surg. Oncol.* 15:67–70.

McGill, H., Geer, J., and Strong, J. (1965). The natural history of atherosclerosis. In *Metabolism of Lipids as Related to Atherosclerosis*, F. A. Kummerow, Ed. Springfield, IL: Charles C. Thomas, p. 36.

Moody, D., Kollias, J., and Buskirk, E. (1969). The effect of a moderate exercise program on body weight and skinfold thickness in overweight college females. *Med. and Sci. in Sports* 1(2):75–80.

Murata, M., Imaizum, K., and Sugano, M. (1982). Effect of dietary phospholipids and their constituent bases on serum lipids and apolipoproteins in rats. *J. Nutr.* 112:1805–1808.

National Academy of Science Committee on Diet, Nutrition and Cancer. (1982). *Diet, Nutrition and Cancer.* Washington, D.C.: National Academy Press.

Noda, M., Takano, T., and Sakurai, H. (1979). Effects of selenium on chemical carcinogens. *Mut. Res.* 66:175.

Nutrition and cancer: cause and prevention. (1984). *CA-A Cancer J. Clin. Res.* 34(2):121.

Offenbacher, E., et al. (1980). Beneficial effect of chromium-rich yeast on glucose tolerance and blood lipids in elderly subjects. *Diabetes* 29:919–925.

Oleske, T., et al. (1983). Plasma zinc and copper in primary and secondary immunodeficiency disorders. *Biol Tr. El. Res.* 5:189–194.

Oliver, M. (1982). Diet and coronary heart disease. *Hum. Nutr. Clin. Nutr.* 36: 413–427.

Oscai, L. (1973). The role of exercise in weight control. In *Exercise and Sports Review*, Vol. 1, J. Wilmore, Ed. New York: Academic Press, pp. 103–123.

Painter, N. (1972). Diverticular disease of the colon and constipation. *Nurs. Times* 68:620–621.

Phinney, S., et al. (1980). Capacity for moderate exercise in obese subjects after adaptation to a hypocaloric ketogenic diet. *J. Clin. Investig.* 66:1152–1161.

Pollitt, E., et al. (1982). Behavioral effects of iron deficiency anemia in children. In *Iron Deficiency, Brain Biochemistry and Behavior*, E. Pollitt and R. Leibel, Eds. New York: Raven Press, pp. 195–208.

Prasad, D., and Edwards-Prasad, J. (1983). Effects of tocopherol (vitamin E) acid succinate on morphological alterations and growth inhibition in melanoma cells in culture. *Canc. Res.* 42:550–555.

Prinz, R., Roberts, W., and Hantman, E. (1980). Dietary correlates of hyperactive behavior in children. *J. Consult. and Clin. Psychol.* 48(6):760–769.

Rabinowitz, M., et al. (1983). Effects of chromium and yeast supplements on carbohydrate and lipid metabolism in diabetic men. *Diabet. Care* 6:319.

Ramirez, J., and Flowers, C. (1980). Leukocyte ascorbic and its relationship to coronary artery disease in man. *Am. J. Clin. Nutr.* 33:2079–2087.

Recker, R., Saville, P., and Heaney, R. (1977). Effect of estrogens and calcium carbonate on bone loss in post-menopausal women. *Ann. Int. Med.* 87:649.

Reiser, S., et al. (1979). Isocaloric exchange of dietary starch and sucrose in humans: effects on fasting blood lipids. *Am. J. Clin. Nutr.* 32:1659–1669.

Roe, D. (1983). *Drug-Induced Nutritional Deficiencies.* Westport, CT: AVI, p. 130.

Ruttenberg, H., et al. (1983). Influence of trans unsaturated fats on experimental atherosclerosis in rabbits. *J. Nutr.* 113:835–844.

Sacks, F., et al. (1983). Dietary unsaturated fats affect blood pressures, platelet thromboxane production, and HDL subfractions in normal subjects. *Arterioscl. Councl. Abstr.* 3:483A–484A.

Saner, G., et al. (1983). Alterations of chromium metabolism and effect of chromium supplementation in Turner's syndrome. *Am. J. Clin. Nutr.* 38:574–578.

Schauss, A., Bland, J., and Simonsen, C. (1979). A critical analysis of the diets of chronic juvenile offenders. Part II. *J. Orthomol. Psychiatr.* 8(4):222–226.

Schlegel, J. (1975). Proposed uses of ascorbic acid in the prevention of bladder carcinoma. *Ann. NY Acad. Sci.* 258:432–437.

Schmeisser, D., et al. (1983). Effect of excess dietary lysine on plasma lipids of the chick. *J. Nutr.* 113:1777–1783.

Schoenthaler, S. (1983a). The Alabama diet behavior program: an empirical evaluation at the Coosa Valley Regional Detention Center. *Int. J. Biosoc. Res.* 5(2):79–87.

Schoenthaler, S. (1983b). The effects of citrus on the treatment and control of antisocial behavior: a double blind cross-over study of an incarcerated juvenile population. *Int. J. Biosoc. Res.* 5(2):107–117.

Schrauzer, G., White, D., and Schneider, C. (1977). Cancer mortality correlation studies. III. Statistical associations with dietary selenium intakes. *Bio. Org. Chem.* 7:23–34.

Scott, R., et al. (1972). Animal models in atherosclerosis. In *The Pathogenesis of Atherosclerosis*, R. W. Wissler and J. C. Geer, Eds. Baltimore: Williams and Wilkins.

Seelig, M. (1983). Vitamin D: risks versus benefit. *J. Am. Col N.* 2:109–110.

Select Committee on Nutrition and Human Needs. U.S. Senate. *Dietary Goals for the U.S.*, 2nd ed. Washington, D.C.: U.S. Govt. Printing Office, p. xxviii.

Shamberger, R., and Willis, C. (1971). Selenium distribution and human cancer mortality. *C Crit. Rev. Clin. Lab. Sci.* 2:211–221.

Shamberger, R., et al. (1973). Selenium in the blood of normals and cancer patients. *N. Natl. Canc. Inst.* 50:867–870.

Simpson, H., et al. (1981). A high carbohydrate leguminous diet improves all aspects of diabetic control. *Lancet* 1(8210) 1–5.

Sirtori, C., Gatti, E., and Mouter, O. (1979). Clinical experience with the soybean protein diet. *JAMA* 247:3045–3046.

Skrobak-Kaczynski, J., and Andersen, L. (1975). The effect of a high level of habitual physical activity in the regulation of fatness during aging. *Internatl. Arch. Occuptl. and Environm. Hlth.* 36:41–46.

ter Well, H., van Gent, C., and Dekker, W. (1974). The effect of soya lecithin on serum lipid values in type II hyperlipoprotemia. *Acta. Med. Scan.* 195:267–271.

Toth, S., Montgomery, C., and Bunn, J. (1984). Weight management: a practical approach. *Pt. Educ. Nslett.* 7(3):3–4.

Tucker, D., et al. (1984). Iron status and brain function: serum feritin levels associated with asymmetries of cortical electrophysiology and cognitive performance. *Am. J. Clin. Nutr.* 39(1):105–113.

Villar, J., Belizak, J., and Fisher, P. (1983). Epidemiological observations on the relationship between calcium intake and eclampsia. *Int. J. Gyn. Obst.* 21:271–278.

Vroulis, G., et al. (1982). Reduction of cholesterol risk factors by lecithin in patients with Alzheimer's disease. *Am. J. Psychiat.* 139:1633–1634.

Webb, T., and Oski, F. (1974). Behavioral status of young adolescents with iron deficiency anemia. *J. Spec. Ed.* 8(2):153–156.

Weinsier, R. (1985). News release from Media Relations Director, Manning, Selvage and Lee, 1250 Eye St., N.W., Washington, D.C. 20005.

Willett, W., et al. (1983). Prediagnostic serum selenium and risk of cancer. *Lancet* 2:130–133.

Wissler, R. (1979). Conference on the health effects of blood lipids: optimal distributions for populations. *Prev. Med.* 8:715–732.

Wooley, S., Wooley, O., and Dyrenforth, S. (1979). Theoretical practice and social issues in behavioral treatments of obesity. *J. Appl. Beh. Anal.* 12:3–25.

Yudkin, J. (1980). Dietary factors in arteriosclerosis: sucrose. *Lipids* 13:370–372.

Zavoral, J., et al. (1983). The hypolipidemic effect of locust bean gum products in familial hypocholesterolemic adults. *Am. J. Clin. Nutr.* 38:285–294.

6

EXERCISE AND MOVEMENT

This chapter discusses the following topics:

- The relationship between fitness, movement, and wellness
- Theoretical frameworks for fitness
- Fitness assessments
- Fitness interventions
- Exercise for special populations
- Overcoming obstacles to exercise
- Body–mind interactions and exercise

Movement is one of the simplest and most effective modes of stress reduction. It also moderates appetite and serves a preventive function against aging and some chronic conditions, including coronary heart disease, obesity, joint and spinal disc disease, fatigue, muscular tension, and depression. When done correctly, movement and exercise can enhance self-image and self-confidence, reduce joint stiffness, increase circulation, improve posture, reduce depressions, positively affect work performance, decrease blood pressure, enhance ability to relate to others, enhance sleep, decrease the need for stimulants, and enhance breathing ability (The President's Council on Physical Fitness and Sports).

SOME WELLNESS THEORETICAL FRAMEWORKS FOR FITNESS

Movement and fitness frameworks that are especially suited to a wellness outlook are Cohen's and Mills' Developmental Movement Theory,

Feldenkrais' Theory of Awareness Through Movement, and Kurtz and Prestera's Body Message Theory.

Mills' and Cohen's Developmental Movement Theory

At the School for Body/Mind Centering in Amherst, Massachusetts, Margret Mills (a fine arts, movement, and theater expert) and Bonnie Bainbridge Cohen (an occupational therapist, neurodevelopmental therapist, and dance therapist) are developing their theory of developmental movement. The thrust of their theory is that the body teaches the brain. Through specific movements, the brain is developed and reshaped, and vice versa.

> In the development of the human infant, including its in utero stages, there is a specific progression which, like a piece from a great hologram, reflects the evolutionary development of vertebrate animals (phylogeny). Thus in examining the development of human beings (ontogeny) we can see a thread that has run through vast periods of evolutionary time, from one-celled amoebas to fertilized egg cells, to swimming fish and bony-finned sharks, to frogs and their relatives who moved up and out of the water to continue on land, where we stretched our limbs down from myriad varieties of vertebrate bodies and learned to live, breathe, and move about the surface of the planet earth. And so we say that ontogeny recapitulates (re-forms or re-pictures) phylogeny. (Mills & Cohen, 1979, p. 1)

In Mills' and Cohen's system, evolutionary development is followed through the course of development of an individual. Thus, the infant moves in ways similar to creatures of a lower evolutionary state such as the worm, fish, etc. As the infant grows, he or she is capable of movements similar to creatures higher up the evolutionary scale, the rabbit, camel, etc.

Mills and Cohen work with the four basic locomotor movement patterns: spinal, homologous, homolateral, and contralateral. The more primitive patterns underlie the more complex ones; thus the spinal patterning must be mastered or the homologous movements will not exhibit their full range of balance, strength, mobility, and dynamics. Development also proceeds from proximal to distal and from push movements to reach and pull movements. In reading the descriptions of movement below, if it is difficult to understand what is involved, stop a minute and picture the creature in action, then duplicate the movement.

Spinal movements include an arching of the body in all directions and flexing and extending the body (concave and convex movements). The fish represents this movement, which assists the brain in differentiating the front from the back of the body and the development of the conception of forward-backward movement.

Homologous movements are those of both upper extremities together and/or both lower extremities together. The phylogenetic stage illustrating this pattern is the frog. (Arms push forward, body moves back; legs push, body moves forward; arms reach, body is pulled forward; legs reach, body moves back.) This movement pattern underlies the conception of vertical up/down relationships.

Homolateral movements include an alteration of movement between one side of the body and the other side. The movements assist in the brain differentiation of the two sides of the body and right/left discrimination.

The *contralateral* movement pattern is the right upper body and left lower body moving together and then the left upper body and right lower body moving together. Movements of the lizard and camel illustrate this pattern, which aids in the diagonal integration of the four quadrants of the body and the relationship of the body in space (3-dimensionality).

If the lower extremities are not developed completely, the trunk will be less stable, and there will be a more static, less mobile support for the extremities. Thus, when walking, kicking, dancing, running, or any movement of the lower extremities is performed, flexibility and strength will be less than possible (Mills & Cohen, 1979, pp. 1–28).

The pioneering work at the School for Body/Mind Centering connects these movements with the nervous system (alertness, thought, precision, condensation) with the endocrine system (intuition, emotions, automaticity, sense of flow and expansion). Mills and Cohen postulate that specific movements involve the use of the endocrine glands for support and initiation serving to stimulate, activate, and strengthen the endocrine gland involved, thereby influencing posture, energy level, and psychological states.

According to Mills' and Cohen's theory, the following movements will stimulate, activate, and strengthen the following endocrine glands:

- Spinal push through the head (worm and fish movements): pineal gland
- Spinal push through the tail (worm and fish backward movements): carotid bodies
- Homologous push (frog hop and rocking on all fours): heart bodies and pancreas
- Homolateral push upper extremities (one side push up, homolateral roll, and diagonal head raising): gonads

- Homolateral push lower extremities (crawling forward, homolateral roll, and hip swing): coccygeal body
- Spinal reach and pull through the head (snake forward and head reaching): mammillary bodies
- Spinal reach and pull through the tail (wagging the tail and tail-leg raising): pituitary
- Homologous reach and pull upper extremities (rabbit hop forward and rope pulling): thyroid
- Homologous reach and pull lower extremities (rabbit hop backward and wall exercise): thymus
- Contralateral reach and pull (forward and backward creep, diagonal roll initiated by the hand or foot, and rope climbing): parathyroids
- Navel radiation (soaring stretch): adrenals
- Breathing (breast stroke and star breathing): thoraco body

(Mills & Cohen, 1979, p. 29)

Feldenkrais' Awareness Through Movement

Physiologists have found that cells in the motor cortex of the brain assemble into a shape resembling the human body that is called the *homunculus*. This is the motor or movement basis for self-image. Feldenkrais contends everyone's self-image is smaller than it might be and that the combinations and patterning of cells may be more important than their number. For example, people who speak two languages make use of both more cells and more combinations of cells. Some people can speak 30 or more languages; this gives a rough idea of the limitlessness of potential for self-image (Feldenkrais, 1977, pp. 14–15).

Everyone has parts of the body for which there is no awareness; for example it is easy for most people to lie on their back and sense their fingertips, but it is probably difficult for many to sense the nape of the neck or the space between the ears.

> The parts of the body that are easily defined in the awareness are those that serve man daily, while the parts that are dull or mute in his awareness play only an indirect role in his life and are almost missing from his self-image when he is in action. (Feldenkrais, 1979, p. 21)

Thus, learning to move parts of the body with consciousness will enhance the self-image, according to Feldenkrais.

> The way a man holds his shoulders, head and stomach; his voice and expression; his stability and manner of presenting himself—all are based on

his self-image . . . it emerges that systematic correction of the image will be a quicker and more efficient approach than the correction of single actions and errors in modes of behavior. (Feldenkrais, 1979, p. 23)

Some important postulates of Feldenkrais' theory are (1979, pp. 33–62):

1. Awareness and self-image are based on movement.
2. Breathing and movement must be coordinated if movement is to be effective.
3. Movement of the eyes organizes movement of the body.
4. When actions are performed correctly, refreshment and relaxation result; when movements are performed too quickly and without attention to breathing, fatigue may result.
5. The body is constantly fighting against the force of gravity unless it is well organized; without appropriate organization, gravity can pull or push the body and affect movement in a negative manner.
6. Individuals can learn to organize their bodies more effectively by practicing slow, gradual movements while breathing correctly and learning to experience the body sensations associated with effective movement.

Kurtz and Prestera's Body Message Theory

Fixed muscular patterns in the body are central to a person's way of being in the world. They form in response to family and early environment . . . Whatever the feeling, it is also expressed physically, and becomes a way of holding oneself, a fixed muscular pattern and a set attitude toward life. . . . These attitudes and fixed muscular patterns reflect, enhance, and sustain one another. (Kurtz & Prestera, 1984, pp. 2–3)

These characteristic patterns inhibit individuals from attaining well-being. When well, the body is:

capable of allowing the free flowing of any feeling. It is efficient and graceful in its movements, aware and responsive to real needs. Such a body has bright eyes, breathes freely, is smooth skinned, and has an elastic muscle tone. It is well proportioned, and the various segments coordinate well with each other. The neck is pliable and the head moves easily. The pelvis swings freely. The entire body is lined up efficiently with respect to gravity; that is, in a standing position, there is no struggle with gravity's downward pull. Pleasure and well-being are characteristic feelings. A person with such a body is emotionally flexible and his or her feelings are spontaneous. (Kurtz & Prestera, 1984, p. 3)

When there is a wholeness to the body/mind/spirit, expression of feelings flows easily; wholeness is disrupted when the flow of energy in the body is disrupted. For example, when an individual experiences anger, but does not express it directly, the breaks in the normally smooth curves of the body can be observed. For example, look at your body right now in the mirror and see if your scapulas are flat and equally so; if not, there is a break in the smooth curve of your back. Likewise, if you look at the front of your body in a mirror, you may see that the right or left side of your chest is more forward, more to the back, wider, longer, or whatever; any of these will look like breaks in the smooth curve of your body. Everyone has some breaks; the difference in magnitude and quantity differentiates all individuals along a continuum from nonmovement and energy blocks to effective movement and energy flow.

In the case of the individual who does not express anger, that unexpressed feeling may be "locked" in a body part; some individuals may lock it in the arms (instead of striking out); others may hold their anger in their abdominal area, leading to digestive upsets and a tight, tense abdomen that may be excessively held in.

Similarly, an infant whose mother constantly grabbed his arm whenever he reached out to explore his environment may turn into an adult with lifeless arms that hang drooping from narrow shoulders; there is no indication of reaching out to life; instead, the infant waits passively for things to come to him.

Infants are born with the capacity for wholeness. Fear can produce blocks. For example, "in blocking the expression of sadness, we tense the jaw, chest, stomach, diaphragm, and some muscles of the throat and face—all the areas which move spontaneously when the feeling is allowed its natural outlets" (Kurtz & Prestera, 1984, pp. 8–9).

Blocks impede the normal flow of energy as muscles tense, circulation is constricted, and skin tone and temperature change. Holding in of feeling is manifested as rings of muscle and fascia tension or breaks in the areas between the major segments of the body: neck and upper shoulders, the diaphragm, the lower back between the abdomen and pelvis, the groin, the knees, and the ankles; feet and eyes can also be held. Figure 4 shows body areas where holding is common.

Gross changes in function, form, color, and development can occur. Hands and feet may be small and cold. The head may be large or the abdomen blown up while the chest is collapsed. As blood supply is reduced due to increased muscular tension, there is a collection of tissue wastes, setting up a mechanism of toxic spasm and stasis. The nervous system responds by firing more signals leading to the pain-spasm-pain-spasm of a headache, backache, or heartache. If this occurs chronically, the tissues harden to splint the area against further attack and structural block develops.

According to Kurtz and Prestera, a backache may be the product of a slipped disc, but the original insult may result in an attempt to hold oneself up or back. A heart attack may be the end result of blocked impulses to love or be loved that become a block in energy flow, a decrease in circulation, a pooling and thickening of blood, and eventually a physiological blockage. Bear in mind that a wellness view considers all dimensions of wellness, thus, in this view, negative nutritional, fitness, stress management, environmental concerns, and negative relationships are more likely to end in chronic difficulties. On the other hand, this book uses a systems approach; in it, one part of the subsystem, such as an increase in fitness or a change to more effective movement, can affect the entire system's functioning. Thus, by working on the body, the entire body/mind/spirit can be affected.

Harmony with gravity aids in reaching up and out in the world; disharmony leads to attempts by the body to compensate; if the chest is going in and down, the belly may go out and up. "The ideal axis for obtaining the greatest balance is that which connects points at the top of the head, middle of the ear, middle of the shoulder, midpoint of the hip joint, center of the knee joint, and center of the ankle joint" (Kurtz & Prestera, 1984, p. 29). Figure 5 shows the ideal axis in person 1 and a compensated balance.

Individuals who are out of balance can express it bodily and emotionally; bodies that are bent forward often express feelings of being overburdened; those bending backward experience life as an unending struggle. Figure 6 shows a person expressing burden through the way the body is held. In Figure 7, the first figure is bowed back and the second is bowed forward.

Tension and stiffness in the lower half of the body, especially the legs and feet, makes balancing difficult; it is as if the person is bracing against a fall. Tightening up may be to protect against being a "pushover," falling down on the job. In Figure 8, the first figure is falling forward a bit; the second has a locked knee indicating bracing.

Feet can reveal how reality is dealt with by the way the ground is contacted; if one foot goes one way and the other another way, this may indicate confusion. Feet rotated outward put added stress on the ankle and knee joints; feet facing forward reduce this stress, allowing more effective weight transfer through the center of the foot. Locking of the knees could indicate an attempt to hold on, hold oneself up, or stand ground. People with rigid legs have difficulty bending their toes forward or back (an indicator of the condition). Figure 9 shows various arrangements for feet.

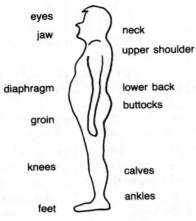

eyes

jaw

neck

upper shoulder

diaphragm

lower back

buttocks

groin

knees

calves

ankles

feet

Figure 4. Common areas of holding.

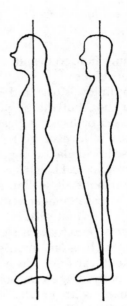

Figure 5. The lateral line and compensated balance.

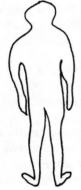

Figure 6. An overburdened individual.

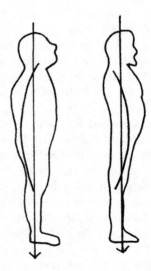

Figure 7. Bowing backward and forward.

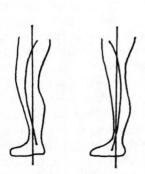

Figure 8. Knees.

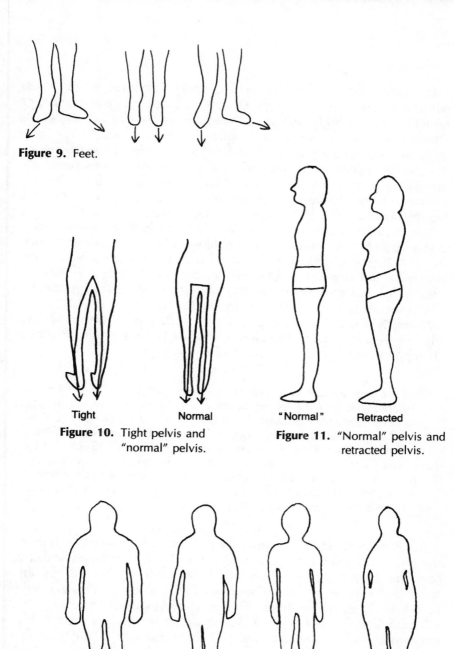

Figure 9. Feet.

| Tight | Normal | "Normal" | Retracted |

Figure 10. Tight pelvis and "normal" pelvis.

Figure 11. "Normal" pelvis and retracted pelvis.

| 1 | 2 | 3 | 4 |

Figure 12. Progression of top to bottom trapped energy.

Limited sexual, anal, and urinary expression is evident in individuals with knees that are quite separate and a space between the thighs terminating in a high peak at the midline, as well as in individuals whose thighs are drawn inward, squeezing the genitals. In the latter case, the chronic contraction of both buttocks and thighs restricts energy flow; if the reader stands up and tries to simultaneously squeeze the muscles in both areas, the degree of tension will be evident. The first person in Figure 10 shows high tension in the genital area; the second figure shows a relatively "normal" configuration.

The position of the pelvis also reveals inner feelings; when tucked under, tight buttocks allow for a "dribbling out of emotion and feeling" (Kurtz & Prestera, 1984, p. 60); when retracted, the individual is unable to release and remains "cocked and ready to fire" (Kurtz & Prestera 1984, p. 61). In Figure 11 the first woman has a pelvis squarely under the trunk; the second woman has a retracted pelvis.

Normally the belly wall expands with each breath. In our society, where exposing "gut" feelings is not rewarded or encouraged, the closest representative of the natural state is the young child.

> There are three areas in which energy streaming can be cut off: the throat, the diaphragm, and the lower abdomen. In the throat area, tightening occurs every time we are asked by our head center to say something emotionally difficult or phony, i.e., not in tune with our internal instinctual life. The diaphragm tightens whenever our gut feelings are supplanted by our head's ideas. The area across the lower abdomen tightens, freezing the pelvis and cutting off genital feelings whenever our head dictates when, how, and where to have sex without harmonizing the dictates of our belly and heart centers. (Kurtz & Prestera, 1984, p. 68)

An overexpanded chest is held in a tight, inflated position at all times; the heart and heart feelings are kept locked up. Individuals with this condition tend to "stay within" the bounds of rules, schedules, attitudes, and logic, emphasizing success and performance (Prestera, 1984, p. 81). In Figure 12 the first man has an overexpanded chest.

The collapsed chest is most closely associated with a basic lack of emotional vitality. The amount of breath taken in is not adequate enough to spark full feeling. In Figure 12 person 4 has a collapsing chest. The illustration depicts a progression from person 1 who has stagnant energy in the upper part of his body to person 4 who has stagnant energy in the lower part of her body. To be balanced, energy must flow up with ideas and creativity and down to produce a firm contact with the ground and reality.

ASSESSING FITNESS

The traditional view of fitness focuses on cardiac fitness. A wellness view contends that fitness is more comprehensive. The recent deaths of a number of world class and other avid runners who were apparently "cardiac fit" provides empirical evidence that a more extensive framework is needed to assess fitness (Koplan, 1979; Thompson, 1979).

When engaging a client from a fitness standpoint, the nurse involves each individual in self-assessment procedures. Some areas of importance include: developmental assessments, structural assessments, flexibility assessments, and aerobic assessments.

Developmental Assessments

When using Cohen and Mills' developmental movement theory, a number of observations and/or questions can serve as assessments of the client's need to practice developmental patterns that will integrate movement with brain and glandular activity. The nurse assesses the client's ability to:

- differentiate the front from the back of the body
- move backwards versus moving forwards
- move up and down in space
- differentiate the top from the bottom of the body
- use the top versus the bottom of the body
- use right/left discrimination (reversal of letters or numbers) (indicates poor right/left integration)
- differentiate the two sides of the body
- move from side to side
- move the body flexibly and comfortably in space
- diagonally integrate the four quadrants of the body
- use trunk mobility when moving (requires good extremity support, trunk stability, and dynamically mobile trunk support)
- walk upright
- run or jog upright
- coordinate hand–eye movements
- show self-love/self-hatred (ability to integrate coccygeal body with homolateral push, lower extremities: L.E.)
- be creative, give and receive, procreate, be organized, show aggression, passivity, sexuality (integrate gonads with homolateral push, upper extremities: U.E.)

- instinct for survival, fight/flight response, strength of stride in walking, courageousness, life force, separate I/ego sense, pain, rage, fear, anxiety (integrate adrenal glands with navel radiation)
- complete transitional activities, power, spatial awareness, appetite, reaching upward and outward, passion, greed, jealousy, anger, boredom, joviality (integrate pancreas with homologous push, L.E.)
- integrate breathing, align the body, be open, defenselessness (integrate thoraco body with breathing)
- love others, center horizontally, width perception (integrate heart bodies with homologous push, U.E.)
- resist infection/cancers, let go, be irresponsible, show fear, have nightmares and fears (integrate thymus gland with homologous reach and pull, L.E.)
- show commitment/conviction, have a full voice, move energy from lower body to head, have a strong heart, endure (integrate thyroid with homologous reach and pull, U.E.)
- show empathy, express self creatively, balance adrenals, manipulation (integrate parathyroids and contralateral reach and pull, U.E. and L.E.)
- show courage, effortless expression of life force, be artistic, express convictions (integrate carotid bodies with spinal push from the tail)
- show compassion, knowledge, integration of personality, conceptual memory (reading, thinking, studying), linear sequential time consciousness, compulsiveness, racism, paranoia, sexism (integrate pituitary gland with spinal reach and pull through the tail)
- show insight, foresight, and hindsight; hallucinations; undifferentiation of the past, present, and future; psychic ability; schizophrenia; realism (integrate mammillary bodies with spinal reach and pull through the head)
- show integration of all experiences, perfectionisms, lack of self-control (integration of pineal body with spinal push through the head)

(Source: Mills & Cohen, 1979, pp. 2–24; Appendix A)

Structural Assessments

Kurtz's and Prestera's theory provides the basic material for developing an assessment tool. Table 33 provides this tool for use with self and clients. Kurtz and Prestera have not developed interventions; however, Feldenkrais and yoga interventions could be used in many instances.

Table 33. Structural Assessments

Front view	Pre	Post
1. Contrast upper body with lower body. Do they appear to fit? Is there a mismatch?		
2. Contrast right side of body with left side for symmetry; is one side more forward or more developed?		
3. Are the eyes of same size and show the same amount of openness?		
4. Is the mouth tight or relaxed?		
5. Is the head tilted to one side or the other?		
6. Are the shoulders level or is one higher than the other?		
7. Is one shoulder longer than the other?		
8. Is the chest concave, hyperextended, or relaxed?		
9. Are both arms the same distance from the body?		
10. Are the hips level or is one higher than the other?		
11. Is the pubic area pulled in toward the center of the body or is the abdomen flat?		
12. Are the knees facing in or out?		
13. Are the knees and lower legs relaxed or tense? The assessor places one hand behind the lower leg and pushes slightly; if knee bends easily leg is relaxed, otherwise it is tense.		
14. Do both feet face forward or does one or the other face out?		
15. Are there any areas where energy appears trapped, that seem over- or underdeveloped? (Look especially at the chest area.)		

Side view	Pre	Post
16. Is the head tilted up, down, or level?		
17. Are the shoulders tilted forward or back?		
18. Are the scapula flat and level on both the left and right side?		

Table 33 *(continued)*

Side view	Pre	Post

19. Is the lower back swayed with the abdomen pushed out or is there a small curve in the small of the back?
20. Is the pelvis tipped out or back?
21. Draw an imaginary line through the ear, shoulder, elbow, hip socket, knee, and ankle; where is the line out of line (unaligned)?

Back view		

22. Look for any areas where energy appears trapped, that seem over- or underdeveloped, especially in the upper back and buttocks.

Additional assessment		

23. What is the ratio of hip to waist size? (Measure waist and hips with a tape measure; divide waist by hip size. For women the average ratio is about .7. A number above .85 shows a threefold increased risk of diabetes. For middle aged men the average ratio is .9 to .95; pot-bellied men above this range had more heart disease and strokes and died earlier than those with small stomachs in one study reported in *American Health*, 1984, 3(May): 45.)

Hunches: Look back at the assessment and hold your body as the person you are assessing does, but exaggerate the posture. What current or potential problems might occur to joints, body parts, internal organs, breathing, circulation, digestion, or elimination based on what you have observed? *Write your hunches down here:*

Now check with the person you are assessing and see if he or she has problems in any of the areas you have hunches about. If problems have not yet surfaced, counsel him or her on potential future issues based on your assessment.

Copyright 1984, Carolyn Chambers Clark.

Flexibility Assessments

There are two major views of flexibility: momentary and chronic. Momentary flexibility can change due to the emotion of the moment. Breathing rises toward the throat, muscles tighten, and a body "stiffness" is visible. Chronic inflexibility develops from years of not using the body appropriately or may be due to accident, surgery, and/or chronic inhibited emotion.

There are several ways to assess flexibility: observe the body in movement, ask clients which areas of the body "feel" tight or stiff, ask clients to complete range of motion or extension exercises. Asking a client to walk away from and toward the nurse will reveal aspects of flexibility. Some questions to pose in this regard are:

1. Does this body move as a solid, shuffling block, or does it give the impression of a spring in the step, a lightness and gracefulness, or something in between? Describe what is observed.

2. Are body movements well defined with arms swinging in opposition to leg movement, knees bending, hips moving with legs, neck and chest moveable, or does the body move as a whole, or something in between? Describe what is observed.

3. Is there a difference in the walk when observed from the front and the back in terms of movement, or do both give similar impressions?

4. Does the person slouch forward or hold the head back behind the center of gravity?

5. Does the person lift the body in an exaggerated manner to move forward? Key indicators of this problem are shoulders hunched up, walking on the ball of the foot, and lack of thrusting forward of the hip.

6. Does the person walk duck-footed or pigeon-toed?

7. Does the person favor one leg? A thump-thump sound indicates favoring.

8. Does the person shuffle or scrape the feet?

A "yes" answer to any of the above indicates a loss of flexibility and could indicate a need for stretching or Feldenkrais interventions.

Marshall (1981), a former chief of sports medicine, suggests the following tests for flexibility:

1. Push the tip of your nondominant thumb back toward the forearm; if the angle between the fingers and thumb is more than 70 degrees, better than average flexibility is present; 60–70 degrees is average; and less than 60 degrees indicates less than average flexibility.

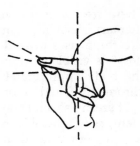

Figure 13. Metacarpal-phalangeal extension.

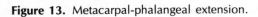

2. Measure metacarpal–phalangeal extension by lifting and holding one arm with elbow bent; with the other hand, push back the index finger; estimate the angle formed from the finger extended to the drop in the wrist. More than 115 degrees indicates high flexibility; 105–115 degrees average; and less than 105 degrees indicates less than average flexibility (see Figure 13).

3. Look at the foot: high arch indicates tight heel cord and tight joints; average arch indicates average flexibility; and flat foot indicates loose joints and extreme flexibility.

Loose-jointed clients are best suited for endurance activities and patterned movements such as dancing, gymnastics, cycling, swimming, or running. They are prone to ligament problems, partial dislocations, and knee problems. Tight-jointed clients are best at explosive activities such as basketball, hockey, tennis, racketball, and sprinting. These clients are most prone to muscle pulls and tears, torn ligaments and cartilage, lower back pain, tendonitis of the shoulder or elbow, and pinched nerves (Marshall, 1981, p. 63).

These three measures are determined by heredity and cannot be changed; there are four other measures of flexibility that can be improved through exercise:

1. Assess shoulder stretch: while standing, hold two ends of a tape measure, belt rope, or towel; stretch the arms straight out in front with arms and wrists straight; continue to hold the tape and bring it over the head and back out behind as far as comfortable; slide hands apart only as much as needed to accomodate the stretching movement, then bring hands forward again, holding the tape the same distance apart; read the number of inches. Under 30 in. is looser than average, 30–40 in. is average, and more than 40 in. is less flexible than average for clients

under 25 years of age; for clients aged 25–45, add 5 in. to each measurement; for clients over 45, add 10 in. to each measurement.

2. Assess thigh stretch: sit on the floor with back straight against the wall; bend knees so bottoms of feet meet and feet are close to groin. Measure distance between knees and floor. For clients under 25 years of age, less than 4 in. is flexible, 4–7 in. is average, and more than 7 in. is tight. For clients 25–45 years add 2 in. to each measurement; for clients over 45 years, add 2 in. more.

3. Assess heel cord flexibility: lie down on a sofa or bed with feet extended off the end and knees straight; flex the ankles to pull toes toward shins; estimate the angle the foot makes to a line extending back through the heel. For all ages, over 105 degrees is flexible, 95–105 is average, and 95 degrees is tight.

4. Assess ability to touch the floor with knees straight and feet together. For clients under 25 years of age, less than 3 in. to touching palms to the floor is flexible, 3–5 in. from palms touching the floor is average, and more than 5 in. is tight. For clients aged 25–45, the measures are less than 4 in., 4–7 in., and more than 7 in.; for clients over 45 years, the measures are less than 5 in., 5–9 in., and more than 9 in. (Marshall, 1981).

Aerobic Assessments

Aerobic exercise involves sustained, rhythmic activity of the large muscle groups. Aerobic exercise uses large amounts of oxygen, causing an increase in heart rate, stroke volume, respiratory rate, and a relaxation of the small blood vessels leading to increased oxygenation. The goal of aerobic exercise is to strengthen the cardiovascular system and increase stamina. Approximately 20 minutes of activity at the appropriate heart rate for each age range produces a training effect without straining the heart unduly.

Aerobic exercise not only conditions the cardiovascular system but can also reduce the amount of body fat. Percentage of body fat can be calculated most easily by pinching the back of the upper middle arm; less than ¼ in. indicates a below average amount of body fat; ¼–¾ in. indicates an average amount of body fat; and more than ¾ in. indicates a high percentage of body fat. For men, 12% of body weight as fat is desirable; for women, 18%. Other methods of determining body fat (in order of complexity and reliability) are calipers and water displacement. When using calipers, the skinfold sites commonly used are: triceps, sub-scapula, suprailiac, and thigh.

Calculating a Safe Range for Aerobic Exercise

A safe rate for aerobic exercise can be calculated in the following manner: 220 (maximum heart rate) – age = maximum attainable heart rate – resting heart rate × 0.6 and 0.8 + resting heart rate = safe range.

e.g.,
$$220 - 44 = 176 - 64 = 112 \times 0.6 = 67.2 + 64 = 131.2$$
$$112 \times 0.8 = 89.6 + 64 = 153.6$$

In the example, a 44-year-old person with a resting pulse of 64 needs to raise the pulse between 131 and 154 to attain a conditioning effect. The pulse can be taken at intervals during exercise to ensure the safe range is not exceeded (clients can take their pulse for 15 seconds and multiply by 4).

Pros and Cons of Stress Testing Prior to an Exercise Program

Stress testing is most commonly accomplished by placing an individual on a treadmill and using an electrocardiogram to measure the effects of strenuous running on heart activity. Some authorities claim stress testing is a useful way of determining whether a strenuous exercise program can be undertaken. Vickery, a physician, claims that the need has been invented based on an excess of cardiologists and a profit motive. Vickery (1978, pp. 109–111) presents the following information to strengthen his claim:

1. The stress test itself has a greater risk of precipitating a heart attack (a risk level of 30–60%) than does unaccustomed, severe exercise (a risk level of 6 to 12%). Based on this information, Vickery calculates that if people gradually work up to a conditioning level, their risk should drop to less than one fifth the risk of a heart attack than if they have a stress test.

2. The stress test is not a reliable indicator of persons at high risk for heart attack. False positives and false negatives abound. In a study of persons without symptoms of heart disease, 47% who tested "abnormal" on the stress test did not have heart disease; in another study, 62% of those who did have heart disease tested "normal" on the stress test. Based on this low level of accuracy, the use of a stress test is questionable.

There are more reliable indicators that can be used to assess client need for medical supervision prior to beginning an exercise program. Vickery

(1978) suggests that a "yes" answer to one or more of the following questions by someone over 35 years of age should result in a visit to the physician; in someone under 35 years old, a call to the physician telling him or her the exercise program planned should be sufficient.

1. Do you have any chest pain when you exert yourself?
2. Do you get short of breath with mild exertion?
3. Do you have pain in your legs when you walk but not when you rest?
4. Do your ankles swell regularly (at times other than when menstruating)?
5. Has a doctor ever told you that you have heart disease?

FITNESS INTERVENTIONS

Developmental Movement Interventions

Crawling, rolling, creeping, hopping, and rocking enhance integration of the lower levels of the brain. Crawling and creeping are especially helpful in integrating the two hemispheres of the brain (Mills & Cohen, 1979, p. xiv). The cross-crawl (a contralateral movement) is especially helpful as a preventive measure for maintaining the normal neurological organization of the brain. Walking with arms swinging freely in opposition to the body, marching in place, crawling on the floor, lying down face up and moving the arms in opposition to the legs, or standing up and doing the dance "the Twist" while touching the right elbow to the left knee all accomplish brain integration (Koenig, 1981). Table 34 shows suggested movements for various endocrine developmental difficulties and/or enhancement of movement. The information in Table 34 can be used with clients who have organic difficulties (e.g., brain damage, stroke, accident, chronic illness, surgery) as well as with clients who wish to enhance their ability in a sport or activity (e.g., move up and back in tennis more effectively; decrease the possibility of a jogging or running injury; enhance immunity; kicking ability; right/left discrimination when driving; transposed numbers when writing; enhanced breathing; or stimulation of various endocrine organs. To integrate, movement actions should be pictured in the mind while moving through the areas described.

Feldenkrais Interventions

Feldenkrais interventions, whether assisted by a practitioner or completed by the client, involve the following principles:

Table 34. Developmental Movement Interventions*

Issues	Intervention
Differentiate front from back of body; forward/back movement; pineal gland; carotid body; heart; pancreas; gonads; coccygeal body; mammillary bodies; pituitary gland, backward movement. (Spinal)	Rolling the body as a unit; rolling the body successively from head, through arms, then legs Roll with arms against chest, head off ground, pushing down the spine through pineal gland and up the spine through the carotid bodies Lie on stomach, initiate movement through head, reaching through mammilary bodies (in midbrain slightly front and above ear) Lie on stomach, reach through tail through pituitary to lift tail and legs off ground Wagging the tail and tail-leg raise through pituitary Lie prone, legs extended; head pushes up through pineal and then tail pushes down through carotid (worm) Lie prone, legs extended, full hip and knee extension as legs reach through the thymus (fish)
Stimulate heart, pancreas, thyroid, thymus. (Homologous)	Frog hop, rock on all fours, rabbit hop backward, rope pulling (with a real or imaginary rope)
Stimulate gonads, coccygeal body. (Homolateral)	Diagonal head raising through gonads; crawling forward simulating elephant and gorilla movements.
Stimulate parathyroids, balance cerebral hemispheres. (Contralateral)	Forward and backward creep on hands and knees, rope climbing; diagonal roll, head off ground, both hands at right or left side, movement initiated through hands; picture moving each hand and arm through the parathyroid (mid-neck level) as roll is accomplished; hands end up at shoulder level.

*Based on ideas presented by Cohen and Mills (1979) and Koenig (1981). For further information see: Mills, M., and Cohen, B. *Developmental Movement Therapy*. Amherst, MA: The School for Body/Mind Centering, 1979.

1. Exaggerate the problematic movement first. For example, if the chest is concave, the client exaggerates that situation.
2. Using very small, smooth, slow movements, move the body in the direction of balance with gravity.
3. Breathe in the abdomen while moving.
4. Center the concentration in the moving and breathing.
5. When difficulty in movement is encountered, imagine breathing into that area while moving.

Specific Feldenkrais interventions demonstrate the ease and power of his technique.

Intervention No. 1: Standing while Sitting. Sit in a chair and pay attention to how you stand up; note which part of the body moves first and which other parts follow and with what degree of difficulty, tension, effort. Write down what happened prior to continuing.

Now sit on the edge of a chair, and let your body rock forward and backward without any sudden increase in effort. Make no attempt to get up. As you continue the movement, grasp the hair at the top of your head so any tensing of the cervical spine can be felt. When tension in the cervical area exists, increase the movement of your head forward and upward by moving your hip joints until the buttocks rise from the chair.

Note the difference in effort in rising when the chest muscles, ribs, and chest are relaxed. Repeat the second part of the exercise, making sure to breathe during it. Summarize your findings.

Intervention No. 2: Increasing Range of Motion in the Neck. Sit comfortably in a chair. Turn the head slowly and easily to the left as far as is comfortable. Note a spot on the wall or ceiling that marks that spot, then return the head to face front. Remember to keep breathing as you complete the exercise. Next, turn the head slowly and easily to the left while keeping the eyes looking forward; return the head to facing front. Now turn the eyes *and* head slowly and easily to the left again. Note how far the head turned this time and compare it with the first time you turned the head to the left.

Almost everyone reports an increase in range of neck motion as a result of this simple exercise. It supports Feldenkrais' theory: use small, slow movements; breathe and concentrate on the movement and its results; break the movement into its component parts and then reconstruct it to attain more efficient movement.

Intervention No. 3: Using Imagery and Movement. Sit comfortably in the chair, breathing in your lower abdomen. When ready, keep your head facing forward, but *picture* your head turning slowly and comfortably as far as possible to the left and then returning to the front facing position. Breathe comfortably and slowly turn your head to the left as far as comfortable to do so. Note the spot on the wall or ceiling and compare it with your other efforts.

Results from this intervention are frequently astounding. Using this series with thousands of participants, the author has found nearly everyone greatly increases their range of motion with this final exercise. This supports Feldenkrais' (1977) theory that imagery alone can affect movement in a positive manner.

Intervention No. 4: Improving Movements of the Lower Back.
This intervention is effective for tightness in the lower back, tension, and for improving efficient use of the lower back. Lie on the floor with knees bent and feet flat on the floor. Cross the right leg over the left knee as if sitting in a chair with the legs crossed. Extend arms out at shoulder level and let them relax. Continue breathing easily while very slowly and smoothly letting the legs drop to the left toward the floor as far as is possible comfortably. Continue breathing and using one slow, continuous movement, return the legs to center and let them drop to the right towards the floor. Continue breathing and repeat the exercise, allowing the legs to move slowly to the right side of the floor and then to the left side of the floor. Then with legs facing front, slowly place legs flat on the floor and observe the sensations in the lower back, pelvis, and legs. Lie still, breathing, and noting changes and sensations.

Intervention No. 5: Increasing Movement in the Shoulders and Upper Back. This exercise is especially useful for people who sit reading or writing for long periods of time or for those who carry their tension in the upper part of their chest or back. Complete all parts of the exercise as if doing so in slow motion.

Lie on the floor, knees bent and feet flat on the floor. With arms extended, and palms meeting one another in front, breathe comfortably and gradually allow the two arms to move toward the left at the level of the shoulder; move as far toward the floor as is easily accomplished. Continue breathing and gradually, and in one continuous movement, allow the arms to move in an arc over the body, directly over the nose and then toward the right side of the body at shoulder level. Continue breathing as the arms sweep to the left side and then return to the right side of the body; use a *very* slow, continuous movement; pay attention to points of resistance, relaxation, tension, etc. Note differences in ability to carry out the movement on each repetition. When relaxation is attained, stop the movement and lie flat on the back breathing easily and noting the effect on the body.

When ready, gradually turn onto the left side of the body with the left leg on the bottom, slightly bent, and the right leg bent at a 75–90 degree angle to the trunk; find the angle of comfort. Continue breathing and slowly bend the right arm and move it across the body, easing (but not in any way forcing) the arm with the left palm on the right elbow moving to the right shoulder as movement continues. Hold the position of easy stretch and breathe easily; continue holding the right arm and picture breathing into the shoulder as if there are tiny lungs located in the shoulder inhaling and exhaling as you inhale and exhale. Continue to *gradually* stretch the right arm (using the left arm to support and assist in the stretch). Holding the right hand in the left gradually (in one slow, continuous movement) move the right arm to the right side of the body and then back to the left side of the body; continue breathing easily throughout. Lie flat on the floor on the back and note sensations in the upper and lower body as a result of the exercise.

Turn to lie on the left side of the body as before. Turn the right shoulder to the left side of the body (assisting with the right arm gradually and continuously while breathing). Hold the shoulder at the point of stretched comfort and move the left hand to the right shoulder. Hold the hand there and breathe into it, moving the left palm after several breaths to another spot on the shoulder when warmth is felt emanating from the shoulder. Closing the eyes and imagining energy and warmth being generated in the shoulder will help to accomplish this feat. After several moments, lie flat on the back and note the effect. Repeat all portions of the exercise using the right side of the body and the left shoulder.

This series can also be completed while sitting in a straight chair. The opposite shoulder/arm is cradled in the other arm. A final component can be added while sitting. Place the left palm on the front of the right shoulder and gradually and firmly push the shoulder back as far as is comfortable while breathing deeply in and out. Hold in the extended position and picture tiny lungs breathing in and out at the point of pressure. Relax and note body sensations. Repeat with that arm several times and then repeat with the other shoulder. For further information see: Feldenkrais, M. *Awareness through Movement.* New York: Harper and Row, 1977.

Deciding on an Appropriate Aerobic Exercise Regime

The aerobic exercises discussed in this section include: running, jogging, walking, swimming, aquadynamics and aerobic dance. Although running and jogging are efficient, inexpensive approaches to increasing cardiovascular fitness and can be begun in stages at any age and by those who have been ill and require rehabilitation, injuries of the ankle, knee, and lower back are common. Some can be prevented by improving posture (see Feldenkrais & Cohen), using appropriate shoes (see Table 35), and strengthening the abdominal muscles (see Table 36). It might also be wise to consider another form of aerobic exercise if low back pain, previous injury, or poor jogging posture already exists.

Pender (1982, p. 260) suggests that a walk–jog program be completed prior to continuous jogging, as follows:

Table 35. Choosing a Shoe for Running or Walking

Five Features to Look for in a Good Running Shoe

1. ¼"–½" heel lift or wedge; the shoe should be thicker and softer in the heel than an ordinary sneaker.
2. The middle area of the sole should be considerably softer than the outer sole to absorb the shock of running on a hard surface.
3. The outer sole should be very flexible at the ball of the foot; test by compressing it with the thumb.
4. The toe should be rounded to allow sufficient room for toe nails and reduce the chance of blisters.
5. The shoes should feel comfortable from the first moment they are tried on, allow at least ¼" room in front and to the side of the toes when standing, and the heels should not slip unduly.

Seven Features to Look for in a Good Walking Shoe

1. The toe area should have sufficient room for toes to wiggle and spread out.
2. The sole should flex at the ball of the foot; bend the shoe and see what force it takes to bend it; that force is equal to the amount needed for the foot to flex the shoe when walking. *A good shoe should not have to be broken in.*
3. The shoe should have a cushioned sole; this is mandatory for walking long distances.
4. The shoe should have an arch support; if it does not, cut out a piece of foam rubber to support the arch.
5. The upper part of the shoe should be made of a material that allows the shoe to breathe; leather and nylon mesh is a good combination. Shoes with laces allow for the best fit.
6. The shoe should be lightweight.
7. The shoe should have a curved sole to facilitate the rolling heel–toe action of correct walking.

Sources: S. Hoag, 1981, Choosing a running shoe; and G. Yanker, 1983, *The Complete Book of Exercisewalking.*

1. Work up to 12 sets for 3 consecutive days of 30 seconds of walking, followed by 30 seconds of jogging.
2. Work up to 12 sets for 3 consecutive days of 30 seconds of walking followed by 1 minute of jogging.

Although jogging and running are popular, walking is still superior in several ways: fewer injuries are reported and walking is better for losing weight *if brisk walking* is maintained. A study at the U.S. Olympic Training Center found that brisk walking burned calories at the rate of 1,012 per hour while running burned only 782 calories per hour. The best way to differentiate brisk walking from jogging is that in walking the feet are always on the ground, never in flight (Clark, 1984).

Yanker (1983, pp. 36–64) recommends the following for achieving proper walking technique:

Table 36. Keeping Your Back Fit

Low back pain affects 80% of the population at some time in their lives. Here are some tips for avoiding the affliction; you can also use them if you have back pain as a way to reduce discomfort.

- Avoid jogging, biking, paddling, rowing, baseball, and softball as regular activities; they all put added, strain on your back (*Sports for Life,* 1979).
- Check your posture whenever you pass a mirror; look to see if your knees are slightly bent, your head is not bent forward, your shoulders are not rounded, and your abdomen or buttocks do not hang out, giving you an exaggerated forward curve to your lower back.
- Enhance your posture by completing the following movements:

    1. Stand in a comfortable position and move your shoulders forward as if trying to get them to touch, then to a middle position, and then to the back as if trying to touch your shoulder blades together. Return to the middle, front, and back several times more.
    2. Sit in a straight-backed chair without arms. Hold your arms at shoulder height with your arms bent at elbows. Twist your body gently to the left and then to the right. Repeat several times.
    3. Get on the floor on your knees; shift your weight back towards your feet. Place your hands out in front of you and walk your arms, using your fingertips, out from your body. This should look as if you're playing a vertical piano keyboard.
    4. Stand with a chair in front of you. With knees bent and stomach muscles tight, keep your shoulders and lower back still while you stick your buttocks out and in and then tilt your pelvis forward. Repeat in a slow continuous movement 8–30 times.

- To stretch the muscles in the lower back and strengthen abdominal muscles, lie on the floor and pull your knees to your chest using only your stomach and arm muscles while pushing your lower back toward the floor.
- When bending over from the waist to brush your teeth or pick up an object, always bend your knees slightly.
- When getting up off a chair or the toilet, bring your feet under you, hold your abdomen in, and straighten up; this lets the legs, not your back, do the work.
- When doing tasks that require long standing, place a foot on a low stool or bench to release back pressure; also move around occasionally and do a few movements such as making circles with your shoulders; tilting your pelvis forward and back while contracting your abdominal muscles; and stand while inhaling as you stretch up on your toes as far upward as you can, then exhale fully as you bend over and let your head move toward the floor.
- Cut back on sugary and fatty foods; being overweight can put added strain on your back.
- Eat sufficient calcium; it can help keep you limber, your spine supple, and can ward off the effects of aging. Be sure to include more or some of the following in your meal plan: sardines, salmon, sunflower seed, tofu, milk, or milk products, dried beans, and green vegetables. Reduce your intake of foods that contain oxalic acid (chocolate, rhubarb), fat, and phytic acid (grains) since they prevent calcium absorption.
- Get enough vitamin C since it seems to aid in calcium mobilization and bone growth. The best natural sources are berries, citrus fruits, green and leafy vegetables, tomatoes, cauliflower, potatoes, and sweet potatoes.

Table 36 *(continued)*

- Learn to relax. Tense muscles can bring on back problems. Purchase or record your own relaxation tape and listen to it twice daily.
- Use mental imagery to picture your back as strong, supple, and relaxed. Conjure up this picture several times each day.
- Think positive thoughts about your body in general and your back in particular. Write these on a 3×5 card and carry them with you; be sure to read them several times a day. Some affirmations to use might be: My back is becoming stronger and more relaxed; it's getting easier and easier to keep my back well and strong.
- If you sit most of the day, devise a system to remind yourself to get up once an hour and walk around, stretch, and take a few deep breaths.

Reprinted permission of *The Wellness Newsletter*, 1983; 4(3):5–6.

- Hold head and back erect, tighten abdominal muscles, tuck buttocks under, and walk tall (image of a golden cord attached and pulling up from the upper chest may help with posture).
- Point toes in direction of travel, reaching out with hip, knee, and heel.
- Plant the back edge of the heel of the forward moving foot at a 40-degree angle to the ground, setting the ankle slightly to the outside, leg and foot at a 90-degree angle.
- Pull forward with the leading leg while pushing back with the back leg.
- Hold hands loosely clenched, arms at a 90-degree angle, just brushing the side; forward movement high as the chest, backward movement near shoulder level. Inhale on left-arm swing, exhale on right-arm swing. Right arm forward with left leg and vice versa.
- Focus eyes 10–15 feet ahead.
- Check out nonparallel leg movements by walking in the snow or sand and observing. For a duck-footed walk, walk with a wider stance and practice the heel walk. To correct pigeon-toed walking, exaggerate pointing the toes before the heel strikes; picture the toes pointing straight. To correct favored-leg walking, concentrate on the forward flow of the legs.

Based on the flexibility/tightness assessment, appropriate exercises can be chosen. See Table 37.

Swimming is an excellent conditioner if bearing weight on the lower joints is contraindicated. However, Diamond (1979, p. 42) has found that swimming the breast stroke, a homologous movement, weakens the thymus.

Table 37. Flexibility Exercises

1–3 Reach left hand over shoulder and clasp right hand for 30 seconds and then switch arms.

4 Stand with feet 3 feet apart, and fingers laced behind back, palms up. Slowly lift arms up and over head while lowering the head gently towards the floor.

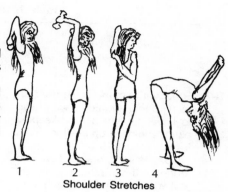

Shoulder Stretches

1–2 With legs wide apart, and palms on the floor, shift hips to the left, bending the left knee; then shift weight to the right, bending the right knee. Repeat 10 times each side in a slow, controlled motion.

3–4 Sit on the floor with soles of feet together; press with hands on the inside of the knees and hold for 30 seconds, then relax. Repeat 20 times.

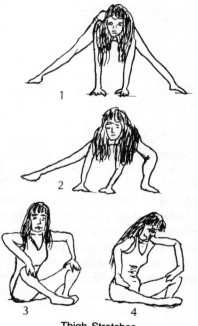

Thigh Stretches

Place hands and feet on the floor, backside up; bend left knee and press right heel to the floor and hold, feeling the pull in the calf. Straighten left leg and bend right knee and press left heel to the floor and hold. Do 20 repetitions each side.

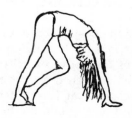

Heel Cord Stretches

Table 37 *(continued)*

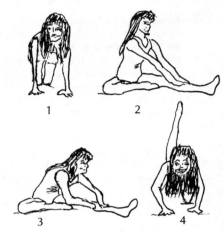

1–2   Squat with palms on the floor directly under shoulders with head to knee; straighten legs, keeping palms and heels on the floor, then lower. Repeat 10 times.

3–4   Sit on the floor, one leg bent into opposite thigh, other leg straight out with foot flexed. Reach arms down the straight leg, lowering chest toward it. Bob very gently 15 times and then switch legs and repeat.

Upper Leg Stretches

NOTE: It is recommended that flexibility exercises of this type be completed *prior to and following* any exercise session.

Besides choosing an aerobic workout that is useful, it is also wise to choose one that is fun or it will not be continued on a lifelong basis. A variant of swimming is aquadynamics or water exercise. The President's Council on Physical Fitness (1983) has produced a booklet detailing the basics and various programs from mild toning to conditioning.

Aerobic dancing is a popular conditioning method. However, there are pitfalls to be aware of. Jones (*The Wellness Newsletter*, 1985), a dance instructor, describes some. Even with an excellent teacher, the student may misread instructor movements and create injuries, overemphasize gross body movement, use the limbs inefficiently, and not take advantage of the neuromuscular enhancement available.

EXERCISE FOR SPECIAL POPULATIONS

Probably the best exercise for clients of all ages and conditions is walking. Exercises for bedridden clients are presented in Table 38.

Most of the above exercises can be adapted for use in a wheelchair or armchair. Even those severely debilitated can approximate some of the exercises or at least rotate the wrists and ankles, flex and stretch wrists and feet, rotate the head in clockwise and counterclockwise di-

Table 38. Exercises for Bedridden Clients

NOTE: Ask client to breathe throughout all exercises.

1. Raise the head from pillow as far as possible; add one raise of the head a week to a maximum of 10 repetitions.
2. Turn the head slowly to the left and then to the right; add one turn of the head per week to a maximum of 10 repetitions.
3. Shrug the shoulders up and back toward the ears as far as possible; add one repetition per week to a total of 10 repetitions.
4. Rotate the shoulders clockwise and then counterclockwise, 5 times in each direction.
5. Bring the right arm (fully extended) over the head, left arm at side; bring down right arm to the side of the body and bring the left arm (fully extended) over the head. Work up to a maximum of 10 repetitions.
6. Cross the wrists at the abdomen and circle both arms at the same time, first clockwise and then counterclockwise; work up to 10 repetitions.
7. Clench the fists tightly and hold for several seconds, then extend the fingers and reach up as far as possible; work up to 10 repetitions.
8. Extend the arms forward and spread the fingers as far as possible; work up to 10 repetitions.
9. Make a fist and rotate the thumbs clockwise and then counterclockwise; work up to 10 repetitions.
10. Raise the right leg up as far as possible and return it to the bed; keep the leg as straight as possible without straining the lower back; work up to 10 repetitions each leg.
11. Grasp the right knee with both hands and very slowly pull it toward the chest while slowly moving the head toward the knee; work up to 5 repetitions with each knee.
12. Grasp both knees with both hands and very slowly pull them toward the chest while slowly moving the head toward the knees; work up to 10 repetitions.
13. With arms at sides of the body, slowly raise the head, shoulders, and legs several inches; hold, then return to lie flat; work up to 3 repetitions.
14. Extend both ankles toward the bottom of the bed; hold, then flex them toward the shins, hold, then relax. Work up to 10 repetitions.
15. Bicycle both legs slowly, completing up to 10 circles.
16. Lie on the stomach with chin resting on hands. Put heels apart and big toes together; squeeze the buttocks together as though trying to prevent a bowel movement; while squeezing, bring the heels slowly together and hold for 2–3 seconds, then relax on the bed. Work up to 5 repetitions.
17. Lie on the left side in a straight line and raise the left leg as high as possible over the other leg; hold, then return it to the bed. Work up to 10 repetitions. Turn on right side and raise left leg up to 10 repetitions.
18. Raise hips 5"–6" off the bed, keeping arms at sides; hold several seconds, then relax into the bed. Work up to 5 repetitions.

rections, and exercise the face by exaggeratedly saying the vowels (A E I O U).

Feldenkrais' movements can be used with the elderly to enhance leg and hip movement. Masters and Houston (1978, pp. 160–167) suggest the following series.

1. Sit halfway forward in a straight-back chair, legs spread a little wider than usual, knees bent, and feet parallel. Rest hands on the chair seat or side, not on the legs.
2. While breathing, let the right leg begin to drop slowly to the right, then bring it back to the middle, paying attention to the sensation in the hip joint.
3. Extend the right leg out in front, resting the heel on the floor. Let the foot fall to the right, keeping the leg straight. Try it again, this time with the knee slightly bent. Repeat 20–25 times while breathing. Rest and observe the sensations in the lower body.
4. Extend the right leg in front, resting on the heel. Let the foot fall easily to the left, keeping the leg straight. Let it gradually return to the middle. Repeat as in no. 3 above.
5. While continuing to breathe throughout, extend the right leg and push the foot along the floor, keeping the leg straight, pushing off and back with the heel. Let the right side of the body follow the movement; hold the side of the chair for balance. As the movement is repeated (20–25 times), notice how the left shoulder goes back as the right shoulder moves forward.
6. Spread the feet and legs a little further apart. Continue breathing regularly while letting the right leg fall toward the other leg. Pay attention to the hip joint and right buttock as the leg falls. Put the right leg out a little further in front and continue breathing and dropping the right leg toward the left leg and returning it to center. Watch as the leg moves and feel what happens in the hip joint and buttock.
7. Turn the right foot toward the left leg and then away from it; notice the pressure on the left buttock when turning the right leg away from the left leg. Let the whole body shift with the foot movement and pay attention to the body sensations. Repeat the movement while breathing for 20–25 times. Rest.
8. Place the right foot parallel to the left foot and let the right leg flop from left to right. As the leg flops to the right, the foot will tilt on its right side; as the leg flops to the left, the foot will tilt on its left side. Experiment with different positions until the point where the leg moves the most freely is found. Rest and breathe.

9. Shift the body weight onto the left buttock slightly so the right buttock rises a little off the chair. Sink into the right buttock and observe the left buttock rising off the chair. Repeat right buttock, left buttock, noticing what happens in the hip joint during the movement and breathing on each movement.

10. Extend the right leg, foot off the floor an inch or so, sitting way back in the chair. Make circles with your foot, keeping the leg stiff, and breathing. Make a few in the other direction, continuing to breathe throughout. Experiment with small circles, large circles, fast and slow circles. Rest.

11. Sit back in the chair with right leg extended and foot off the floor a few inches. While breathing, move the foot and leg as a piece from left to right several times. Continue to breathe and flop the foot left and right, keeping the leg straight. Rest.

12. Lean forward and extend the right leg, placing the heel on the floor. Slide the foot backward and forward along the floor, keeping the knee straight. Note how differently the hip joint is being used now. Let the whole body move as the foot slides forward and back. Place the right hand on the right hip and feel the movement as the right foot and leg are moved to the right and to the left. Sense where the socket is that connects the leg into the hip and notice what is happening to the left side of the rib cage. Rest.

13. Place the two feet side by side with the legs bent. Move the right knee from left to right and see how it moves. Breathe in as the right knee is moved from left to right. Do the same movements while breathing out. Note which movement is easier. Repeat the movement using the breathing that is easiest. Rest.

14. Extend both legs and lift the right leg several times and then the left one. Note which feels lighter. Get up and walk around. Turn to the right and then to the left. Note in which direction it is easier to turn.

15. Lift the right leg in front and then the left leg; note which leg made the larger movement. Rest and note the sensations in both sides of your hip, and in both legs.

16. After a rest, or the next day, repeat nos. 1–15 above using the left leg. Continue doing the exercise daily, alternating legs.

Those with diabetes can benefit greatly from exercise. Exercise increases insulin sensitivity. "The effect is most pronounced in muscles, which are a major customer for the circulating blood sugar. As muscles are conditioned, they seek to increase their stores of glycogen, and . . . call for more sugar from the bloodstream. After a bout of exercise, insulin and glucose levels fall for a day or so, and can be seen before any loss of weight or fat" (Brownell & Stunkard, 1980).

Those who participate in a regular exercise program show enhanced insulin action and reduced plasma glucose levels. The relationship between degree of physical conditioning and ability to metabolize glucose holds despite differences in age, sex, or ratio of body fat to total body weight. Elevated levels of blood glucose may be associated with many of the physical problems experienced by people with diabetes. Thus, exercise may ward off problems and enhance wellness for them.

Studies conducted in Sweden by Dr. Ralph A. DeFronzo of Yale University support the beneficial effect of exercise. The researcher found that 85% of body glucose uptake occurs in the skeletal muscles. This explains why people with diabetes show improved control over their disease when they participate in physically conditioning exercise (*Research Resources Reporter*, 1983).

Exercise is beneficial to those with arthritis, too. Researchers at the University of Michigan Medical School in Ann Arbor asked women with the affliction to pedal on a stationary bicycle from 15 to 35 minutes 3 times a week. After 12 weeks the women reported higher energy levels, less pain and swelling, increased ease in doing household chores, and heightened interest in social activities. Those who pedaled for 15 minutes showed more improvement than those who pedaled for 35 minutes.

Exercise can have a positive effect on bone mineral loss. Smith reported studying a group of 30 elderly women for 3 years. Eighteen did nothing special in terms of exercise, while 12 participated in a 40–45 minute exercise program 3 days a week. They did exercises from the sitting position in a straight-backed chair. At the end of 3 years, the control group had a 3.2% loss in bone mineral measurements while the physically active group showed a 2.29% increase. Physical activity plays an important role in preventing loss of flexibility and bone mass. Thus effects of aging need not include bone aging.

Overly vigorous exercise is not needed. In fact, female marathon runners showed a decrease in bone mass in a study conducted at the University of California in San Francisco. Most had stopped menstruating, yet their estrogen levels were not different enough from nonrunners to explain the loss in bone mass. Thus, marathon running, at least for women, may not ward off the effects of bone aging as well as chair exercises.

Memory loss effects of aging can also be warded off with exercise. Researchers at the University of Utah divided volunteers (average age 61) into three groups: one that exercised aerobically, walking up to a target pulse of 120 beats per minute for 40 minutes; a group that did pushups and lifted weights; and another that remained inactive. After 4 months of training, the aerobic group improved their oxygen intake by 25% and showed improvement in six of eight mental tests; the weight lifting group improved their oxygen intake by 9% and improved in only one of eight mental tests; the inactive control group remained the same in oxygen intake and mental agility. An English study by psychologist Patrick Rabbit corroborates this study; he found that of 1,200 elderly people, the 10% who showed no memory loss at all had intact cardiovascular systems. His findings support the idea that good memories need sufficient oxygen. Exercise is probably the best way to ensure that sufficient oxygen reaches the brain to keep the mind active (Clark, 1983).

Children, too, can benefit from exercise, but certain kinds may reduce their level of wellness. According to Bob Arnot, M.D., Sports Medicine Specialist, football, weight lifting, running, or jogging can be bad for children who have not reached adolescence yet. They can damage growth plates and may incur physical and emotional damage in these activities if pushed too hard. Ballet is not a good exercise either because feet can be deformed by walking on pointed toe too frequently.

On the other hand, lacrosse, gentle stretching, situps, side-to-side hopping, soccer, and swimming are good, especially if properly supervised. The International Athletic Association Federation echoes the refrain. They discourage intensive competition and strenuous training in puberty and prepuberty age groups because separation of growth plates may occur in the pelvis, knee, or ankle. Although these separations can heal with rest, it is not known whether harmful effects might turn up later. The Medical Committee of IAAF suggests that up to the age of 12 children should not run more than 800 meters in competition. Russell Pate at the University of South Carolina is researching the topic of marathon running for children (The Department of Physical Education, Columbia, SC).

OVERCOMING OBSTACLES TO EXERCISE

Attrition in exercise programs is a major problem (Jordan-March, 1985). Davis, McKay, and Eshelman (1982) contend there are two major obstacles to overcome in undertaking and keeping at an exercise program: making exercise part of a life style and avoiding injury. Suggestions for making exercise a safe part of a life style include:

1. Start small and keep it fun.
2. Keep records of daily and weekly progress; include both subjective reactions and objective measures: weight, blood pressure, pulse.
3. Focus on the rewards of exercise; keep a record of moods and

compare differences in relaxation, energy, concentration, and sleep patterns.

4. Post goals, mottos, pictures of the ideal self, affirmations, and notes of encouragement.
5. Use visualization daily to picture successful attainment of exercise benefit, e.g., looking toned, radiant, graceful.
6. Work with a peer facilitator or join a structured exercise class, running club, or fitness center. Spend more time with people dedicated to wellness.
7. Reward and congratulate yourself for working toward exercise goals as well as attaining them. For example, after a month in an exercise program, buy a new pair of running shoes or treat yourself to a meal out.
8. Use proper equipment and clothing when exercising.
9. Include at least 10 minutes of warm-up and cool-down exercises in an exercise program. Avoid running up to the front door, going inside, and sitting down; complete stretching exercises, shower, and change to dry clothes.
10. Stop exercising or at least slow down and consult with a practitioner if any unusual, unexplainable symptoms occur.
11. Avoid exercising for 2 hours after a large meal and eating for 1 hour after exercising.

BODY/MIND INTERACTIONS AND FITNESS

Many investigations of mind/body connections examine the effects of the mind on the body. The discipline of psychosomatics is an example. Sime (1984) approaches mind/body interactions looking at the effect exercise has on the mind. His article includes an extensive review of the literature. Although many studies prior to 1979 examined the effect of exercise on mood, many had methodological flaws. Three studies since 1979 used experimental designs, including control groups, but lacking randomization. In one study 128 elderly females, 65 to 90 years of age, participated in an exercise program. They reported significantly lower state (situation-specific) anxiety, better sleep patterns, and less tension than a comparable group that participated in arts and crafts activities (Reiter, 1981).

In a related study the participants were 18 to 27 years old. The study compared running and exercise classes with a social group that met during lunch. The control group was higher in anxiety before treatment; this illustrates the selection-bias problem—those who are highly anxious may be the least likely to choose exercise voluntarily. All groups tested significantly lower on anxiety, indicating that some of the benefits of exercise programs may be of a diversionary nature (Wilson, Berger, & Bird, 1981).

A third study compared a college swimming class with a lecture group. Swimming produced significant decreases in anxiety, tension, anger, depression, and confusion and an increase in vigor; no changes were noted in the lecture class participants (Berger & Owen, 1982).

Another topic of interest is the comparison of exercise to other non-drug anxiety-reducing techniques. In one study, vigorous activity, meditation, and diversion all showed equal ability to reduce anxiety (Bahrke & Morgan, 1979). This suggests that time-out or diversion may be a useful intervention for those antagonistic to exercise as a tension-reducing measure.

Benson and his colleagues have demonstrated the positive effects of combining exercise with relaxation procedures (Benson, Dryer, & Hartley, 1978). DeVries (1972) has shown clearly that exercise of the appropriate type, duration, and intensity can bring about a significant tranquilizer effect.

Recent evidence indicates that the wide variation in perception of pain is due to the level of endorphin in the bloodstream (Willer, Dehen, & Cambier, 1981). The level of beta-endorphin has been shown to be higher following exercise, as intensity of exercise increases (Colt, Wardlow, & Frantz, 1981). Endorphin remains in the blood for at least 2 hours following prolonged, intense exercise (Appenzeller, 1981). These results support empirical observations of regular exercisers' findings that anxiety levels decrease for 30 minutes to several hours after exercise, then increase progressively until exercise is resumed (Sime, 1985). The "high" runners (and others who engage in conditioning exercise) report is probably a reflection of the endorphin level.

Exercise seems to be most useful in reducing anxiety when combined with cognitive strategies (see Chapter 5) and when breathing is synchronized with exercise (Sime, 1982). Synchronization keeps pace and effort at a comfortable level and also distracts the person from any negative sensations associated with intense exercise.

Two studies of runners suggest that the greater the distance and the more intense the exercise, the less the level of depression (Wilson, Berger, & Bird, 1981; Kavanaugh et al., 1977). Studies have shown that exercise is equally as effective as time-limited psychotherapy (Greist et al., 1978). Another large study (600 self-selected students) provides support for the efficacy of exercise as a treatment for depression (Brown, Ramirez, & Taub, 1978).

Goldberg and Fitzpatrick (1980) reported the use of movement therapy as a treatment for low morale and low self-esteem in a population of institutionalized aged. They found movement therapy group members demonstrated greater improvement in total morale and attitudes toward aging. Thus, movement and exercise can be used as an intervention to enhance normal growth and development in aging and self-esteem and morale.

When using exercise as a treatment for depression, the following practical considerations should be kept in mind:

1. Use a slow, graduated exercise program. It fosters a sense of mastery; a new, positive self-image; and cathartic relief.
2. Run with a companion who runs at about the same speed and is not competitive. (An indicant of noncompetitiveness is the ability to make complimentary comments regardless of fitness level.)
3. Monitor pace with the talk test (never exerting beyond the capacity to maintain a conversation with one's peer). Keep moving even if fatigue necessitates a slow walk.
4. Keep a log of activity for self-motivation, reinforcement of the activity, and to chronicle progress.
5. Make a contract with a peer or practitioner providing a substantial bonus for success and a meaningful penalty for failure.
6. Teach clients to synchronize breathing with movement. (Feldenkrais and yoga (see Chapter 7) are possible interventions to combine with an exercise program.)
7. Provide more extrinsic rewards for novice runners; in time, runners get intrinsic reward from running. Until then, reinforcement for running may need to be provided by a peer or practitioner.

INTEGRATIVE LEARNING EXPERIENCES

Beginning Level

1. Assess yourself using the following measures:

   A. Cohen/Mills' developmental movement theory
   B. Kurtz and Prestera's structural assessments
   C. Aerobic conditioning (calculate safe ranges)
   D. Marshall's flexibility tests

2. Develop and try out appropriate interventions based on the above assessments; use Table 23, p. 108, to organize the data.
3. Calculate your safe aerobic exercise range and cross check yours with a peer.
4. Role play responses to the following client responses using assertiveness criteria to evaluate your efforts:

A. "Cancer is due to a virus. What good can thinking or imagining do?"
B. "I don't want to exercise; I'm too depressed."
C. "I have diabetes and I have to take it easy or I'll need more insulin."

Advanced Level

1. Complete an assessment of one child, one young adult, and one senior client using assessments based on the frameworks of: Cohen/Mills, Kurtz/Prestera, aerobic conditioning, Marshall's flexibility criteria.
2. Develop appropriate interventions for the three clients assessed; organize the information gathered using Table 23, p. 108.

REFERENCES

Appenzeller, O. (1981). What makes us run. *NE J Med* 305:578–580.
Bahrke, M., and Morgan, W. (1979). The positive effects of swimming on mood: swimmers really do feel better. Paper presented at the Annual Conference of the North American Society for Psychology of Sport and Physical Activity, University Park, Maryland, May.
Benson, H., Dryer, T., and Hartley, L. (1978). Decreased O_2 consumption during exercise with elicitation of the relaxation response. *J Hum Stress* 4(2):28–42.
Brown, R., Ramirex, D., and Taub, J. (1978). The prescription of exercise for depression. *Physician Sports Med* 6:34–49.
Brownell, K., and Stunkard, A. (1980). Physical activity in the development and control of obesity. In *Obesity*, A. Stunkard, Ed. Philadelphia, PA: W.B. Saunders, pp. 300–324.
Clark, C. (1983). Exercise—the way to keep young and pain free. *The Wellness Newsl.* 4(3):2.
Clark, C. (1984). Walking better than jogging for losing weight. *The Wellness Newsl.* 5(2):1–2.
Colt, E., Wardlow, S., and Frantz, A. (1981). The effect of running on plasma-endorphins. *Life Sci* 28:1637–1640.
Davis, J. (1963). Review of scientific information on the effects of ionized air on human beings and animals. *J Aerospace Med* 34(1):1.
Davis, M., McKay, M., and Eshelman, E. (1982). *The Relaxation and Stress Reduction Workbook*, 2nd ed. Oakland, CA: New Harbinger Publications, p. 201.
deVries, H. (1981). Tranquilizer effect of exercise: a critical review. *Am J Phys Med* 60:57–66.
Diamond, J. (1979). *Behavioral Kinesiology.* New York: Harper and Row.
Feldenkrais, M. (1977). *Awareness Through Movement.* New York: Harper and Row.
Goldberg, W., and Fitzpatrick, J. (1980). Movement therapy with the aged. *Nur Res* 29(6):339–346.

Greist, J., et al. (1978). Running through your mind. *J Psychosom Res* 20:41–54.
Hoag, S. (1981). Choosing a running shoe. *The Minn Wellness J* (July), pp. 1, 4.
Jones, D. (1985). What's missing in aerobic dance? *The Wellness Newsl* 6(3):2.
Jordan-Marsh, M. (1985). Development of a tool for diagnosing changes in concern about exercise: a means of enhancing compliance. *Nur Res* 34(2): 103–107.
Kavanaugh, T., et al. (1977). Depression following myocardial infarct: the effects of long distance running. In *The Marathon: Physiological, Medical, Epidemiological and Psychological Studies*, P. Milvy, Ed. Annuals of the New York Academy of Science, p. 301.
Koplan, J. (1979). Cardiovascular deaths while running. *JAMA* 242:2578–2579.
Kurtz, R., and Prestera, H. (1984). *The Body Reveals*. New York: Harper and Row.
Marshall, J. (1981). How to get good looks, top performance and staying power for your body. *Self* (March), 56–72.
Masters, R., and Houston, J. (1978). *Listening to the Body*. New York: Delta.
Mills, M., and Cohen, B. (1979). *Developmental Movement Therapy*. Amherst, MA: The School for Body/Mind Centering.
Pender, N. (1982). *Health Promotion in Nursing Practice*. E. Norwalk, CT: Appleton-Century-Crofts.
President's Council on Physical Fitness and Sports. (n.d.). *An Introduction to Running: One Step at a Time*. Washington, D.C.: HEW.
President's Council on Physical Fitness and Sports. (1983). *Aquadynamics*. Washington, D.C.
Reiter, M. (1981). Effects of a physical exercise program on selected mood states in a group of women over age 65. *Diss Abstracts Intnatl* 42, no. 81-23283.
Research Resources Reporter. (1983). Washington, D.C.: National Institute of Health, n.p.
Sime, W. (1982). A new look at the association/dissociation in long distance running. *Running Psychol* (May), 5–6.
Sime, W. (1984). Psychological benefits of exercise. *Advances* 1(4):15–29.
Thompson, P., et al. (1979). Death during jogging or running. *JAMA* 242:1265–1267.
Vickery, D. (1978). *Life Plan for Your Health*. Reading, MA: Addison-Wesley, pp. 10–11.
Willer, J., Dehen, H., and Cambier, J. (1981). Stress induced analgesia in humans: endogenous opioids and naloxone reversible depression of pain reflexes. *Science* 212:689–691.
Wilson, V., Berger, B., and Bird, E. (1981). Effects of running and of an exercise class on anxiety. *Percept Motor Skills* 53:472–474.
Yanker, G. (1983). *The Complete Book of Exercisewalking*. Chicago, IL: Contemporary Books.

7

SELF-CARE, TOUCH, AND WELLNESS

This chapter discusses the following topics:

- Theoretical frameworks for touch and healing
- Self-care assessments
- Touch and healing assessments
- Smoking cessation: an example of a self-care intervention
- Touch and healing interventions

This chapter is closely related to Chapter 6: both deal with aspects of the wellness dimension of fitness. This chapter is focused on self-care and touch and their relationship to wellness. Theories, assessments, and interventions for behavioral kinesiology, therapeutic touch, yoga, massage, acupressure, reflexology and psychoneuroimmunology are provided. Additionally, information and skills to enhance self-care skills are presented.

THEORETICAL FRAMEWORKS FOR TOUCH AND HEALING
Diamond's Theory of Behavioral Kinesiology

I have come to believe that all illness starts as a problem on the *energy* level, a problem that may exist for many years before it manifests itself in physical disease. It appears that a generalized reduction of body energy leads to energy imbalances in particular parts of the body. If we become aware of these energy imbalances when they first occur, we have a long grace period in which to correct them. We will then be practicing primary prevention. (Diamond, 1979, p. 2)

Diamond developed his theory after years of working as a traditional psychiatrist, investing huge amounts of his own energy to bolster up the clients who were not really interested in changing. "I could never get it through to them that their well-being was really their responsibility" (Diamond, 1979, p. 4).

Noting that the longer his clients remained in therapy, the more depressed therapist and client became, he searched for a broader framework from which to practice—one that included nutrition and various physical and postural therapies. *Diamond's Behavioral Kinesiology*

> uses the basic testing techniques of Applied Kinesiology, but focuses on the factors in the . . . surroundings and life-style that are raising and lowering body energy. Many of the factors that lower energy are products of the technological revolution: the poisons and noises in our environment, the overrefined and unnatural foods we find on the supermarket shelves, the synthetic fabrics from which so many of our clothes are made. Other factors are individual habits or tendencies, such as posture, ability to handle stress, and human relationships. (Diamond, 1979, p. 7)

The thymus gland is of great import in Diamond's work. He points out that until recently (most prevalent around the period from the 1920s to the 1950s), the thymus gland was irradiated (to make it smaller) and thought to have no function in adult life. It is now known that the thymus gland is crucial to the immunity mechanisms in the body. Hormones in the thymus influence lymphocytes to mature and give rise to lymphocytes called T (thymus-derived) cells that protect the body from foreign cells by the process of immunological surveillance. Thus, the thymus is a true endocrine gland. During severe stress, injury, or sudden illness, the thymus shrinks to half its size as millions of lymphocytes are destroyed (Diamond, 1979, pp. 8–13).

Diamond has developed a muscle test using the deltoid muscle as an indicator of the body's energy supply. "A device that measures muscle strength, called a kinesiometer, shows that strong muscles can withstand up to 40 pounds of pressure, whereas a muscle that is weak can resist a pressure of about 15 pounds" (Diamond, 1979, p. 17). His research suggests that it is the thymus that is being tested by having subjects who test weak chew a tablet of thymus extract and upon retest the indicator muscle becomes strong.

Chi is the term used by the Chinese to describe energy. They developed an ancient and accepted treatment in the United States called acupuncture. In this system of thought, energy is believed to flow along pathways called meridians that do not appear to follow any *known* anatomical pathway. Behavioral Kinesiology is not testing "the mechanical strength of the muscle, but rather the energy in the meridian associated with that muscle and the ability of the body to replenish energy" (Diamond, 1979, pp. 27–28). In Diamond's theory, the thymus gland monitors and regulates energy flow in the meridian system.

According to Diamond, if the thymus monitors and balances energy, well-being occurs; if not, physical damage and ultimately organic disease occur. Various stressors have been found to decrease muscle strength in the indicator muscle, indicating impairment of thymus function and a lack of balance in the left (rational, logical) and right (holistic, creative) hemispheres of the brain.

Krieger's Theory of Therapeutic Touch

Dolores Krieger, R.N., Ph.D., theorizes that prana (Sanskrit term for energy) is transferred in the healing act. She draws on Eastern literature, finding apt analogies in Western thought. For example, the source of prana in Eastern thinking is the sun; likewise, the source of energy for photosynthesis is the sun. Eastern thinking contends that well people have an excess of prana; Western physiology texts state there is a great deal of redundancy in the human body. Krieger pictures the healer as a person with excess prana or energy who has a strong sense of commitment and intention to help people. "The act of healing, then would entail the channeling of this energy flow by the healer for the well-being of the sick individual" (Krieger, 1979, p. 13). Healers do not become depleted of energy, however, because they are in a constant state of energy input-throughput-output. Healers become depleted of energy only if they become too closely identified with the process or try to draw on their own energy (rather than being a channel for energy). Healers are thought to accelerate the healing process by giving the healee an extra boost to his/her recuperative system (Krieger, 1979, pp. 15–17).

Krieger presents physiological data to back up her theory. There is evidence that Therapeutic Touch raises hemoglobin levels and influences EEG patterns; the healer's EEG changes to a high amplitude beta state, indicative of deep concentration similar to meditation, and the healee's brain waves are typically low amplitude alpha waves, correlated with a state of calmness and well-being. There are indications that the "highly personalized interaction invokes in the healee a sense of self-responsibility for his or her health" (Krieger, 1979, pp. 16, 17, 75).

According to Krieger (1979, pp. 89–90), Therapeutic Touch works well with all stress-related diseases, having a significant effect on the autonomic nervous system, thereby influencing nausea, dyspnea, tachycardia, pallor, and peristalsis. Borelli and Heidt (1981) report the use of therapeutic touch with children and their families, with the terminally ill person, in the operating room, in jails, and with clients hospitalized in a cardiovascular unit of a general hospital. Signs that Therapeutic Touch has occurred in the client include a deepening of voice level; slowing and deepening of respirations; a sigh, deepened breathing, or comment such as "I feel relaxed"; peripheral flush or pinking of the skin due to dilation of peripheral blood vessels, first noticed in the face (Krieger, 1979, pp. 75–76).

The healer centers and uses the hands (placed 2–3 inches from the client's skin) to move quickly over the body, reading signals of congestion or blockage of energy flow. The feeling of pressure sensed in the hands when congestion or blockage is present can be explained biophysically; as the healer moves the hands over the body, positive ions are picked up; this pressure sensation is related to atoms that have lost an electron. Positive ions are associated with feelings of lethargy, headache, irritability, and inflammations of the mucosal tissues; negative ions have been noted in areas that may induce a feeling of well-being, such as waterfalls and mountains (Davis, 1963; Robinson & Dirnfeld, 1967).

Krieger refers to the pressure as a "ruffling in the field"; the healer can remove the positive ions by shaking or wiping the hands. When the healer's hands are placed in the area of a "ruffle" and then the hands are moved away from the body in a sweeping gesture, the pressure is reduced and the feeling of energy flow is sensed; this is called "unruffling the field" (1979, p. 54). The unruffling motion can be used to soothe babies or reduce pain and tension. A 2- to 3-minute treatment is sufficient for children or the debilitated. With others the healer stops when the body feels balanced.

The object of Therapeutic Touch is to balance the healer's "field" so that symmetry of energy flow is restored. With practice the hands begin to move toward areas of unbalanced energy flow as they become more sensitive to changes in the field of another person's body.

Krieger reports that prana can be transferred to objects, especially cotton. By holding a piece of cotton in one hand and placing the other hand above the cotton and imagining reaching down to the hand under the cotton, energy can be transferred. In this way energy can be stored to be used at a later date when less energized or to prepare for clients' use when they feel fatigued (Krieger, 1979, pp. 28–29).

Yoga

The word *yoga* means to unite, implying the balance or harmony that can exist within the individual. Yoga is an Indian philosophical system that emphasizes the practice of special techniques to attain the highest degree of physical, emotional, and spiritual integration. Hatha yoga is the branch that emphasizes physical postures (asanas) and breathing practices (pranayama) to attain body/mind balance.

Studies of the effects of Hatha yoga have shown it especially beneficial to optimal functioning of the endocrine, circulatory, musculoskeletal, respiratory, and nervous systems (Iyengar, 1966; Udupa, Singh, & Settiwar, 1971). Yoga has been demonstrated to reduce blood pressure, lower pulse rate, reduce serum cholesterol, regulate menstrual flow and thyroid function, increase range of motion in joints, reduce joint pain, and increase feeling of well-being (Lasater, 1984, p. 296).

Massage

Message has had a long and checkered history. It has been alternately extolled as a panacea for an extensive list of ailments and rejected as a therapeutic procedure. Despite extravagant claims for and against it, for millennia, massage has been employed successfully. In contemporary times we are witnessing a renaissance in its popularity, possibly the result of a growing public disillusionment with modern depersonalized clinical practices that emphasize surgery and drugs rather than personal contact and self-responsibility or preventative maintenance . . . (Knaster, 1984, p. 247).

In ancient Greece and Rome, massage was used for many conditions. With the rise of Christianity, the habit of bathing, touch, nakedness, and concerns with the body were deprecated because religious teachings scorned the body as a repository of sin (Knaster, 1984, p. 249). During the nineteenth century, Per Henrik Ling, originator of the Swedish movement-cure, and Johan Georg Mezger, a Dutch physician whose classification of massage movements led to acceptance by clinicians, did much to reestablish massage as a valued treatment.

The effects of massage are psychological, mechanical, physiological, and reflexive. Massage is an art (a unique way of communicating without words and showing caring) and a science; systematic manipulation of the body tissue produces beneficial effects on the nervous and muscular systems, local and general circulation, the skin, viscera, and metabolism (Knaster, 1984, p. 247).

During massage, "the hands stimulate the sensory receptors of the skin and subcutaneous tissues, causing a series of reflex effects . . . some of these effects are capillary vasodilation or constriction, relaxation or stimulation of voluntary muscle contraction, and possible sedation or stimulation of pain in an area remote from the area being touched" (Tappan, 1984, p. 262).

Ruth Rice (1975), a nurse psychologist and specialist in early child development, has researched sensorimotor stimulation of premature infants. She developed a specific stroking and massage technique. Her research demonstrated that touching, movement, and sound stimulate the nerve pathways and increase myelination (speeding up neurological growth), increase the release of the growth hormone somatrophin (leading to faster weight gain), and increase the output of the hypothalamus (general arousal center) leading to increased cell activity and endocrine functioning.

Acupressure

Acupressure is the predecessor of acupuncture. It grew from the instinctual response of massaging sore muscles by pressing sore spots on the body and noting the positive effects. Currently, the term is applied to a number of techniques of applying pressure to stimulate acupuncture points on the body.

Acupressure releases tension and relieves pain. It is a preventive treatment used to balance energy. Chinese medicine contends that the vital force, chi, that controls the functioning of the body systems permeates living tissue circulating along clearly defined pathways called meridians. There are 12 organ meridians; each one takes its name from the organ to which it is connected. Energy is believed to flow through each of the 12 meridians, flowing into one another, forming a continuous pathway for energy. When energy is blocked, it can be balanced by applying pressure to specific points.

Theory of Reflexology

Reflexology is based on the premise that body organs have corresponding reflex points on other parts of the body. The reflex points are believed to be up to 20 times more sensitive than the corresponding organs. The foot is viewed as one of the scanner screens that records body functions. Working the reflexes in the feet helps rebalance organs that are functioning properly by releasing blocks that impede the smooth flow of body energy. Reflex points also influence functional relationships to that organ. For example, stimulating the heart reflex on the foot helps balance energy flow to the heart as well as the rest of the circulatory system (blood vessels, lymphatics, etc.) (Berkson, 1977, pp. 1–2). There are other areas with reflex points (wrist, hand, ear, neck, abdomen, face, head, arms, legs, nose, and iris), but the feet are the most effective because:

1. They link with energy from the earth and are strong energy poles of the body.
2. Working on feet is relatively nonthreatening and noninvasive.
3. Feet accumulate deposits of acids and tensions (due to the effects of gravity, pressure, and the normal wear and tear of walking upright), causing tissue degeneration which can easily be felt, seen, and treated.
4. Touching the feet is a soothing gesture that can deeply affect others; for example, agitated children can be calmed by rubbing their feet.
5. Clearly charted representations of the body organs on the foot are available.
6. Because feet are usually covered with shoes and socks, they remain tender to the touch and more sensitive than some other reflex points. Additionally, there is less body musculature that might interfere with assessment and intervention than in most other parts of the body.
7. Feet are a symbolic representation of the infinite energy in the universe. Jesus washed the feet of his disciples, linking, cleansing, protecting, and blessing their whole being (Berkson, 1977, p. 7).

Berkson has developed the Integrated Treatment from her study of reflexology, nutrition (she has a master's degree in the subject), acupressure (she is a certified shiatsu therapist), yoga, massage, and polarity. Her method combines diet, exercise, and healing visualization and affirmations to broach the physical, mental, spiritual, and artistic. Blocks are released and deposits are thrown off, increasing vitality of the whole person and increasing relaxation and activity potential (physical). The act of reflexology is a giving and receiving, a sharing of communication resulting in confidence and calming (mental). Together, healer and healee call upon the healing energy of the universe to surround, uplift, and permeate; the use of affirmations and the projection of a positive healing environment is a spiritual act of being of service to others (spiritual). The Integrated Treatment calls for knowledge, skills, and a personalized interaction between healer and healee to produce healing (art) (Berkson, 1977, pp. 7–8).

Theory of Psychoneuroimmunology

The new field of *psychoneuroimmunology* focuses on the links between the mind, brain, and immune system. The latter is a very complex system consisting of about one trillion cells called *lymphocytes* and about one hundred million trillion molecules called *antibodies*. The immune system has a special capability that allows it to patrol the body and guard its identity. Many immune functions may be impossible to understand if the classical scientific method is used—reducing the system to its simplest elements and attempting to predict the behavior of the whole from its parts (Institute of Noetic Sciences, 1984).

A number of studies by David McClelland at Harvard University examined the role of correlation between the levels of one immune substance in saliva (Immunoglobulin A or IgA, a measure of defense against respiratory infection) for individuals with different motivational styles. He found those driven by an inhibited power motivation had lower IgA levels than those concerned with forming warm, close relationships (1985).

In an interview with Joan Borysenko (1985), McClelland revealed the findings of his latest research. Working with movies of healers such as Mother Teresa, McClelland found that although not everyone reacted the same *consciously* to caring and loving, all their bodies reacted by secreting more IgA. At the conscious level, some reported intense dislike for religiosity, discounted the healers' ability to help, and/or described the movie as phony in written stories about the film. The subjects' opinions of the movie had no correlation to whether their immune function improved. Salivary IgA increased even in people who intensely disliked Mother Teresa. McClelland states these findings support the premise that it is not necessary to believe in the healer (placebo effect) in order to benefit. "At the conscious level, a person may not believe at all, but at the unconscious level, something in the person may still respond to the healer" (Borysenko, 1985, p. 36).

To examine the differences between those watching the films whose immune function improved and those whose did not, McClelland coded the watchers' thoughts and fantasy patterns to find what correlated with increased salivary IgA secretion. He found the most positive correlation with a "kind of affiliative connection in which a person is doing something positive involving another person, trying to help someone, or to establish a love relationship, or a friendly relationship; the curious part of it is the person is not invested in the outcome . . . on the goal of the activity" (Borysenko, 1985, p. 36).

McClelland describes the concept of unconditional love that has relevance for nursing; when using a wellness framework it is important for nurses to ensure they are acting based on true caring, not on a need to have power over others.

People with the need for power often express it by helping others, even when it isn't required. In that case, giving help isn't motivated by a true expression of caring but is used as a means to achieve importance or control . . . noninvolved striving is the highest level of activity, because if you are concerned about the outcome, that's your ego. In a way it correlates with self-love, with self-esteem, in the sense that the state of being egoless comes from recognizing that you're okay within yourself. You don't have to prove that you are worthwhile by looking for reflections of your goodness in the activities that you pursue (Borysenko, 1985, p. 37).

In the interview with Borysenko (1985, pp. 37–38), McClelland reports a study of students who were developing colds and were sent to a local healer. With one of the groups, the healer actively spent time, touching them and telling them how wonderful they were. The second group (control group) was told by the healer to see someone else to whom he had given his power. Among those the healer attended to, 11 of the 13 did not come down with a cold; in the control group, 11 of the 13 did. Students who did not show cold symptoms had a much higher concentration of IgA. Some of the strategies the healer used were: comment on their positive physical attributes, use testimonials (e.g., show people letters from somebody just like them who had persevered and done well). "Studies tell us that's important—just to know that someone else has succeeded in whatever it is you want to do. It supports choice, and that freedom counteracts helplessness" (Borysenko, 1985, p. 38).

Type A behavior and the inhibited power motive syndrome are connected with the increased secretion of catecholamines, which suppress some aspects of the immune function . . . too much of the catecholamine norepinephrine is associated with decline in immunoglobulin A, which thereby makes the body less able to fight off certain viruses. (Borysenko, 1985, p. 38)

Studies done two decades ago demonstrate that hypnotic suggestion can alter some aspects of immunity. Other studies have shown that warts (virus-induced) can be removed by hearing or repeating a suggestion specific to removing warts while in a deeply relaxed, hypnotic state. As holism and wellness become more accepted approaches, these findings may be applied with the same enthusiasm and scientific sanction that some surgical and chemical treatments are receiving today.

At Georgetown University, Nicholas Hall, a biochemist, is examining the physiological basis for imagery's affect on immunity. Focusing on the hormone thymosin, he has demonstrated a correlation between use of imagery and an increase in thymosin and white blood cell count (an immune system measure).

Psychoneuroimmunology provides a first step toward an "affirmative science" that makes quality of life as important as traditional science's attempts to achieve "value-free" inquiry. This shift in emphasis raises new kinds of questions, including (Institute of Noetic Sciences, 1984):

- What changes occur in the body as a result of being given a non-treatment (placebo)?
- What are the physical changes that take place when positive emotions occur?
- When there is a build up of positive emotion, does well-being occur?
- Is human touch vital to the will to live?
- Can the ability to enhance the immune system be learned, thereby eliminating the need for medication and surgical treatment?

McClelland cautions against the use of drug short cuts to enhance immunity:

> A second possible pitfall is that people will look for short cuts. They will look particularly for drug short cuts, because if we find that certain psychological conditions do something to the hormones, people will say, why go to all this trouble to change psychological characteristics, you can just give a pill that will produce the same hormonal effect . . . I think you almost always run into side effects when you do things that way. . . . When people go through programs in which they learn how to use meditation-based therapies and realize why they have their individual approaches to things and discover different choices, not only does all that frequently make their immediate symptom go away, it also leads to larger life changes. They have learned something fundamental about themselves—and of course, you don't learn that from a pill. (Borysenko, 1985, p. 39)

SELF-CARE ASSESSMENTS

A wellness view engages the client in self-assessment and in learning to examine family members and determine when professional assistance is needed and when it is not. Such a view not only demystifies the process, but leaves the nurse free to teach, discuss outcomes with clients, and enhance independence.

Tables 39–45 present information that can be used to teach clients self-assessment procedures relevant to prevention and self-knowledge. Additionally, the nurse can teach the client vital sign procedures. Studies have shown that when clients take their own blood pressure at home the findings are more reliable than when a professional takes it in a physician's office; the factor of anxiety probably interferes in these cases to lower reliability.

Table 39. Directions for Breast Self-Examination

1. Examine your breasts by looking in the mirror at them. First, place your arms at your sides, then place both your arms over your head. The breasts should look about the same, although many women have one breast that is a little larger than the other. Look especially for dimpling of the skin, bulges in one breast, or any *change* in size or shape.

2. Examine your breasts while lying flat. Examine each breast with the hand from the opposite side of the body. Press the breast tissue gently against the chest wall, using the inner fingertips. Roll the tissue between your fingers and the chest wall, moving your fingers in a circular massage motion. Do not pinch the tissue, because all breast tissue feels lumpy then. Examine the inner half of each breast while holding the same-side arm over the head. Examine the outer portion of each breast while holding the same-side arm down at your side. Examine underneath the nipples and over to and including the armpit.

Source: C. C. Clark, *Enhancing Wellness: A Guide for Self-Care,* p. 109. New York: Springer Publishing Co.

Screening as a Preventive Measure

Screening for a disease does not provide primary prevention; it may prevent further complications once an illness is present. Screening can also create problems by stigmatizing those tested; for example, children labeled as having heart murmurs became psychologically damaged while they grew out of the condition physically (Abrams, 1979; Bergman, 1977; Napodano, 1977).

The use of screening is currently being reevaluated. Physicians who used to recommend yearly checkups are now saying they are no longer needed. The American Cancer Society (ACS) has revised its recommendations for screenings, finding that there is no correlation between checkups and survival for several cancers; instead, prevention is being recommended for lung cancer, including smoking cessation. Examination of the breast by a physician is now recommended every 3 years (instead of yearly) until age 40, when yearly exams are recommended. (Since women can learn to examine their own breasts, it is not clear why physician examinations are needed for those properly prepared. It is possible to envision a future where women practice preventive measures and screening becomes totally obsolescent.) Table 46 presents detection tests and prevention measures for major illnesses; Table 47 lists questionable screening procedures.

Table 40. Directions for Examining Some of the Lymph Nodes

Neck glands

1. Relax jaw and neck muscles.

2. Place the first three fingers of each hand immediately below the ears, and move the fingers in a smooth circular motion.

3. Move the fingers down a short distance and a little to the side, and repeat the circular motion.

4. Continue moving the fingers down and toward the front of the jaw little by little, until the fingers of one hand are very close to the fingers of the other hand.

5. Note enlarged glands.

Underarm glands

1. Drop one arm to the side and relax it.

2. Use the opposite arm to feel for gland under the arm, with the thumb on the chest and the fingers using a circular movement under the arm, including high into the underarm region.

3. Note enlarged glands.

Groin glands

1. Place fingertips in the groin area, and move the fingertips from side to side, using firm pressure.

2. Move fingertips downward toward the thigh.

3. Note any enlargement.

Source: C. C. Clark, *Enhancing Wellness: A Guide for Self-Care*, p. 110. New York: Springer Publishing Co.

TOUCH AND HEALING ASSESSMENTS

Behavioral Kinesiology Assessments

Diamond's behavioral testing technique requires two people: the assessor stands facing the client, who is asked to stand erect with the right arm relaxed at the side and the left arm held straight out to the side. The assessor places his or her left hand on the right shoulder and the right hand on the client's wrist. The client is then asked to resist as the assessor pushes his or her arm down. Neither smiles during the pro-

Table 41. Directions for Examining the Abdomen of Another Person

1.	Make sure the room temperature is warm enough.
2.	Ask the other person to lie on his or her back on a firm surface such as a mat on the floor.
3.	Have the person remove any clothing that covers the area from their chest to the hair line of their pelvis, and to place both arms comfortably at the sides of the body or at the back of the head.
4.	Ask the other person to bend his or her knees slightly, to take a few deep breaths, and to concentrate on relaxing the abdominal area.
5.	Place one hand on top of the other, both palms down, and fingertips touching. Use the top hand to provide pressure, and the bottom hand to feel the abdomen.
6.	Move your hands over the entire abdomen, pressing lightly. Ask the other person to signal whenever pain is felt.
7.	Note when the person tenses up when you examine an area and ask, "What did you feel?"
8.	If the other person complains of being tickled, use slightly firmer pressure.
9.	Note and record any areas of tenderness or areas that are rigid to the touch.

Source: C. C. Clark, *Enhancing Wellness: A Guide for Self-Care*, p. 111. New York: Springer Publishing Co.

cedure as this can affect the outcome. The assessor is measuring the spring of the muscle and does not push to muscle fatigue. Clients whose thymus is weakened by stress will not be able to hold their arm up.

Clients are then instructed to thump the sternomandibular joint 10–12 times (on the skin over the point where the second rib joins the breastbone), and the assessor retests. Diamond's research shows the client will now test strong and be able to hold the arm with a great deal more resistance than prior to tapping over the gland.

Clients who test strong are called "centered" by Diamond: "his energies are centered and he is invulnerable to stress" (1979, p. 32). The centering effect has a physiological analog in the concept of right-brain (holistic, creative) and left-brain (rational, logical). Diamond has developed a test for cerebral imbalance that tests magnetic, not electroencephalographic, activity. The client and assessor stand as before, but this time the client bends the right elbow, holding the right palm to the side of the head at ear level (not touching the head or hair and keeping the head straight) at the left side of the head. If the client is cerebrally

Table 42. Directions for Two Methods of Examining the Thyroid Gland

Examining the thyroid gland through touch

1. Feel for the band of cartilage (soft, bonelike material) running down the middle of your throat.

2. Place the thumb of the right hand on the right-hand side of the cartilage and the three fingers of the right hand on the other side, about 2 inches below the chin.

3. Swallow, and feel the connection between the two parts of the thyroid as it glides beneath your fingertips. When this happens, you are in the correct place to feel for your thyroid gland. If you do not feel the gliding action, the fingers can be moved up or down slightly and you can swallow again.

4. Once the correct spot is found, keep the three fingers where they are and move the left hand and place the three fingers of that hand on the same level as the other hand, but slightly to the side of the throat.

5. Then the fingers of the right hand move around slowly in a circular motion, searching for the thyroid.

6. The same process is repeated (with the hands reversed) for the right half of the thyroid.

Examining the thyroid gland through inspection

1. Look in the mirror, searching for any sign of enlargement on either side of the cartilage.

2. Elevate your chin and look in a small hand mirror for any enlargement while swallowing.

Source: C. C. Clark, *Enhancing Wellness: A Guide for Self-Care*, p. 112. New York: Springer Publishing Co.

balanced, the indicator muscle will remain strong when the assessor pushes down on the wrist; the client will also test strong when the right hand is placed at the right side of the head.

Therapeutic Touch Assessments

Krieger suggests that both telereceptive and personal field assessments be completed by the nurse (1979, pp. 23–51). Prior to approaching a client, the nurse centers to ensure a fully integrated, unified, focused assessment. Centering also protects the nurse from picking up negative energy from the client and/or bringing his or her negative energy into

Table 43. Fitness Record

Directions

Monitor and add data as often as suggested in the text, or if there are symptoms suggesting the need for more examination.

PHYSICAL EXAMINATION

My blood pressure at rest is: My *height* is:

My *pulse* at rest is: My *weight* is:

My normal *temperature* is:

From observing my *skin*, I noticed the following:

From observing my *eyes*, I noticed the following:

From examining my *lymph nodes*, I found:

From examining my *breasts* (woman)—*testicles* (man)—I noticed:

My *abdominal* area is:

RECORD OF IMMUNIZATIONS

I have had the following basic immunizations:

yes   no

.... DPT (diphtheria, pertussis, tetanus) and oral polio virus

.... measles

.... rubella (only for females whose blood test shows no immunity to rubella)

I have had the following boosters:

yes   no

.... diphtheria dates:

.... tetanus   dates:

Table 43 *(continued)*

ADDITIONAL INFORMATION

Age 7-11 (with symptoms of extreme thirst, frequent urination, and weight loss):

I test my urine for sugar regularly and find:

Sexually Active:

I use the following method of birth control:

I protect myself from VD by:

Those who have been exposed to tuberculosis:

I had a PPD or Tine Test most recently on: (date)

Those who are over 40 or over 30 and have a family history of glaucoma:

I had a Schiotz tonometer test done on: (date)

Those who have a history of genetic disease or who are over 40 and thinking of becoming pregnant:

I plan to tackle the problem of genetic difficulties by completing the following actions:

EXPOSURES TO HARMFUL SITUATIONS

I was exposed to the following illnesses:

1.   date:

2.   date:

3.   date:

I had x-rays of the following kinds:

1.   date:

2.   date:

3.   date:

I was exposed to the following other situations:

1.   date:

2.   date:

3.   date:

Table 43 *(continued)*

MENTAL HEALTH EXAMINATION

Check *Yes, No,* or *S* (*Somewhat* or *Sometimes*) for each statement

		Yes	No	S
1.	I think I handle stress pretty well at work (school)	......	.....	......
2.	I like my coworkers (peers)	......	.....	......
3.	I think I handle stress pretty well at home	......	.....	......
4.	I get out of the house enough to "do my own thing"	......	.....	......
5.	I seem to share a great deal with my family, and I look forward to being with them	......	.....	......
6.	I have the right numbers (for me) of close friends I share things with	......	.....	......
7.	I feel comfortable in social situations	......	.....	......
8.	I seem to have enough energy to do the things I want to do	......	.....	......
9.	I usually get along pretty well with people	......	.....	......
10.	I get enough respect from others for work I do	......	.....	......
11.	I am able to fully utilize those activities for which I have been trained	......	.....	......
12.	I live pretty comfortably	......	.....	......
13.	I seem to be financially secure	......	.....	......
14.	I feel at ease about spending money	......	.....	......
15.	I participate in activities that give me a boost	......	.....	......
16.	There are people or organizations I can turn to in times of trouble	......	.....	......
17.	I know my strengths	......	.....	......
18.	I know my weaknesses or limitations	......	.....	......
19.	I am willing to take reasonable risks to get what I want	......	.....	......
20.	I feel good about persevering and working toward a goal, even if I don't always get what I want	......	.....	......
21.	I structure my day so I am satisfied with its outcome	......	.....	......
22.	I have some long-term goals, and I am working toward them	......	.....	......

Table 43 *(continued)*

23.	I can change my routine once in a while, without undue discomfort	......	.....	......
24.	I try continually to learn or do new things	......	.....	......
25.	I see illness as part of the challenge of living	......	.....	......
26.	I believe that I can help to cure myself when I am ill	......	.....	......
27.	I believe I have some choice in what happens to me	......	.....	......
28.	If I were going to die this evening, I would not change my life	......	.....	......
29.	I have spent my life choosing what I do, not only in being swayed by peers, bosses, teachers, family, friends, or health care workers	......	.....	......
30.	I have confidence in my future	......	.....	......
31.	My life spreads around me, a series of connected experiences	......	.....	......
32.	I believe there is a reason for my being here	......	.....	......

Source: C. C. Clark, *Enhancing Wellness: A Guide for Self-Care,* pp. 113–116. New York: Springer Publishing Co.

the assessment process. Although Krieger does not suggest it, the nurse can use imagery to place a shield of light (or some other substance) around the nurse that allows energy to be picked up and sensed, but not to personally affect the nurse.

Telereceptive assessments include:

- What do clients' voices tell me about their emotional level?
- What do clients' gaits tell me about their locomotion, guarding of body parts, hesitancy, tension level?
- What do clients' facial expressions tell me about their level of involvement with me?

Human field assessments are completed standing, facing clients, moving from the head quickly to the feet while holding the hands 2–3 inches away from their bodies. The back of the body is assessed while standing behind clients and moving in the same manner over the area until

Table 44. Communicating about Our Sexual Experiences

Directions:

Ask yourself the questions in the left-hand column and your partner those in the right-hand one. Share the information you gain and use is to enhance your sexual relationship.

Questions to ask self	*Questions to ask my partner*
"How can I tell you when I want to make love and when I want to cuddle or hug?"	"How can I tell when you want to make love and when you want to cuddle or hug?"
"How can I help you tell me you're interested in sex so I don't feel threatened, forced, or used?"	"How can I tell you I'm interested in sex without threatening or forcing you?"
"How can we work it out when I want sex and you don't?"	"How can we work it out when you want sex and I don't?"
"What pleases me sexually?" "How can I let you know this?"	"How can I best tell you when what you do pleases me sexually?"
"How could I guide you or tell you so you know how to please me sexually?"	"How can I guide you or tell you so you know how to please me sexually?"
"What do I know about what pleases you sexually?"	"What can you tell me about what pleases you sexually?"
"What is sexual turn-off for me?"	"How can I tell you about what turns me off sexually?"
"What method of birth control do I think we should use?"	"How can I talk to you about birth control methods we plan to use in a way that enhances our sexual relationship?"
"How pleased am I with the method of birth-control we are currently using?"	
"Do I think about sex as if performance is the most important or as if pleasure is?"	"Do you think about sex as if performance is the most important or as if pleasure is?"
"How can I focus more of my attention on pleasure than on performance?"	"How can I help you to focus more on pleasure than on performance?"
"Do I want to introduce some new experiences or position into our sexual relationship?"	"Do you want to introduce some new experience or position into our sexual relationship?"
"What interferes with me letting go and enjoying a sexual experience?"	"What interferes with your letting go and enjoying a sexual experience?"

Source: C. C. Clark, *Enhancing Wellness: A Guide for Self-Care*, p. 249. New York: Springer Publishing Co.

Table 45. Vaginal Self-Examination

One of the areas least accessible to women is their vagina; many women have never seen what their vagina looks like. Learning to examine one's own vagina is not a substitute for a pelvic exam, but it can help integrate the vagina into self-image, alert the owner to potential problems, check birth control equipment and natural birth control methods (cervical texture, color, os, mucus, and shape change indicate ovulation; adequacy of diaphragm coverage and correct placement of an IUD can be assessed), fertility (mucus is liquid and thin when close to or at time of ovulation), and pregnancy (blueing or purpling and softening of the cervix and increased vaginal secretions).

Before Beginning

1. Purchase a plastic speculum or, during your next pelvic exam, ask for the one used.
2. Find a flashlight with a high-intensity light.
3. Find a hand mirror; a self-supporting one is best because it leaves one hand free.
4. Find a firm surface to lie on and a private place for your exam.
5. Make sure you have time so you won't have to rush.
6. *Optional:* Have some K-Y jelly handy to make insertion of the speculum easier. Vaseline is not recommended: it closes vaginal pores and isn't sterile.
7. Practice using the speculum with one hand, holding it upside down. (Hold the speculum with the bill pointed away; thumb on level which opens the blades; push level in and up to lock the speculum; pull down to close the blades for entry and withdrawal.)

Examining the Vagina

1. Get into a reclining position with equipment nearby.
2. Put K-Y jelly on the bill of the speculum *(optional)*.
3. Hold the speculum in the right hand (if right-handed) and spread the labia with the fingers of the left hand.
4. Take a few deep breaths and wait until you are comfortable prior to proceeding; if anxiety is encountered, use imagery or a relaxation exercise to become calm. Use the measure at any time during the examination that discomfort or anxiety is experienced. Ensure a pleasant, meaningful exploration.
5. Gently insert the speculum to the base of the blades and turn it so the handle is up; open the blades and lock them open.
6. Reach for mirror and flashlight and look for the ridges of the vaginal walls and on the back wall, a smooth, pink, muscular ring that is the cervix. (If the cervix is not readily visible, bear down for a moment.) The color of the walls should look like the inside of the mouth (pink, not red); look for any sores, reddened irritated areas, unusual discharge or bleeding, and growths or bumps on the walls.

Note: For further information on vaginal self-exam and interpreting vaginal discharges, see nurse practitioner Carol Berry's "Doing Your Own Vaginal Self-Exam," *Medical Self-Care,* 1980, pp. 281–284.

Table 46. Detection Tests and Preventive Measures for Major Illnesses

Illness	Detection tests	Preventive measures
Heart disease	blood pressure checked at least once per year have infants age 1–6 months examined for heart malformations	have a throat culture when you have a *very* painful sore throat that lasts longer than a few days; if culture is positive, take antibiotic to reduce chance of rheumatic heart disease stop smoking exercise lose weight or maintain ideal weight cut down on fat, sugar, and highly processed foods
Cancer	self-examination of breasts by women self-examination of the thyroid (for women over 18 years of age who are sexually active) obtain a Pap smear yearly until 2 negative results are obtained, then obtain smears every 3 years to age 35 and every 5 years from age 35–60 examination of the skin for changes—for example, increase in size, number, or look of moles self-examination of the testicles by men	do not get an x-ray without questioning why it is necessary; refuse those that seem unnecessary stop smoking and being near smokers do not participate in sexual activity at an early age and/or with many different partners know environmental chemicals that are cancer-producing, and work to eliminate them and your exposure to them limit drinking alcohol

225

Table 46 *(continued)*

Illness	Detection tests	Preventive measures
Cancer (cont.)		limit exposure to the sun and/or use PABA cream to block exposure
		increase fiber intake
		try to eat foods not sprayed with dangerous pesticides
Stroke	none, except some strokes are preceded by temporary clumsiness and numbness in hand or foot, temporary blindness in one eye, or slurring of speech: these should be immediately brought to the attention of a physician	same as for heart disease
Diabetes	self-test for sugar in the urine, using Tes-Tape, Clinistix, Clinitest Tabs, Diastix, or similar products available in pharmacies; especially useful for juveniles who have extreme thirst, frequent urination, and weight loss	lose weight
		increase exercise
		eat proper diet
		to date it is not known that anything can be done to prevent juvenile diabetes
Tuberculosis	PPD or Tine Skin Test every year or two for ten years after exposure to tuberculosis	avoid exposure to people who have it

Arthritis	none, except for ankylosing spondylitis; in this case, you should check with a physician if you answer yes to four or five of the following: Have you had back pain for three months or more? Has your back been stiff in the morning? Did the problem start before you were 40? Did the pain and stiffness begin slowly? Does the problem improve with exercise?	some experts think taking dolomite (calcium and magnesium) will ward off osteoarthritis
Gout	possibly uric acid blood test in middle-aged, overweight men with a family history of gout	control weight avoid alcoholic drinks
Venereal disease (VD)	having a culture made from the cervix (opening) to the uterus or penis is useful only for people who have large numbers of sexual partners having a blood test (VDRL, FTA) one to three months after exposure	avoid contact with infected persons use condoms use discretion in choice of sexual partner
Glaucoma	having the eye pressure measures with an instrument called a Schiotz Tonometer once every four years after the age of 40, or once a year after age 30 if anyone in your family has glaucoma	
Anemia	an occasional microhematocrit (not a complete blood count) is reasonable for *children* especially if they are *not* eating an adequate diet	a balanced diet that includes vitamins and iron

Table 46 *(continued)*

Illness	Detection tests	Preventive measures
Thyroid problems	self-examination for small lump to the side of the Adam's apple those who *have* had radiation treatments for acne or ringworm to the head or neck or for enlarged tonsils or adenoids should have their thyroid examined yearly and learn to do a self-examination of the thyroid	refuse x-rays to the head or neck for acne, ringworm, enlarged tonsils, or adenoids
Mental retardation	if you are pregnant and know of a genetic disease that causes mental retardation in your family, see a genetic counselor, think about getting amniocentesis (test of fluid from uterus or womb); likewise, if you are over 40 if there is phenylketonuria (PKU) in your family, have your baby tested immediately after birth and start him or her on the special PKU diet	if there is genetic illness in your family, get genetic counseling prior to marriage
Kidney disease	urine test for pregnant women	

Source: C. C. Clark, *Enhancing Wellness: A Guide for Self-Care*, pp. 101–104. New York: Springer Publishing Co.

an assessment is completed. The nurse does not hesitate in a spot, but continues moving the hands; if sensations are unclear, the nurse moves body and hands to the side of or away from clients and repeats the downward movement until an assessment is clear. The nurse searches for differences in energy flow and uses the following questions to assess blocks:

- What does the area around clients tell me about them?
- Which areas of the body "feel" hot, cold, like shocks, pressure, tingling, pulsating, or dead to me?
- What sensations can be picked up on my hands on the right side of the body vs. the left, top vs. bottom, and back vs. front?

Clients can also be assessed while they are sitting in a chair or on the floor; the nurse stands, kneels, or sits, depending on which position allows for the most complete assessment of the client.

In preparing to assess a client, the nurse first enhances hand sensitivity by rubbing the palms together and gradually separating them until energy flow between the hands is noted. By experimenting, the distance between the two palms at which sensations are most evident is probably the distance from the client's body at which the nurse's hands should be placed during assessment.

Yoga Assessments

An assessment for the utilization of yoga postures includes a determination of whether the following conditions responsive to specific movements exist:

- low back pain
- nausea
- indigestion
- tension/worry
- pregnancy
- morning sickness
- pelvic congestion
- menstrual cramps
- osteoarthritis
- spinal disc problems
- thyroid dysfunction
- prolapsed uterus
- varicose veins
- depression
- upper respiratory conditions

Table 47. Questionable Screening Procedures

1. rectal exams

2. xeromammography (x-ray) of the breast (unless you are over age 40 and your sister or mother has breast cancer)

3. proctosigmoidoscopy (looking into the rectum and lower bowel through a tube) prior to age 50

4. x-ray to detect lung cancer

5. test for hidden blood in the stool prior to age 40

6. glucose tolerance test if elderly (77 to 100 percent will test positive for diabetes when they may not have the illness)

7. coronary arteriograms (they are very complex and have a significant chance of causing disability or death)

8. electrocardiograph stress tests (findings are inconclusive unless you have symptoms of heart disease; the test itself may be disabling)

9. screening for heart murmurs in children (the vast majority of murmurs do not indicate disease; children and parents' reactions may cause them to act *as if* there is a disease when there is not)

10. screening for high levels of uric acid for gout (unless you are a middle-aged, overweight man, with a family history of gout)

11. tests to determine whether you have a high cholesterol level (there is no definitive study to show that lowering the cholesterol level will prevent atherosclerosis or coronary heart disease)

12. tests to determine abnormalities through such procedures as chest x-rays, rectal, gastrophy, urine and sputum cytology

13. x-ray examinations to evaluate lower-back pain

14. tests to identify carriers of sickle cell anemia

15. abdominal x-ray to judge liver size or gastrointestinal bleeding

16. x-ray to detect ankle sprain

17. routine barium enemas for hernia

18. urograms and arteriograms for people with high blood pressure

19. daily (portable) x-rays of all patients in coronary care units (CCUs)

20. bone survey x-rays of people with hyperparathyroidism

21. preemployment x-rays of the chest and spine

22. use of CAT scanner in inappropriate situations

23. any x-rays during pregnancy

Massage Assessments

An assessment for the use of massage includes a determination of whether the following conditions or needs exist that are believed to be responsive to the approach:

- parent/infant bonding
- muscle spasm/soreness
- headache
- buildup of toxins and wastes

- inadequate healing
- fatigue
- tension
- premature infant development

Acupressure Assessments

An assessment for the use of acupressure includes identifying the existence of the following conditions or needs that have been found to respond to the technique:

- headache
- arthritis
- back tension and lower back pain
- menstrual discomfort
- labor and delivery
- morning sickness
- deficient lactation or mastitis
- overall balance
- appetite balance
- circulation balance
- digestion balance
- elimination balance

- fainting
- fracture healing
- inflammation
- mood elevation
- motion balance
- muscle balance
- pain control
- sciatic relief
- substance abuse
- throat
- strains, sprains, and their prevention

NOTE: It is important to keep in mind that besides questioning screening procedures, laboratory tests are also at question due to the large percentage of false positives and false negatives that occur. No test is 100% sensitive or able to distinguish between those who have the condition and those who do not (Galen, 1974). Additionally, laboratory testing has been found to be up to 50% inaccurate by the Center for Disease Control that monitors and regulates testing (Mendelsohn, 1979). Finally, a large number of tests may be performed at teaching hospitals because residents must perform a minimum number in order to have a residency program approved; this increases the likelihood of performing tests when they may not be warranted. These factors interact to produce unreliable results. Probably the best protection is to obtain as much information as possible from qualitative procedures rather than relying on laboratory tests. Observing the client and asking pertinent questions is certainly more humanistic and can provide more useful information if the nurse is well prepared in observation and communication skills.

Source: C. C. Clark, *Enhancing Wellness: A Guide for Self-Care*, p. 105. New York: Springer Publishing Co.

Figure 14. Foot reflexology points.

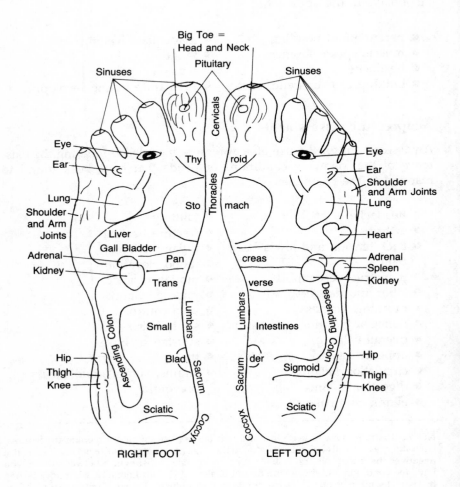

Sources: The Foot Book, D. Berkson, New York: Harper and Row, 1977; *The Massage Book,* G. Downing, New York: Random House, 1972.

Reflexology Assessments

Figure 14 presents the foot reflexes used for assessment and treatment. Berkson (1977) suggests the following assessments be made:

- What does the skin color tell me?
- Are the heels of the shoes worn evenly?
- Are the eyes clear?
- Is the tongue coated?
- Are the nails strong and the hair shiny?
- What do the client's voice and posture tell me?
- Which joints rotate easily?
- Which reflex points are the most tender or the most difficult to relieve?
- How does bone feel under the skin?
- How do muscles feel?
- What temperature differences are there? (an even, warm temperature indicates balance)
- What differences in texture are there? (bunions and callouses can indicate imbalances)
- What areas on the foot indicate a hard resistance? (indicating tension, deposits, or degeneration, unless a bone, tendon, or ligament resides there)
- What areas feel hollow or recessed? (indicating lack of nutrition and energy imbalance)

SMOKING CESSATION: A SELF-CARE INTERVENTION

Table 48 provides suggestions for smoking cessation. A recent intervention for smoking cessation is the use of nicotine gum. Although originally thought to be a panacea, recent research shows it is most effective when used in combination with other approaches (Clavel & Benhamou, 1984). Additionally, nicotine chewing gum is suggested primarily for smokers who are heavily addicted to nicotine (Glantz, 1984).

Table 48. Smoking Cessation Suggestions

- Keep a notebook of current and past successes. Use the list as a reminder of your ability to succeed in new ventures.
- Identify a personal reason for quitting, not a "should" do because it's bad for me.
- Make a list of things that are personally pleasurable; choose one as a reward (instead of a cigarette) when feeling uncomfortable or bored.
- Make a list of reasons smoking began and compare with a list of current reasons for smoking.
- Write down all the missed opportunities that are regretted; choose one that is reachable and take action on it.
- Keep a log of each cigarette lit, including: purpose (to get up, to get to work, to relax, to appear calm, to celebrate, to quell hunger, after sex, after eating, etc.);

Table 48 *(continued)*

focus on smoking the cigarette and sensations occurring during and after smoking.

- Write a list of stress enhancers; learn structured relaxation and stress reduction approaches to deal with each stressor.
- When using cigarettes as an energizer, substitute six small high-protein meals, sufficient sleep, a glass of milk, a piece of fresh fruit, fruit or vegetable juice, exercise or movement, or a relaxation exercise.
- End all meals with foods not associated with smoking, e.g., a glass of milk or half a grapefruit rather than a cup of coffee or a drink.
- Switch to noncaffeinated coffee or tea, or bouillon.
- Eat a couple of sunflower seeds instead of having a cigarette.
- Have carrot sticks, celery, and other crudités ready to chew instead of smoking a cigarette.
- Eat more foods that leave the body alkaline and reduce the urge to smoke: vegetables, seeds, fruits.
- Use affirmations, such as, "I no longer smoke," "I can quit," "It's getting easier and easier to quit smoking," or "It's getting easier and easier to think about quitting smoking."
- Use deep breathing or breath for unity when the urge for a cigarette appears.
- Work with a peer who can be called for positive feedback when the urge for a cigarette occurs. Be sure the peer is positive about ability to quit and does not nag or induce guilt.
- Stay away from friends who smoke and from places where people smoke.
- Buy different brands of cigarettes and avoid smoking two packs of the same brand in a row.
- Buy cigarettes only by the pack, not by the carton.
- Smoke with the opposite hand from the one usually used.
- Brush the teeth right after eating.
- Put cigarettes in an unfamiliar place.
- Every time a cigarette is reached for, ask: "Do I really want this cigarette?"; "Do I really need a cigarette?"; "What can I do instead of smoking this cigarette?"
- Develop and prepractice responses to peer pressure to smoke, including: "Come on, one won't hurt," "Smoking makes you independent, like an adult," "Here, have one," "Are you a sissy?" Take an assertiveness course if necessary to develop the skill of saying "NO."
- Tell six people, "I've quit smoking, and it was easy."
- Ask friends and co-workers not to leave cigarettes around or offer them.
- When the urge for a cigarette occurs, picture the word "STOP" in big red letters.
- Ask for a hug instead of having a cigarette.
- Choose a time to stop smoking when a peak mental or physical performance is not expected.
- Write a contract and sign it with a trusted person so continuing to smoke will prove embarrassing or will result in great loss.

- Read articles and books by people who have successfully quit smoking or helped others to.
- When feeling depressed, talk with people who have successfully quit smoking and ask for information about why they are glad they quit.
- Chew Nicorette (nicotine) gum to quell the urge to smoke.
- Go to the morgue and look at someone who died from lung cancer.
- Talk to someone in the hospital who has incurable lung cancer about the course of the disease; get to know what that individual is like as a person.

Note: Programs for children have been most successful when they are focused on showing smokers losing control and on teaching kids how to take control. For further information, contact: Clearinghouse on Drug Abuse, P.O.B. 416, Kensington, MD 20795, Tel.: (301) 443–6500.

Sources: J. Rogers, *You Can Stop,* New York: Pocket Books, 1977.

D. Van Deusen, "Kicking the Cigarette Habit: Some Reflections from an Old Pro," *The Wellness Newsletter* 5(2):3–4, 1984.

National Institute on Drug Abuse, "Life Skills Program," Clearinghouse on Drug Abuse: Kensington, MD, 1984.

TOUCH AND HEALING INTERVENTIONS

Behavioral Kinesiology Interventions

Diamond's research (1979, pp. 33–124) suggests the following activities may be helpful in balancing the cerebral hemispheres and activating the immune response, via thymus stimulation:

1. Center and balance the hemispheres by placing the tongue on the roof of the mouth. This intervention can be used to regain balance when threatened by an event.

2. Activate the thymus 3–4 times a day as a preventive measure; tap at the level of the sternomandibular joint 10–12 times in a rhythmic manner.

3. Read poetry in a rhythmical manner; this is a dual-brained activity: reading is a left-brained activity and rhythmical qualities require the right hemisphere.

4. Take an energy break to look at a landscape painting (beautiful scenes in nature strengthen thymus muscle tests) or read poetry.

5. Tap the thymus and change ears frequently when listening on the telephone (listening with the left ear encourages left-brained activity and listening with the right ear encourages right-brained activity).

6. Practice contralateral walking and crawling to balance brain hemispheres.

7. Practice thymus thumping after homologous or homolateral movements such as jumping jacks, weight lifting, rowing, bicycling.

8. Concentrate on turning negative emotions (hate, envy, suspicion, and fear) which weaken the thymus into positive emotions (love, faith, trust, courage, and gratitude) which activate the thymus. Diamond does not suggest suppressing negative thoughts and emotions; people expressing negative emotions tested weak using the thymus test in Diamond's studies. (See Stress Management for suggestions regarding how to change negative thoughts and feelings into positive ones.)

9. Use facial expressions (smiles) and gestures (outstretched arms, nodding the head yes) to strengthen the thymus; avoid frowns and shaking the head no; they weaken the thymus. For those who cannot smile: tweak the cheek, and the smile muscle (zygomaticus major) linked to the thymus will activate the mechanism.

10. Avoid listening, reading about, or watching violence (hijackings, floods, fires, murders, and other disasters) that adversely affect the thymus.

11. Avoid being around people who use negative comments, e.g., "You're ugly," "I hate you," "You're stupid!" Such statements weaken the thymus response.

12. Avoid attempting to be "therapeutic" with a client if under stress; stress subtly distorts speech via the hyoid bone and this distortion is picked up by the listener. When under stress, use a centering technique or thump the thymus prior to working with a client.

13. Avoid the following or at least test individually, as Diamond has found them to produce weakness in the thymus for many individuals:

- tinted sunglasses
- electronic pulse and quartz-crystal watches (varying the position in which they are worn may not disturb thymus function; individualized testing is necessary to determine response)
- hats made of synthetics weaken the activity of the thymus gland
- synthetic wigs
- high-heeled shoes (the brain is confused by sensory messages from the ankle signalling that both feet are at the end of a forward step)
- synthetic clothing and bedclothes
- disposable diapers
- toiletries
- ice cold drinks or showers
- fluorescent lighting
- fiberglass insulation
- household fuel and chemicals (e.g., cooking gas, cleaning agents)
- smoking, smoke filled rooms, watching someone smoke, or viewing a picture of someone smoking

- auto exhaust
- not breathing equally through both nostrils; if this cycle has been disturbed, breathing through the left nostril (increasing negative ions necessary for well-being)
- x-rays, electrical generators, and microwaves; Diamond's studies found the walk-through screening device did not weaken the thymus, but anyone within 10 ft of the carry-on baggage machine tested weak; even microwave ovens that operate safely weaken the thymus; CB radios affect thymus, but only for a short distance; microwave transmitters and electrical transmission lines weaken the thymus
- Viewing certain symbols weakens the thymus, including the pitchfork, crosses (only those that have vertical arms longer than horizontal arms), swastikas (depending on which cerebral hemisphere is dominant; clockwise or counterclockwise swastikas weaken the thymus). Diamond found that a circle with four intersections and a dot in the middle balanced the hemispheres and reduced stress.
- Rock music with an anapestic beat that stops at the end of each bar or measure is correlated with cerebral imbalance and weakens the thymus. Listening to specific sounds strengthens the thymus: running water, bird sounds, cats purring, and classical music strengthen.
- Refined sugar and additives weaken the thymus. Over 90% of Diamond's clients tested weak with beef, wheat, and dairy products.

14. Good posture stimulates the thymus; metal folding chairs and soft, comfortable chairs weaken; firm chairs with straight backs do not. Crossing the legs while sitting weakens, and driving while sitting on a soft seat also weakens. Diamond recommends sitting on a firm board or sheet of hard plastic when driving or flying to counteract fatigue.

15. The Alexander Horizontal Position aligns the body and permits the free flow of energy, enabling the thymus to correct imbalances. (Lie supine on the floor, knees bent, feet flat, with a book or two under the head so the neck is at about a 45-degree angle to the body.)

For further information see: Diamond, J., *Behavioral Kinesiology*, New York: Harper and Row, 1979.

Therapeutic Touch Interventions

The main therapeutic touch intervention is "unruffling the field." As the nurse sweeps the hands down the client's body, any areas that feel like pressure or congestion are "unruffled."

Prior to any intervention, the nurse centers and holds the intention to heal. This is accomplished by placing the hands "with palms facing away from the body at the area where you felt the pressure and then move the hands away from the body in a sweeping gesture . . ." (Krieger, 1979, p. 54). Energy can also be directed from a higher energy area to a low energy area by moving the hands in the appropriate direction in a brushing movement.

Another use of therapeutic touch is to act as a channel for energy to bring it to the client from a universal energy source. This is particularly helpful if the client is fatigued or needs concentrated energy to heal. In this case, the nurse centers, protects herself or himself, and pictures an energy source such as the sun, God, or another light or energy source. With eyes closed, the universal source of energy can be pictured being channeled through the nurse's hands to the area in need of healing or energizing. For further information, see Krieger, D., *The Therapeutic Touch*, Englewood Cliffs, NJ: Prentice-Hall, Inc., 1979.

Yoga Interventions

Yoga is a discipline devoted to balance; all forward bending postures are recommended to be balanced by a backward bending one. Forcing, straining, or stretching to the point of pain is the opposite of the needed approach. Postures are meant to be performed slowly, almost meditatively, while breathing consciously. Postures should be done on a cushioned floor, before eating, and while wearing loose clothing. Breathing should be in and out through the nostrils.

1. *The Bow.* Reported useful for gastrointestinal disorders, constipation, upset stomach, sluggish liver, abdominal fat. While lying flat on the stomach, grasp ankles, inhale, and lift legs, head, and chest, arching the back into a bow. Hold, then exhale and lie flat. Repeat 3–4 times, resting in between to note effects.

2. *Cobra.* Reported to tone ovaries, uterus, and liver, relieves constipation, limbers spine; excellent for slipped discs. WARNING: not recommended for those with peptic ulcer, hernia, or hyperthyroid. Lie on the stomach, arms at shoulder level; push the upper body up with the arms, arch the back and look up while inhaling; hold and exhale while lowering the upper body slowly to the floor.

3. *Corpse Pose.* Reported to stimulate blood circulation, alleviate fatigue, nervousness, neurasthenia, asthma, constipation (enhance by visualizing increased circulation and movement of material through the intestines), diabetes (enhance by visualizing circulation to and from

pancreas), indigestion, insomnia, lumbago (enhance by visualizing enhanced circulation to nourish back muscles), mental concentration, and generalized relaxation. Lie flat on the back, legs and arms a comfortable distance from the body; let the body sink into the floor. During the second and third trimester of pregnancy, lie on the side using pillows as necessary.

4. *Knee to Chest.* Reported to relieve stiffness and soreness of back and extremities, constipation, diabetes, flatulence. Lie flat on back and bring knees to chest; rock back and forth gently, massaging the spine. Lower the legs one at a time slowly. Bring one leg to the chest, pulling it in in a controlled stretch with interlocked fingers. Hold the position and breathe. Slowly bring the head toward the knee, hold and exhale. Inhale and bring knee to nose and hold for a count of 10; exhale and repeat 5–10 times. Repeat with other leg. Draw up both legs so knee moves toward the nose; hold while breathing and exhale. Return legs to floor and rest, noting the effect.

5. *Kneeling Pose.* Reported to increase circulation to prostate gland and uterus. Sit on heels, keeping back straight. While breathing through nostrils, separate the feet and slowly sink in between, moving buttocks toward the floor. Move gently, avoiding straining knee ligaments. Keep feet facing straight back.

6. *The Lion.* Reported to relieve sore throat; stimulates circulation to throat and tongue (enhance by visualizing relaxation of throat and improved circulation to the area). Sit on the heels, palms on knees, fingers fanned out. Protrude the tongue as far as possible, open eyes and mouth as far as possible, roll eyeballs upward. Exhale saying "Ahhhh" and feeling the sensation in the back of the throat.

7. *Locust.* Reported to relieve problems of abdomen and lower back. WARNING: not recommended for those with hernia or acute back problems. Lie flat on stomach, head facing ahead, chin on the floor; relax and breathe. Keeping arms close to the body, palms up, slowly raise one leg toward the ceiling using the lower back muscles. Hold briefly and then exhale while lowering the leg to the floor. Rest. Repeat with the other leg. Repeat 2–3 times but not to point of fatigue.

8. *The Mountain.* Reported to strengthen lungs, purify blood, improve digestive system, tone nervous system. Sit cross-legged on the floor; stretch arms up toward the ceiling, fingertips together. Stretch up while breathing slowly and deeply 5–10 times; exhale and lower arms.

9. *Neck and Eye Exercises.* Reported to relieve headache and eyestrain, improve eyesight, relax neck and shoulder tension. Sit cross-legged on the floor, wrists at rest on knees. Nod head forward slowly 3–4 times; nod toward the left and right shoulder 3–4 times, allowing the mouth to fall open. Inhale and shut the eyes tightly; hold, then exhale, opening

the eyes wide and blinking rapidly 8–10 times. Hold the eyes open wide while looking around the entire circumference of the eyeballs; reverse the circle. Look diagonally from left upper to right lower and vice versa. Look up and down 10 times. Remember to breathe throughout. Rub palms together, close the eyes, and cover them with the palms, while completing 5 slow breaths. Repeat until eyes relax. Visualize energy and brightness moving into the eyes.

10. *Uddiyana.* Reported to alleviate constipation, indigestion, gastro-intestinal problems, diabetes, and obesity. WARNING: Avoid if pregnant or hypertensive. Stand with feet apart, knees slightly bent; lean forward and arch the back. Keep hands on thighs. While exhaling, suck abdomen toward the spine and hold for several seconds. Relax and repeat on exhalation. Work up to 20 repetitions with one exhalation.

11. *Cat Stretch.* Reported useful in relieving back pain of pregnancy and aids in generalized relaxation. While on all fours on the floor, arch the back and then concave it.

12. *Spinal Twist.* Reported to increase spinal flexibility, aids in the return of the uterus to its nonpregnant size, strengthens oblique abdominals (stretched during pregnancy), and stimulates elimination from the intestines and bladder. Sit on the floor, right knee bent at a 90° angle to left leg. Bend left knee and place the left foot in front of the right knee. Place right hand directly behind right hip. Place left hand directly behind right hand. While exhaling, move the left hand in a circle (feeling spinal stretch) to rest on the floor behind left hip; hold, then rest. Return the left hand to the position behind the right hand by completing a slow semicircular movement in front of and to the side of the body. Switch legs and repeat, twisting first to the right and then to the left.

13. *Triangle Pose.* Reported to prevent degenerative arthritic changes, tone the sides of the body, and maintain joint health in the feet, ankles, knees, and hips. Stand with feet 3–5 feet apart, right foot at a 90° angle to left foot. Gradually reach down with right hand to grasp right ankle; hold left arm straight up in the air directly above right arm; eyes watch left hand while breathing and holding the pose. Repeat on left side of the body.

14. *Shoulder Stand.* Reported to regulate the thyroid, increase flow of venous blood from the lower extremities to the heart, prevent varicose veins, and reduce gravitation pressure on internal organs. WARNING: contraindicated in cases of hypertension, neck problems, ear, throat, or eye infection and obesity. Lie on the back, palms facing the floor; press palms down and lift legs up and over the head, supporting the back with the hands and resting so the chin is on the chest. Align the chin with navel and big toes. Relax, breathe, and enjoy.

15. *Sun Salutation.* Reported to invigorate, calm, exercise arms and spinal cord, prevent and relieve stomach ailments, reduce abdominal fat, improve digestion and circulation, limber spine, tone abdominal, thigh, and leg muscles, strengthen nerves and muscles of arms and legs, shoulders, arms, and chest. An all around preventive posture that should be done at least every day by everyone.

Figure 15 provides directions for the Sun Salutation (Berkson, 1977; Lasater, 1984; Lowe & Nechas, 1983).

For further information see: Lowe, C. and Nechas, J., *Whole Body Healing*, Emmaus, PA: Rodale Press, 1983, pp. 508–552; or, Weiss, K., (ed.), *Women's Health Care: A Guide to Alternatives*, Reston, VA: Reston Publishing Co., pp. 294–309.

Massage Interventions

Mechanical pressure is used in massage to:

> . . . rid the muscles of toxic products by "milking" these acids into the lymphatic and venous flow toward the heart. As the muscles relax, fresh blood flows into them, bringing necessary nutrition to the area. It is obvious that massage should *not* be given if there is a possibility of spreading inflammation; or of dislodging a thrombus; thus causing embolism; or if there is such obstruction that the mechanical assistance of massage could not improve the blood flow. However, massage given *first* to the proximal aspects of an injured limb will ensure that these circulatory pathways are open enough to carry the venous flow along toward the heart. (Tappan, 1984, p. 260)

There are five basic massage strokes:

1. *Effleurage* is the stroke that glides over the skin on the surface. It is the most common stroke. Effleurage is often used to begin a massage to explore for areas of tenderness or tightness. The hand is molded to the skin, stroking with firm and even pressure, usually upward.

2. *Petrissage* strokes lift the muscle mass and wring or squeeze it gently. Kneading manipulations are completed with the hands or fingers pressing and rolling the muscles. It stimulates muscular and nervous tissue, frees adhesions, and stretches adipose tissue to release toxins, pesticides, and additives stored there.

3. *Friction* with the heel of the hand, thumb, or fingertips (according to the area to be covered) penetrates into deeper tissue. The tissue under the skin is moved, not the fingers on the skin. The stroke is used to

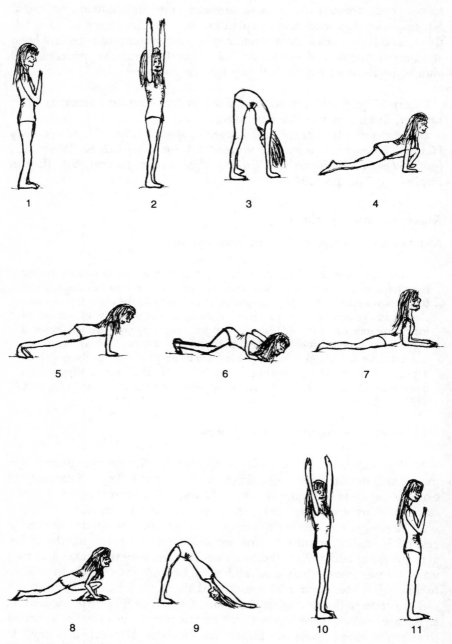

Figure 15. Sun salutation.

massage deep into joint spaces or around bony prominences, and can break down adhesions; it cannot affect a deep abdominal fibrositis, however.

4. *Vibration* is a fine, tremulous movement, sometimes only fluttering above a body part. It is used for its soothing effect which can also be accomplished via an electrical vibrator.

5. *Tapotement* is the use of the fists, or cupped palms, or the loose flinging of the hands to percuss a body area. The movement is done parallel to the muscle fibers to prevent trauma or spasm. This stroke is especially effective on tight shoulders or necks.

Experiment with a peer, friend, or family member with the various strokes and their effects prior to working with a client.

When practicing massage, it is wise to communicate with the client, asking where tense or tight spots are, experimenting with different strokes and asking for client input, and teaching the client self-massage measures. A massage is not a good time for general conversation, but nurse and client should be focused on the massage experience. It is not unusual for clients to experience strong positive or negative feelings during massage; the body work releases unresolved feelings. If this should occur, stop the massage and use listening skills until the feelings and thoughts have been expressed. Resume when the client is ready.

There is little agreement about oil use; some practitioners recommend it for its reduction of friction; vegetable (not mineral) oil is suggested because it is easily absorbed by the skin, whereas mineral oil tends to clog the pores. Practitioners who do not recommend the use of any oil believe oil interferes with energy exchange and finger sensitivity.

The best surfaces for giving a massage are: a massage table, a water bed, the floor. Most beds are too soft to offer the support needed to apply the appropriate amount of pressure. When giving a massage on the floor, it will of necessity be shorter in duration to prevent damage to the nurse. To counter some of the fatigue and stress, use foam knee padding or several sleeping bags to kneel on. A single mattress taken from a bed and placed directly on the floor will work, but its height is inconvenient. Working outside on the grass is a beautiful, serene experience for nurse and client. A massage is best received in the nude, but if the client is uncomfortable, negotiate this item.

The nurse's hands should be clean and fingernails trimmed down so the fingerpads are available for massage. Warm them if cold; either use warm water or rub them together vigorously. Be sure the client removes all jewelry, contact lenses, glasses, etc. The nurse removes wristwatch, rings, and anything that will detract from the massage for the client.

Approach the client's body slowly, gradually working up to stronger strokes. Always keep at least one hand on the client; stopping and starting touch is disruptive to the flow of massage. Use body weight rather than hand and arm muscle to apply pressure. Use good body mechanics, bending the knees and relaxing into massage movements; breathe regularly, avoid holding the breath.

Begin a massage by holding the palms lightly against the client's forehead for a few moments, applying no pressure. Center and then begin massage. Table 49 gives information concerning massage.

Table 49. Massage

1. Ask the client to lie down on his or her back. Stand, sit, or kneel in back of the client's head. Massage the forehead with the balls of the thumbs ending at the temples.
2. Use the tips of the forefingers to press against the bony rims of the eye sockets.
3. Massage the chin between the thumb and forefinger.
4. Use the palms to massage both sides of the face.
5. Bring both hands under the neck (be careful of the ears); hold the head firmly and straight out from the neck. Knead the neck with one hand with the other hand moving from the bottom of the neck to the nape. Cradle the head firmly in your hands and pull out with a moderate pressure, hold the head, and begin making a cloverleaf (see Figure 16).
   This is an integrating brain movement that also releases tension. As you work, watch the client's chest for breathing changes; note skin color changes and sighs indicating relaxation. After completing the butterfly pattern, hold the head cradled in the hands for several nurse and client breaths. Slowly place the client's head on the work surface and slowly move hands to the shoulders.
6. Push down on both shoulders with moderate to heavy pressure using body weight; hold the shoulders down through several slow breaths and then release the push, but keep the hands on the shoulders. Press in on the trapezius shoulder muscles looking for tight, hard, sore spots and lumps (muscle knots). When any is found, very gradually apply pressure with the ball of the thumb until reaching a point where it is sore; ask the client to tell you "when it's sore." Stop increasing the pressure at that point and hold the pressure you have. Wait for the client to relax; this can be enhanced by asking him or her to "breathe into my finger." Observe for signs of relaxation (muscle loosens, breath deepens and moves lower in the body) and then increase pressure with the ball of the thumb until another sore layer is reached. Repeat above. Move to locate and relax other sore areas in the shoulders.
7. Place the fingertips under the shoulders and move down to the shoulder blades, moving slowly if resistance is encountered, allowing the client to breathe in and out prior to moving the hands down. Watch for change in breathing and an opening up of the chest. When noted, go to number 8.
8. Place one hand on each side of the neck; turn the head to the left and to the right until resistance is met. If the neck is extremely tight, ask the client to "breathe into my hands" and gradually work the neck to the right and then to the left.
9. Holding the upper, back part of the head in both hands, lift the head as far forward as is comfortable. Stop when resistance is met, then gently nudge the head an inch farther forward. Slowly return the head to flat again.

10. Place the heel of the hands on the upper chest and push down and hold through several of the client's breaths, then release.

11. Place the hands under the client's armpits and gradually and firmly pull back and hold through several client breaths, then release.

12. Make fists of the hands and start at the middle of the chest below the collar bone and slide the knuckles out and down the torso following the ribs. Do successive movements until the entire rib cage has been covered. Avoid the abdominal area. Go lightly.

13. Move to the right side of the client and make a firm, circular motion several times, radiating out from the navel and down toward the bladder. Knead the abdominal area.

14. Grasp the client's right arm with both hands; pull the arm firmly and slowly toward the foot, keeping it in proper alignment with the shoulder; hold through several client breaths, then release.

15. Starting at the wrist, knead up the forearm and upper arm; glide the hands down to the wrist. Knead the hand and down each finger, pulling each finger out with firm, strong pressure (you will get some resistance and/or hear a crack as pressure is released).

16. Repeat no. 14 and no. 15 with the other arm and hand.

17. Move to the client's feet. Grasp the right ankle with both hands and exert firm, even pressure by leaning back; this will release tension in the hip joint. Knead up from the ankle to the hip. Glide the hands down to the ankle.

18. Make a fist with the right hand and make circles on the bottom of the foot. Knead the rest of the foot and pull out firmly on each toe.

19. Complete no. 17 and no. 18 on the left leg and foot.

20. Ask the client to turn over on the stomach. Use pillows to support the abdomen, neck, etc. Knead up the back of the right leg. Grasp both ankles with the hands, lean back, and hold for one or two breaths, releasing any additional tension in the hip.

21. Knead up the back of the other leg.

22. Move to face the client's head. Using the weight of your body, push the client's shoulders down, hold through several client breaths, release.

23. Move to the right side of the client. Drum the outer edges of the hands lightly, but rapidly across the right shoulder and back several times. Drum down the spine and the leg and up the other leg to the top of the spine, down the spine and down the other leg, and back up to the top of the spine.

24. Place the heel of the right hand at the middle of the right shoulder and the heel of the left on the middle of the left buttock; alternately rock the body, pushing down first with the right heel (hand) and then with the left heel (hand). Complete this rocking motion 2–3 times. Then place the heel of the left hand in the middle of the left shoulder and the heel of the right hand in the middle of the right buttock; rock 2–3 times, remembering to breathe and bend (see Figure 17).

25. Place the right hand underneath the lower abdomen and the left hand directly above on the lower back; push up with three fingers with the right hand and work down all five meridians (see Figure 17).

26. Right (or lower hand) pushes on the coccyx (sitbone) towards head; upper hand works from the spine outward, working one vertebra at a time (see Figure 17).

Table 49 *(continued)*

27. Find coccyx, then go 2" out to the right from it; client will feel some pain/ pressure; when area has been located, release the pressure and work on the left shoulder and neck area with the other hand (keep the hand in place on the coccyx). Repeat, reversing hands and moving 2" out to the left from the coccyx (see Figure 17).

28. Stand on the left side of the client, left hand to the left of the cervical spine, right hand just below it; work down the side of the spine with fingertips of both hands, making two clockwise circles into each spinal process; this soothes. Work around the coccyx and up the other side of the spine making two counterclockwise circles, up and into the spinal processes; this stimulates.

29. Place the hands on the client's head and quickly run both hands down the head, shoulders, arms, legs, and off the end of the feet. Return to the head and repeat until the entire back of the body has been covered with this quick, light movement.

30. Ask the client to slowly turn over when ready. Place the hands lightly on the client's cheeks and hold for a minute or two.

31. Move to the right side of the client, facing his or her head, and repeat the quick movement of the hands from the head down and off the body until every spot on the body has been covered.

32. Let the client rest for a few minutes while you meditate or close your eyes and relax.

Note: If, during the massage, any muscle knots are found, use deep, hard pressure with the thumb; if that does not release the muscle, use acupressure, pushing straight in with the thumb for 8–10 seconds, release, and repeat until muscle relaxes. Additionally, ask the client to picture that muscle relaxing.

For further information, see: Downing, G., *The Massage Book*, New York: Random House, 1972.

Schneider (1979) advocates the use of *infant massage* as a relaxation and *bonding* procedure.

> The most important elements that form the bond between mother and child include skin-to-skin contact, prolonged and steady eye-to-eye contact, and the soothing high pitched sounds of mother's voice in response to her infant's cry. Infant massage which serves as communication between parent and infant helps cement that bond. Baby learns to enjoy the wonderful comfort and security of loving and being loved. She acquires knowledge about her own body, as mother shows her how to relax a tense arm or back, or helps her release some painful gas. (p. 17)

Fathers are encouraged to learn infant massage. It is an excellent tool, providing quality experience for father and infant. The infant learns father can touch gently and lovingly and can be counted on to satisfy physical and emotional needs. The father learns to satisfy his infant and enhance his self-esteem and self-confidence.

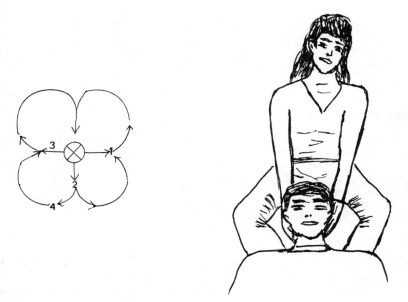

Figure 16. Integrating and relaxing the brain.
Sitting on the floor facing the back of the client's head, or standing behind the head of the massage table or bed, the nurse exerts a slight, equal pull straight back with both hands from underneath the neck. Beginning and ending at midpoint **X**, the head is guided through two loops on the right side of midpoint and then two on the left side of midpoint. The head is gently placed on the floor, table, or bed, and hands are very slowly released from underneath the neck.

Schneider (1979, p. 25) suggests the first 9 months is the ideal time to start. Daily massages up to 6 or 7 months of age are recommended. As the child becomes more active, once or twice a week is sufficient, but "growing pains" can be reduced through a pre-bedtime massage. Children who are not introduced to massage until age 3 or 4 can be offered a brief, gentle back massage at bedtime; in time, children begin asking for a massage. Older children can be taught to give their brothers and sisters a massage; this will increase bonding between the children, enhance the older child's self-esteem, and help resolve being replaced when a new infant is born. Rolling, milking, and circular strokes can be used with the infant. The arms and legs can be kneaded just as in adult massage.

All babies will fuss and cry at some times during massage; this is expected. It may be that parts of their bodies they were not aware of are sore to the touch; a gentler massage in these areas will relax the infant.

For the first 3 months of life, infants may resist having their arms massaged since moving the arms so far from the body may seem un-

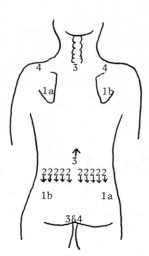

Figure 17. Back massage.
1a = rock
1b = rock
2 = work down meridians
3 = right or lower hand on coccyx/
sitbone, other hand works up and outward from spine
4 = right or lower coccyx, left hand
works opposite shoulder and neck area

natural; gentle shaking and patting movements are suggested in this case. Back massage is usually enjoyed at this time.

From 4 to 7 months, soreness and tension often moves to the back (crawling and sitting begins) and face (sucking and teething). At the end of the first year, tension may move to the legs. Infants who have been massaged from infancy will help by massaging themselves and by one and a half years will massage their dolls and teddy bears, and often their mothers.

Schneider (1979, pp. 31, 76) suggests the following interventions when the infant fusses:

1. Breathe deeply and relax. Use affirmations including, "I now let go of tension. My body is relaxed. I now let go of thoughts. My mind is open and free. I am the gentle power of love, flowing through my hands to (baby's name)."
2. Stop in the middle of the massage to cuddle, hold, or walk the baby.
3. Give the baby a teether or small toy to play with or chew on.

Acupressure Interventions

The palms of the hands, the thumbs, or the four fingers apply 3–5 kg of pressure to the client's body for 3–5 seconds in acupressure. Pressure is gradually increased until the maximum pressure is reached; then it is decreased. The direction of pressure is toward the center of the client's body. The weight of the whole body, not just the hands, is used (Serizawa, 1972, pp. 24–25).

Figure 18. Preventive acupressure
(increases circulation to the most commonly injured areas)

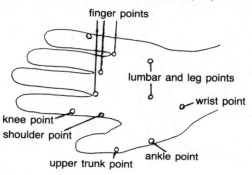

finger points

lumbar and leg points

wrist point

knee point

shoulder point

upper trunk point   ankle point

Apply firm pressure with ball of thumb; five seconds on and five seconds off for 30 seconds. Do both hands.

(*Source:* Nickel, 1984, pp. 24–73.)

Nickel (1984) suggests preventive acupressure for sport activities. (See Figure 18). Areas of common injury are focused on prior to engaging in the activity, thus strengthening the body against injury during play. Nickel (1984) also suggests an overall balancing point using ear acupressure techniques; see Figure 19. The points suggested in the two illustrations can also be used once an injury is incurred; acupressure should not be used to avoid the pain associated with a strain, tear, or fracture in order to continue with vigorous exercise, but can be used in conjunction with other treatments.

Lowe and Nechas suggest specific acupressure points for relief of pain. The Hegu point is the key to relieving pain in the head, neck, and arms. To locate the point:

. . . lay your left hand on a flat surface. Position the thumb so that it forms a right angle with the index finger. Now feel along the bone that extends back from the knuckle of the index finger. Along the index finger bone is the Hegu point. The point actually lies a little down and under the index finger bone. If you press down right alongside the bone, you have to press sideways, after you reach a sufficient depth, to reach a point under the bone . . . As you press harder you should feel the pressure radiating along the nerves in your hand. This sensation signals that you are on the Hegu point. (p. 15)

Early morning stiff necks, dental pain, and headaches respond well to hard pressure on the Hegu point.

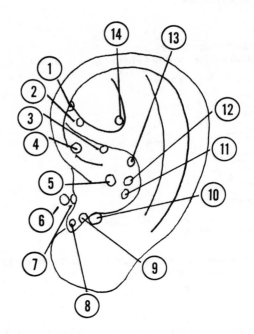

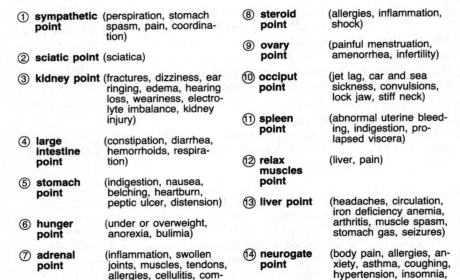

① **sympathetic point** (perspiration, stomach spasm, pain, coordination)

② **sciatic point** (sciatica)

③ **kidney point** (fractures, dizziness, ear ringing, edema, hearing loss, weariness, electrolyte imbalance, kidney injury)

④ **large intestine point** (constipation, diarrhea, hemorrhoids, respiration)

⑤ **stomach point** (indigestion, nausea, belching, heartburn, peptic ulcer, distension)

⑥ **hunger point** (under or overweight, anorexia, bulimia)

⑦ **adrenal point** (inflammation, swollen joints, muscles, tendons, allergies, cellulitis, common cold, fatigue, respiration, fever, frostbite, sinuses)

⑧ **steroid point** (allergies, inflammation, shock)

⑨ **ovary point** (painful menstruation, amenorrhea, infertility)

⑩ **occiput point** (jet lag, car and sea sickness, convulsions, lock jaw, stiff neck)

⑪ **spleen point** (abnormal uterine bleeding, indigestion, prolapsed viscera)

⑫ **relax muscles point** (liver, pain)

⑬ **liver point** (headaches, circulation, iron deficiency anemia, arthritis, muscle spasm, stomach gas, seizures)

⑭ **neurogate point** (body pain, allergies, anxiety, asthma, coughing, hypertension, insomnia, itching)

Figure 19. Overall balancing: ear acupressure.
Apply firm pressure with thumb ball and index finger for 1 minute, in 5-second-on and 5-second-off intervals. Use right ear.
(*Source:* Nickel, 1984, pp. 83–103.)

Another location for headache is the Fengchi points on the back of the head, in the depressions on either side of the cervical vertebrae below the occipital bone. Pushing hard up and into the skull will relieve some headaches. One or the other points, or a combination of Hegu and/or Fengchi works for most people; experimentation is necessary. Tenderness of a meridian point is the best indicator the point has been located.

A point that brings backache relief is Xuehai, located on the inside of the thigh, just back of the knee cap. The Liangqui point is located on the outside of the thigh behind the knee cap. The Tiantu point can help asthma; it is at the base of the throat right above the suprasternal notch; pressing this point on children may cause a slight choking sensation that may frighten the child.

The Yuyao point in the middle of the eyebrow eases fatigue, and Taichong, at the place where the big and second toe meet, energizes. Zusanli, about 3″ below the knee, relieves abdominal pain and motion sickness as well as energizes. Yongquan, located just behind the ball of the foot, energizes and revives after a faint (Lowe & Nechas, 1983, pp. 1–29).

Patterson (1984) suggests the following accupressure points for specific problems: all points in Figure 20, Neck and Shoulder Release.

Reflexology Interventions

Prior to attempting reflexology, sensitivity of the fingers must be developed. Placing a thread under the page of a book is a good exercise. When that can be sensed, try two pages, three, and so on. Using different materials, dental floss, rubber bands, and seeds of different sizes also works. As with other body therapies, it is not wise to practice them when feeling depleted or ill oneself since it is possible to drain energy from the client. Protecting oneself, using energizing affirmations, and attending to other dimensions of wellness (nutrition, stress

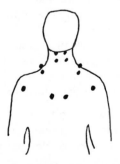

Figure 20. Acupressure for neck and shoulder release.

management, relationships, environment) will tend to make depletion an uncommon happening.

Pressure in reflexology should evoke a "good hurt" or pressure that is comfortably tolerated. To estimate the pressure needed, practice pressing a bathroom scale to 20–25 lb. of pressure. Very sore spots may require a build-up to this amount of pressure. Once the appropriate amount of pressure is found, hold it until a rhythmic pulsation is felt or until the client experiences a release (observe for change to a deeper breathing pattern, change to a better skin tone, relaxation in facial expression, and/or the client's words). For very painful spots, return to them again and again rather than trying to relieve the pain all at once; too much work all at once may bruise the capillaries.

Practice strengthening and using the *thumb*, for it is the most sensitive of the fingers. Continued experimentation with reflexology will strengthen them. As with other body work, working with the fingertips in reflexology promotes the nurse's physiological balance; every time the foot is pressed, spinal and brain energy are activated in both nurse and client (Berkson, 1977, p. 33).

Preparation for reflexology with a client:
1. Remove nail polish from fingernails and cut nails so nail pads are exposed. Shake, stretch, squeeze, and wash hands so they are relaxed and warm.
2. Find a quiet spot and ask the client to assume a comfortable sitting or lying position. Avoid music, disruptions, and any conversation except that related to the effects of the strokes.
3. Assume a relaxed position; a relaxation exercise can assist both nurse and client to prepare for a reflexology session. Visualizing a protective covering of light and affirming that no negative energy will be transferred from client to nurse is a safety measure.
4. Ask the client to relax and let go and avoid trying to assist.
5. Hold the client's feet in the hands for a few minutes while centering to orient both to the physical contact. Remember to breathe throughout the session.
6. Begin with the right foot. Avoid removing the hands from the foot until all steps have been completed. Each petrissage stroke (releases toxins) should be followed by an effleurage stroke (encourages removal of toxins to the bloodstream).

   A. Take the foot in both hands and stretch the sole gently, toes toward ankle and toes toward sole several times; note callouses, bunions, degree of flexibility, etc.

B. Hold the front of the foot in the left hand (reverse if left-handed) and the heel in the right hand; rotate the heel slowly and gently clockwise and then counterclockwise; note resistances and range of motion.

C. Grab hold of the foot and wring it like a sponge, one hand above the other, twisting in opposite directions; continue up and down the foot from ankle to toes, using steady, firm pressure. In this movement as in many others, the tendency for novices is to be too gentle; a firm pressure is needed to counteract tickling and to obtain results.

D. Stimulate the lymphatic drainage by pressing the lymphatic drainage point between the big and second toe (Figure 14). Use the thumb to stretch the skin from the heel along the outside of the foot to the toes using 20–25 lb. of pressure. Remember to breathe.

E. Sandwich the foot in between the two hands; use the knuckles to rub over all points on the foot. Breathe.

F. Start at the end of the big toe and use the thumbs to stretch the tendons toward the ankle up into the lymphatic area. Do all toes and the spaces in between. Breathe.

G. Anchor the heel with one hand and push on the ball of the foot with the other palm to the client's limit; hold for 15–30 seconds, then release. Breathe.

H. Anchor the heel with one hand and press the toes and foot toward the floor with the other to the client's limit and hold for 15–30 seconds, then release.

I. Rotate the foot laterally and hold and then medially and hold. Rotate the whole foot clockwise and counterclockwise.

J. Hold heel firmly in left hand and firmly press all inside and outside ankle reflexes for 3–5 seconds on each spot (see Figure 14). Rub ankle in an upward movement (effleurage).

K. Stabilize the foot with one hand, using the other to grasp the big toe firmly with thumb on top and forefinger on the back; make stretching movements from the base to the top of the toe; repeat on each toe. Work each toe medially, laterally, forward, and back. Breathe.

L. Hold the big toe close to its base, thumb on top where it meets the foot and forefinger beneath the joint connecting the toe to the foot. Support the foot well with the other hand and pull the toe straight out to the toe's maximum stretch for 10 seconds, then use a firm jerk straight back, listening for a cracking sound; some toes will "crack," while others will not; avoid forcing it. Jerk once or twice on each toe and then move on to the next one; return later to release tension; this movement stimulates tendons and clears the head and neck of congestion since all meridians and nerve endings for the brain and neck are stimulated (Berkson, 1977, p. 47).

M. Begin with the big toe; hold each toe in succession firmly and work down its corresponding tendon toward the ankle.

N. Begin with the big toe and rotate each toe three times in a full circle clockwise and then counterclockwise; observe for resistance and gritty sounds (indicating crystal formation).

O. With the fingers of one hand on the top of the toes and the other hand anchoring the heel, push forward firmly, hold a stretch, go a bit further, then release (toe extension release).

P. Grasp the toes firmly with hand, thumb on top of toes and fingers underneath in the lung area. Quickly bend the toes downward while pushing up from underneath at the lung reflex; this movement will release tension in the shoulder girdle. Optional: flex and extend each toe individually.

Q. Hold the big toe firmly and pull it towards the other foot; smack the side of the thoracic reflex (bony ridge beneath the toes) with the top of the palm as if clapping the hands; repeat 8–10 times. Releases tight shoulder blades, clears the neck, throat, eye, and ear, and reduces bunions (Berkson, 1977, p. 49).

R. Press firmly on all points of the big toe, front, back, side, and top. Repeat with each toe using very firm thumb pressure. Stimulate the web of each toe with the thumb and forefinger, top and bottom; use a pinching movement. Effective for eyes, ears, and sinuses.

S. Inch along the top of all toes with fingernail and flick each toenail up and away from the toe. Nails store electromagnetic current; flicking and stimulating the periphery stimulates meridians and releases energy (Berkson, 1977, p. 52).

T. Stimulate the eye and ear points at the base of the toes and stretch the skin from the small toe to the inside of the big toe; this will drain the sinuses and soothe the eyes and ears (Berkson, 1977, p. 52).

U. Stimulate venous drainage by rubbing each toe from its tip to its base.

V. Start with the spinal points on the sole of the foot (Figure 14), working the sacral and lumbar area by the heel up to the cervical area by the big toe, then work down the other side to the heel; follow with friction and effleurage.

W. Press all points on the lateral, medial, and top of the foot and ankle using knuckles; follow with effleurage.

X. Use a wringing motion up the leg; push the middle three fingers under the tibia from the ankle to the knee. Observe for swelling, granular tissue, and deposits; work them out with rubbing and pressure.

Y. Support the leg and use the middle finger or knuckle to press up the center of the calf from the Achilles tendon to the knee, stimulating the endocrine glands; highly stressed clients are tender there (Berkson, 1977, p. 56).

Z. Push firmly all the way up the leg from the ankle to the thigh, increasing the lymphatic and blood flow. Close by clapping the foot from heel to toe, and then brushing the hands down the legs several times from the knee off the end of the toes and then several inches away from the body. Repeat A–Z with left foot.

Figure 14, p. 232, can be used to treat specific conditions, e.g., pancreas for diabetes; small intestines area for digestive or assimilation difficulties; stomach for heartburn, nausea, bad breath, vomiting, or tightness under breast bone. Working on the toes will assist with headache, tension, congestion, sinus trouble, weak eye muscles, fatigue, etc. Although reflexology can be used this way, it is recommended the steps from A–Z be completed daily as a preventive measure. For further information, see: Berkson, D., *The Foot Book: Healing through Reflexology*, New York: Harper & Row, 1977.

INTEGRATIVE LEARNING EXPERIENCES

Beginning Level

1. Assess yourself using the following measures:

   A. Breast/vaginal self exam or testicular exam
   B. Sexual communication (Table 44)
   C. Diamond's behavioral kinesiology
   D. Krieger's Therapeutic Touch

2. Develop and try out appropriate interventions based on the above assessments with a peer; also ask your peer if she/he has any symptoms that you have not assessed via the above assessments, and develop and try out interventions for those. Use Table 23, p. 108, to organize the data.

3. Work with a peer to complete a therapeutic touch assessment of each other.
4. Work with a peer to complete a reflexology assessment and appropriate interventions.
5. Complete a massage with two peers using Table 49; compare your results.
6. Role play responses to the following client responses with a peer using assertiveness criteria to evaluate your efforts:

   A. "Doesn't yoga have something to do with winding yourself up like a pretzel? How can that be healthy? Sounds harmful to me!"
   B. "Thump my thymus! What good can that possibly do?"
   C. "How can my feet affect my heart? Hogwash!"
   D. "I let my doctor examine me; I don't want to know what's happening with my body unless there is something really wrong."

7. Role play a discussion with a client (using a peer to play the client) regarding which detection tests she should have so she will not miss an illness process. Use assertiveness criteria to evaluate the outcome.

Advanced Level

1. Complete assessments of one child, one young adult, and one senior client using assessments based on the frameworks of:

   A. Diamond
   B. Krieger
   C. Berkson (reflexology)
   D. Yoga
   E. Acupressure

2. Develop appropriate interventions for the three clients assessed. Organize your results using Table 23, p. 108.

REFERENCES

Abrams, H. (1979). The "overutilization" of x-rays. *NE J Med* 300:1213–1216.
Bergman, A. (1977). The menace of mass screening. *Am J Pub Health* 67(7):601–602.
Berkson, D. (1977). *The Foot Book: Healing The Body Through Reflexology.* New York: Harper and Row.

Berry, C. (1980). Doing your own vaginal self-exam. In *Medical Self-Care*, T. Ferguson, Ed. New York: Summit Books, pp. 281–284.

Borysenko, J. (1985). Healing motives: an interview with David C. McClelland. *Advances* 2(2):29–41.

Downing, G. (1972). *The Massage Book*. New York: Random House.

Galen, R. (1974). False-positives. *Lancet* (Nov. 2):1081.

Institute of Noetic Sciences. (1984). The new field of psychoneuroimmunology. *Investigations* 1(1):n.p.

Iyengar, B. (1966). *Light on Yoga*. New York: Schocken Books.

Knaster, M. (1984). Massage: the roots of women's healing. In *Women's Health Care: A Guide to Alternatives*, K. Weiss, Ed. Reston, VA: Reston Publishing Co.

Koenig, S. (1981). Touch for health. In *The Holistic Health Lifebook*, E. Bauman et al., Eds. Berkeley, CA: And/Or Press, pp. 44–51.

Krieger, D. (1979). *The Therapeutic Touch*. Englewood Cliffs, NJ: Prentice-Hall.

Lasater, J. (1984). Hatha yoga for women's health. In *Women's Health Care: A Guide to Alternatives*, K. Weiss, Ed. Reston, VA: Reston Publishing Co.

Lowe, C., and Nechas, J. (1983). *Whole Body Healing*. Emmaus, PA: Rodale Press, pp. 508–552.

McClelland, D., et al. (1985). Stressed power motivation, sympathetic activation, immune function and illness. *Advances* 2(2):43–52.

Napodano, R. (1977). The functional heart murmur: a wastebasket diagnosis. *J Fam Prac* 4(4):637–639.

Nickel, D. (1984). *Accupressure for Athletes*. Santa Monica, CA: Health AcuPress.

Patterson, A. (1984). Acupressure for women's health. In *Women's Health Care: A Guide to Alternatives*, K. Weiss, Ed. Reston, VA: Reston Publishing Co., pp. 270–283.

Rice, R. (1975). Premature infants respond to sensory stimulation. *APA Monitor* 6(11):8–9.

Robinson, N., and Dirnfeld, F. (1967). The ionized state of the atmosphere as a function of meteorological elements and the various sources of ions. *Int J Biometerol* 11(11):279–288.

Schneider, V. (1979). *Infant Massage*, 2nd ed. Aurora, CO: Vimala Schneider.

Serizawa, K. (1972). *Massage the Oriental Method*. Elmsford, NY: Japan Publications, Inc.

Tappan, F. (1984). Massage, reflexology and women. In *Women's Health Care: A Guide to Alternatives*, K. Weiss, Ed. Reston, VA: Reston Publishing Co., pp. 258–269.

Udupa, K., Singh, R., and Settiwar, R. (1971). Studies on physiological, endocrine and metabolic response to the practice of yoga in young normal volunteers. *J Res Indian Med* 6(3):345–353.

8

ENVIRONMENTAL WELLNESS

This chapter discusses the following topics:

- Environmental factors influencing wellness
- Assessing environmental wellness
- Environmental interventions

ENVIRONMENTAL FACTORS INFLUENCING WELLNESS

Researchers have found many environmental factors influencing wellness, including: waste disposal and transport, air quality, smoking, drinking water, crowding, radiation, consumer products, occupation, noise, acid rain, ions, light, and color. Many of these factors interact to enhance or detract from wellness.

The Environment and Cancer

Of current interest is the relationship between the environment and cancer. "It has been estimated that 50–90 percent of human cancer is due to known or unknown environmental factors. It is necessary to regard all agents demonstrated to be carcinogenic in animals as potentially carcinogenic in man, since present information precludes any reliable distinctions" (NIH, 1980, p. 33). Specific environmental risk factors include: cigarette smoking, personal habits, occupation, drugs, food, water pollutants, atmospheric contaminants, and some household products.

Solid Wastes

According to the National Institute of Health (1980, p. 27) 8 billion gallons of municipal waste are produced daily, industry dumps 20 million tons of waste materials annually into the environment, and 2 billion tons of solid waste are produced by farm animals in the United States. In the recycling of municipal waste, it can be contaminated by industrial, hospital, research, wastes, and pesticides; all these can enter plants grown on the soil using recycled sludge or waste water and be consumed on the dinner table (NIH, 1980, p. 28).

Air Quality

A major factor influencing environmental wellness is the quality of indoor and outdoor air. Some variables lowering the quality of outdoor air are: industries that vent dangerous chemicals into the air (both the areas nearby are affected and those far away due to high smokestacks and acid rain that falls many miles away), vehicle exhaust (especially from diesel engines), emissions from toxic waste dumps, nuclear plants, and nuclear testing areas. A major factor in air quality is the presence of smokers. Smoking not only affects those who smoke in terms of increasing risk for lung cancer and heart conditions; it also affects the passive smoker.

Known harmful effects of maternal smoking on the fetus include retarded fetal growth in utero, premature labor, mental retardation, hyperkinesis in childhood, higher perinatal mortality, spontaneous abortion, congenital neural tube defects, other birth defects, cardiac effects, higher breathing frequency, and elevated hemoglobin and hematocrit. Pathophysiologically, it is reported that smoking causes (1) lowered arterial pressure of the mother; (2) permanent damage to the uterine arteries; (3) lowered uteroplacental perfusion; (4) lowered caloric intake of the mother; (5) uterine artery vasospasm; and (6) fetal carboxhemoglobinemia. In normotensive mothers, smoking one cigarette raises arterial blood pressure (both systolic and diastolic), producing decreased placental blood flow; normal flow is restored only after 15 minutes. (Voldman, 1983)

Additionally, children of smoking parents are apt to have more upper respiratory ailments (Bryce & Enkin, 1984), lower scores on spelling and reading tests, shorter attention spans, more hyperactivity (Naeye & Peters, 1984), and infantile colic and ear inflammation twice as frequently as children of nonsmokers (Forskningsroen, 1984). Cancer risk in adulthood may also be increased (Sandler et al., 1985).

Indoor air pollution is a relatively new problem. Older homes, offices, hotels, and hospitals were not hermetically sealed. Prior to the interest in energy conservation, buildings were not composed of double-glazed windows, sealed windows, and synthetic materials, and there were sufficient cracks and leaks in walls and windows to let stale air out and fresh air in. Synthetic building materials and equipment and gas and kerosene stoves give off irritating gases and fumes. When combined with cigarette smoke and the fungus growth and spread of organic matter through air conditioning and humidifying equipment, air to breathe is severely compromised (Ager & Tickner, 1983; Epstein, 1978, pp. 450–453; George, 1985; Indoor air pollution and S. 1198 fact sheet, 1985). The problem is compounded in hospitals where bacteria, viruses, particles of fecal material, etc. are circulated to distant parts of the building via the air conditioning, plumbing, and laundry shute systems. The problem of hospital-acquired infection is growing and requires control (Mendelsohn, 1979, pp. 72–73; NIH, 1980, p. 26).

Smoking

There is a 62.5% mortality rate in hospital fires due to cigarette ignition. Measures to limit rather than eliminate smoking by clients have proven unsatisfactory, since most burn-related deaths occur while the clients are unattended (Bongard et al., 1984).

Smoking affects the quality of life in other ways; for example, it is correlated with higher absenteeism and health costs, excess office maintenance, increased ventilation needs, and lowered employee morale (Weis, 1984).

Drinking Water

Water quality is another factor affecting environmental wellness. Drinking water contains contaminants of varying harm: perhaps the most insidious are the organic compounds from sewage treatment plants and industrial discharge. Keough (1980, p. 10) states that an estimated 500–1,000 new chemicals are introduced into industry yearly, leading to increased drinking water contamination. Preliminary studies suggest a link between cancer and some organic and inorganic contaminants in drinking water. The higher incidence of heart disease in soft water areas may be due to the cadmium leached from plumbing by the corrosive action of the water. Soft water may also leach lead from the plumbing and contribute to mental retardation in children (NIH, 1980, p. 23).

Measures to destroy organisms found in drinking water also present potential hazards. Drinking chlorinated water is associated with cancer, high blood pressure, and anemia. Chloroform is formed in the chlorination process; this chemical is rapidly absorbed in body fat and tissues. Other potentially dangerous offshoots of the chlorination process are tribromomethane and chlorobenzene, a CNS depressant.

Several authors have noted the potential dangers of water fluoridation, including the possibility of surpassing the acceptable level of
fluoride by using substances containing natural fluoride (e.g., tea) and
drinking fluoridated water (Keough, 1980, pp. 22–33). Diesendorf
(1980) has reviewed the scientific studies on fluoridation and found that:
(1) The use of fluoridated water in kidney dialysis may lead to severe
bone disease. (2) There is evidence of low tolerance to fluoride. In one
study 1% of the study group of 1,100 suffered dermatological, gastrointestinal, and neurological symptoms from receiving a daily tablet of
approximately 1 mg/day of fluoride. (3) There is no guarantee that
adding a fixed concentration of fluoride to the water supply delivers a
controlled dose to individuals. Measurements in Canada found that
workers received 2 to 5 mg daily with a 1 mg fixed concentration;
skeletal fluorosis has been observed in concentrations of 0.8 to 4.0
mg/liter. A major study in an American hospital found 3.6 to 5.4 mg
with a mean of 4.4 mg. Additionally, a review of the studies used to
support fluoridation reveals statistical and methodological problems.

In addition to the dangers of consuming drinking water, a recent
study (Brown, Bishop, & Rown, 1984) showed that the skin route of
exposure to chemicals in drinking water accounted for 29–91% (64% on
the average) of the total dose of chemicals received by the individual.
The following compounds found in drinking water samples were studied: toluene, ethylbenzene, and styrene. Although not studied by the
researchers, Regna (1984) points out toxics like benzene, carbon tetrachloride, vinyl chloride, and trichloroethylene are commonly found in
surveys of drinking water supplies completed by the Environmental
Protection Agency (EPA).

Personal Space

Amount and type of personal space is an environmental wellness factor.
Crowding increases stress and contributes to the "spread of acute and
contribution to the chronic disease morbidity and mortality" (U.S. Dept.
of Health, Education and Welfare, 1977, p. 29). There is a variation in
personal space required and individual and ethnic parameters must be
assessed.

Radiation

Radiation can decrease personal wellness. The U.S. Academy of Sciences has confirmed that radiation exposure changes the electrical
charge of atoms and molecules in cells and that there is no level considered safe since even very low levels affect the body and its processes and

its effects are cumulative (Dickson, 1979). Toxic agent and radiation control is one of the 15 health priority areas addressed by the Public Health Service's Objectives for the Nation. Cancer is the chief concern of the overuse of diagnostic x-rays in medicine and dentistry. Diagnostic x-rays account for more than 90% of the total human-controllable ionizing radiation exposure for the U.S. population. Because of this problem, the Public Health Service has developed the following objective: By 1990, the number of medically unnecessary diagnostic x-ray examinations should be reduced by some 50 million examinations annually (Rall, 1984). Additionally, radiation is produced by microwave ovens, long-distance telephone microwave relay towers, police, weather, and airport radar systems, nuclear-generating stations, atom bomb tests, fluoroscopes, diathermy, radioactive isotopes, electron microscopes, some types of computers and office machines, high voltage electrostatic air filters, and AM-FM radio and TV broadcasting stations.

Consumer Products

Many consumer products can affect wellness negatively, including: foods in cans with leaded seams (increase lead toxicity); drugs (interact with pollutants to increase their toxic effects; estrogens and chemotherapeutic agents increase the risk of additional cancer); cosmetics (many contain carcinogenic substances); pesticides (many have been linked with cancer and contaminate soil, surface water, animals, and fish); toys (accidents result most commonly from choosing toys that are not age appropriate); cleaners (can cause burns and eye and lung irritation); aerosols (can irritate lungs and affect ecological balance); waxes (irritation of lungs and nasal passages); cleaning fluid (irritation and cancer); deodorizers (allergic reactions); insect repellents (skin irritation); formaldehyde fumes released from new products including pressed wood materials, urea-formaldehyde foam insulation, permanent press fabrics, and wet strength paper towels (eye, nose, and throat irritation, difficulties in breathing, headaches, fatigue, memory loss, nausea, and cancer in laboratory animals); decorated glassware (lead decals are toxic); ice cube trays if cadmium-coated (this heavy metal can leach into sherbet if the trays are used to produce it); silver polish if not adequately rinsed from kitchen utensils contains the heavy metal cadmium; pesticide treated shelf liners (toxic and volatile); and plastic food wraps containing PVC (a carcinogen).

Occupation

A number of workers are at high risk. Hospital workers are at high risk for cancer due to occupational hazards related to handling laundry (liver cancer) and exposure to ionizing radiation (leukemia) (Mancinon, 1983). Other substances in hospitals linked with cancer include: anesthetic gases, benzene, formaldehyde, ethylene oxide, sex hormones, and alkylating agents used to treat cancer. Hospital workers are at risk for exposure to ethylene oxide, a sterilant linked with dermatitis, burns, eye irritation, pulmonary edema, leukemia, lymphoma, and possibly stomach cancer, miscarriage, birth defects, and reproductive conditions.

The manufacture of consumer products increases the negative effects for those employed in certain work. Workers in high risk industries (asbestos, rubber, chemical, plastic, PVC/VC, steel, smelting, and some mining operations) have increased rates of cancer, respiratory, and gastrointestinal disorders (Epstein, 1978, pp. 435–458).

Those who work with pesticides and grain workers (who must unload incoming cargoes of fumigated grain) are at high risk for short-term effects: nervousness, tremors, difficulty breathing, nausea, vomiting, skin irritation, collapse, coma, and death; and long-term effects: liver, kidney, CNS, and eye damage; allergic skin reactions, sterility, birth defects, stillbirths, and cancer (Fumigants used in the food industry, 1983).

Asbestos poses a major threat to 2.5 million workers in diverse occupations. Those at especially high risk are construction workers, brake mechanics, maintenance employees, and shipyard workers. Mt. Sinai Environmental Sciences Laboratory projects that there will be 200,000 excess cancer deaths from asbestosis by the year 2,000.

Benzene is a major cancer hazard for 3 million workers in the chemical industry. A risk assessment by scientists from OSHA and the National Toxicology Program estimate that between 44 and 152 of 1,000 workers will contract leukemia if they are exposed to the current legal limit for 45 years.

Roofers and waterproofers are exposed to asphalt and coal tar pitch fumes laden with hydrocarbons known to cause cancer in laboratory animals including lung, skin, bladder, and gastrointestinal cancers. More than half a million workers employed in cotton agriculture and yarn and fabric manufacture are at risk for brown lung, a chronic, irreversible respiratory condition worsening with exposure. It is estimated that 30,000 workers in the South Atlantic region are already totally disabled by the condition and that 83,000 will be afflicted in the future.

Industrial workers and gas station attendants are at risk from exposure to EDB, which is known to cause cancer in animals and is suspected of causing reproductive problems.

Up to 2.6 million workers may be exposed in the manufacture, installation, and use of formaldehyde products. Inhalation or skin contact has been linked with cancer since the mid-1970s. It is estimated that 6 million workers have work-related hearing loss and 15 million are currently exposed to hazardous noise levels.

Approximately 835,000 workers in diverse occupations are exposed to lead; exposure to the metal is known to cause intoxication, loss of appetite, constipation, nausea, tremors, weakness, numbness, colic, and kidney disease; long-term exposure has been linked with CNS and brain damage, reproductive conditions, and possibly heart disease (OSHA Standards: 1981–1984, 1984).

Nurses are at especially high risk for radiation exposure. Spills from sites or drainage tubes of implants (evidenced by blue, red, or purple stains on dressing or bedclothes) and contamination from the client's urine, vomitus, feces, or blood are sources of radiation exposure. Holding clients for x-rays or standing too near x-ray equipment during its use are other sources. Working with clients receiving cobalt teletherapy exposes the nurse to further dangers since the client is radioactive. Nurses who work in ICUs or other areas where portable x-rays are commonly used are at risk also.

Although nurses interested in environmental hazards relevant to nursing did not believe they received adequate acceptance as late as 1980 (Is AJN relevant to nursing?, 1980), by 1982 the American Nurses' Association had passed several resolutions relevant to the environment. The resolution relevant to health hazards in the workplace was (Tedesco, 1982):

WHEREAS, Nurses for decades have dedicated their careers to promoting the health and welfare of their own clients, to the extent that consideration of the nurses' health and welfare has been neglected; and

WHEREAS, Nurses are among health care workers in hospitals who routinely face exposure to toxic chemicals, gases, infectious diseases, radiation and other hazards that have been shown to cause cancer, acute and chronic illness, spontaneous abortion and birth defects; and

WHEREAS, Nurses are among health care workers in the community who face exposure to physical harm from infectious disease, violent crime and other environmental hazards; and

WHEREAS, Documentation in order to plan preventive and corrective action regarding nurses' health hazards is inadequate; and

WHEREAS, Without further epidemiological evidence, employee prevention and safety programs will remain ineffective and non-goal directed; therefore be it

RESOLVED, That the American Nurses' Association assist nurses to identify and to report health hazards to appropriate government, health and nursing agencies or associations; and further

RESOLVED, That the ANA continue to encourage research and investigative activities into occupational risks and health hazards encountered by nurses in the workplace.

Noise

Continued exposure to sound at high decibels (noise) is correlated with hearing loss, elevated blood pressure, tension, nervousness, and imbalance in the fluid, electrolyte, and hormonal systems. The Environmental Protection Agency's rule of thumb is that if an individual has to raise his or her voice to be heard, the noise is too loud and should be avoided. Although it is believed hearing is lost during the aging process, a remote Sudanese tribe living in a noise-free culture has near perfect hearing past 80 years of age. Being exposed to daily rapid-transit trains, V-8 engines, or aircraft can result in psychological, psychosomatic, and cardiovascular symptoms. Some sound levels that create risk to hearing loss include live rock bands, jackhammers, heavy duty trucks, and living next to a freeway; a jet takeoff (100 meters away) or a jet engine (25 meters distance) can be harmful to hearing (Raloff, 1982).

Acid Rain

A byproduct of high smokestack emissions is acid rain. Deaths of fish and entire ecological systems have been traced to industrial emissions hundreds of miles away. Weathering is accelerated and there are possible effects to human skin and hair (Rosenfield, 1978).

Ions

The air is filled with ions; "pos-ions" or positive ions are produced by various kinds of friction which tends to "knock off the negative electrons and produce an overdose of positive ions. On a dusty or humid day this overdose may be massive because the neg-ions promptly attach themselves to particles of dust, pollution, or moisture and lose their charge" (Soyka, 1977, p. 21). An overdose of "neg-ions" or negative ions seems to be beneficial to well-being while an overdose of pos-ions leads to fatigue, tension, and hyperactivity. Probably due in part to the overproduction of serotonin as well as interfering with the normal clotting mechanism, ". . . Pos-ions stimulate the metabolism and that alone could be responsible for an increased flow of blood from an open surgical wound. Whether the problem is thrombosis or hemorrhage depends on the patient" (Soyka, 1977, p. 63).

Neg-ions are associated with the calm after a storm (the pos-ions have been washed away), mountain areas (sun, clean air, and rock strata interactions), seashore (waves bounce on beaches and rocks), waterfalls, and showers. Pos-ions are associated with tall buildings, air conditioning systems, enclosed areas (e.g., riding in a car with the windows closed and vents open or spending hours in hermetically sealed buildings where windows cannot be opened), storms, certain desert winds, full moons (number of pos-ions close to the earth's surface increases as the negative outer face of the ionosphere is repelled), synthetic fibers (static electricity potential is high compared to natural fabrics), pollution, smoking, and any other situation setting up friction resulting in the loss of neg-ions.

Light

Full spectrum light is associated with well-being, whereas less than full-spectrum light, e.g., fluorescent lighting, is associated with decreased wellness. Full spectrum light enters the eye and stimulates the pituitary. Studies of bird and animal migration and hen egg production "has led to strong evidence that mammals respond to particular wavelengths of *visible light* as well as other areas of the *total spectrum,* including the longer wavelengths of ultraviolet that penetrate the atmosphere" (Ott, 1973, p. 13).

One of Ott's experiments provides evidence for the effect of different types of light on well-being. Thirty pairs of mice were kept in a room lighted by white fluorescent bulbs; 30 other pairs were kept in another room lighted with pink fluorescent bulbs; a control group (of eight pairs) was kept in a room receiving daylight filtered through window glass. All mice were of the C3H strain, which is highly susceptible to spontaneous tumor development. The mice in the control group developed cancer 2 months later than the mice in the white fluorescent light and 3 months later than those under the pink fluorescent lighting.

In later experiments with larger numbers of mice (over 2,000 in all), not only tumor development, but necrosis of the tail, calcium deposits in heart tissues, smaller litters, and behavioral problems were associated with pink fluorescent lighting. The effect of tinted pink glass on behavior was also noted by Ott. Mink placed behind deep pink glass became increasingly aggressive, as did students who wore "hot pink" sunglasses (Ott, 1977, pp. 155–157).

Ott (1977, pp. 192–202) reports studies of the effect of light on well-being. In one study, four first-grade classrooms in a windowless school in Sarasota, Florida showed dramatic reactions in hyperactive children when new, full-spectrum fluorescent tubes (that duplicate natural light) were used in two of the classrooms. Under the standard cool white fluorescent lighting, some first-graders demonstrated nervous fatigue, irritability, lapses of attention, and hyperactive behavior. When the new full-spectrum fluorescent tubes were installed, a marked improvement occurred in the children's behavior. Films of classroom behavior for 4 months showed the children in full-spectrum light remained calm and more interested in their work while those in rooms with the standard cool white fluorescent light were observed fidgeting to an extreme degree, leaping from their seats, flailing their arms, and paying little attention to their teachers. Similar results were reported in studies in two schools in California. Additionally, the number of cavities and the extent of tooth decay in new teeth showed significant differences; the children in the improved lighting had one third fewer cavities.

Ott (1977, pp. 195–196) contended that since several conditions are treated with specific wave lengths of light (jaundice with blue light and psoriasis with black light), living under artificial light lacking these wavelengths might logically contribute to causing the condition original-ly. Contrarily, too much direct exposure to the sun (full-spectrum light) is correlated with skin cancer; however, it is not necessary to be in the sunlight to obtain full-spectrum light. Being outdoors during daylight hours (preferably not in direct sunlight), sitting in a room flooded with natural light, or using full-spectrum fluorescent lighting will all produce wellness enhancement without increasing the risk of skin cancer.

Dr. Richard J. Wurtman, Director of the Neuroendocrine laboratory at M.I.T., sheds further light on the benefits of full-spectrum light. "Light striking the retina stimulates the optic nerve, which . . . in turn sends out impulses to the hypothalamus, a part of the brain with a great influence on emotions. From there, stimulation travels through neuro-chemical channels to the pituitary and pineal glands, which release the hormones that control body chemistry" (Houck, 1979).

> In Russia, daily exposure to low dosages of ultraviolet is prescribed by law for coal miners as an aid in fighting black lung. Researchers believe that ultraviolet light stimulates enzyme reactions, increases the activity of the entire endocrine system and increases immunological responses. And the U.S. Navy has been irradiating its personnel on submarine duty. There has been less illness among irradiated crewmen, the navy reports, and full-spectrum lighting has had a definite beneficial effect on the sailors' emotion-al lives. (Houck, 1979, p. 34)

Color

Each color has its own wave length in the spectrum of light. Although working in red light has been shown to increase productivity and reduce fatigue, people tire more easily and are more prone to accidents than if they work in a green light vibration (Don, 1977, p. 17). Color can be used to decorate the environment, chosen in color of dress, used in serving attractive meals, and has been used as a treatment for various conditions; thus color can enhance or detract from the quality of life.

ASSESSING ENVIRONMENTAL WELLNESS

Assessments of environmental wellness can be made for the following issues: indoor and outdoor air pollution, crowding, radiation, consumer products, noise, ions, and use of light/color.

The reactions of household plants to toxic radiation and harmful gasses is one way to assess whether the environment enhances wellness. Impatiens, Petunia, Clematis, Nicotiana, and Tradescantia have all proven useful as detectors. In the case of Tradescantia, the petals change color from blue to pink (a sign of mutagenesis) when the flower has been exposed to radiation or a gas that is harmful to humans (Liberati, 1982).

The National Cancer Institute found that in certain locales the incidence of canine bladder cancer is an early identifier of human cancers: it takes 20 years for the development of cancer in humans, but only a decade for it to develop in dogs (Watchdog, 1981).

The questions below can be used to assess indoor air pollution problems:

- Does the room seem stuffy and humid?
- Do odors linger for a long time?
- Do eyes get irritated when spending time in the room?
- Are headaches a common complaint after spending time in the room?
- Is there a complaint of difficulty with breathing in the room?
- Is there a complaint of sleepiness while in the room?
- Are cardiovascular symptoms present (associated with cellophane, plastics, extreme temperature changes, hazardous art and hobby supplies)?
- Is asbestos or formaldehyde used in building or consumer products?
- Are aerosols used?
- Are any cleaning agents or solvents used containing carbon tetrachloride, trichlorethylene, perchloroethylene, or benzene?
- Does the individual work in a high risk industry?
- Does the individual handle contaminated clothing belonging to other family members?
- Does the individual (or family member) use chemicals in arts and crafts pursuits?

- Are ventilation and air circulation systems inadequate?
- Does anyone in the work area smoke?

Additional information about assessing indoor air pollution and a free subscription to the newsletter *Indoor Air News* can be obtained by writing: Edith Furst, Consumer Federation of America, 1424 16th Street, N.W., Washington, D.C. 20036, or calling (202) 387-6121.

Outdoor air pollution can be assessed by asking the following questions:

- Does the individual live near a major expressway or high risk industry?
- Are pesticides sprayed on the lawns or in the air?
- Are toxic waste dumps, nuclear plants, or nuclear testing nearby?

Assessing Water Quality

Water quality can be assessed in a gross manner by eyeballing a glass of it. Some questions to ask are:

- Does the water foam as it splashes into the glass? (can indicate detergent residue)
- Is the water murky? (could indicate clay, silt, metals, synthetic or natural chemical compounds, plankton, microorganisms, sewage, industrial waste, asbestos, soil, or rusty pipes)
- Is the water colored? (indicates the water has not been properly treated or decaying plant matter is entering the water source)
- Does the water have a peculiar taste or odor? (could be due to anything from industrial solvents to a dead animal in the cistern; chlorine adds an unpleasant taste and smell to water)

Most people become accustomed to the taste of their drinking water and may find it difficult to discriminate between good and bad quality water. If drinking water *suddenly* tastes bad, it is an indication that a water test should be completed. Water can be tested by state departments of public health, county health departments, or regional departments of environmental resources.

Crowding

Adverse effects from crowding must be assessed on an individual basis. Individuals of different ethnic groups, ages, or socialization processes may have different needs for personal space; these need to be assessed with each client.

Radiation

Exposure to radiation can be assessed by keeping a record of dental and medication x-rays and frequency of contact with microwave ovens, long distance telephone microwave relay towers, airport radar, nuclear-generating stations, atom bomb tests, fluoroscopes, diathermy, radioactive isotopes, electron microscopes, computers, office machines, high voltage air filters, and radio broadcasting stations.

Consumer Products

Many consumer products can create symptoms. Again, individual differences must be assessed. The listing on page 262, "Consumer Products," provides a starting point. Symptoms which appear to have no organic basis may be due to a hazardous substance. The Health Systems Agency of New York City (111 Broadway, New York, NY 10006) prepared a quick reference guide to the health effects of hazardous substances. The following information may assist in assessing whether symptoms are due to hazardous substances.

Skin Problems. Rashes, irritation, redness, or itching may be due to having touched a metal-cleaner, wood, or food, preserving chemical, a household soap or chemical, or could be a reaction to a food or cosmetic.

Respiratory Problems. Difficulty breathing or lung conditions may be due to exposure to construction or insulation materials, meat wrappings, paint, materials used in textile manufacture or arc-welding, radiological (x-ray) materials, improper ventilation and heating, traffic exhausts, animals, dust, industrial air pollution, or inflight airline services.

Heart and Circulatory Problems. May be due to exposure to traffic exhaust, diesel engine operation, sewage treatment, cellophane, the manufacture of plastic, repairing a motor vehicle, extreme temperature changes, pesticides, or hazardous art and hobby supplies.

Digestive Problems. The most common ones are pain in the abdomen, vomiting, diarrhea, blood stools, or liver disease. May be due to exposure to jewelry making materials, dry cleaning fluid, refrigeration manufacturing, food or printing processing, contact with lead based paints, batteries and electrical equipment, or improperly handled food.

Nervous System Disorders. May be due to exposure to wood-working materials, paints, traffic exhausts, fireproofing, plumbing materials, soldering, manufacture of textiles and petrochemicals, pesticides, or improperly prepared food.

Eye Irritation or Cataracts. Could be due to exposure to petroleum refining, chemical handling, paper production, laundering materials, photographic films, or glass blowing.

Reproductive Problems. May be due to exposure to operating room procedures, pesticides, or battery components.

Blood Disorders or Cancer (especially leukemia). May be due to exposure to dye manufacturing, dry cleaning, chemical handling, hazardous art or hobby materials, or rodent bites or excretions.

Nose or Sinus Problems (especially inflammation and tumors). May be due to exposure to welding, photoengraving, glass, pottery, linoleum or textile manufacturing, wood or leather products, or battery components.

The Consumer Product Safety Commission (CPSC) distributes guidelines for selecting safe consumer products, including toys. The Commission can be reached at 1111 18th St., N.W., Washington, D.C. 20207, (202) 634–7780.

The relatively new field of clinical ecology examines the effect of the environment on well-being. According to Randolph and Moss (1980), the physical environment can be responsible for conditions ranging from fatigue to headaches, arthritis, colitis, hyperactivity, and depression. Randolph and Moss suggest that clients maintain a 4-day period between eating foods of the same family; the pulse before and after eating offensive foods is used as a measure of allergic response to it. (Pulse either increases or decreases after eating an allergen.) Diamond's (1979) behavioral kinesiology assessments can also be used to determine negative reactions to consumer products.

Assessing Occupational Risks

The list of high risk occupations appears in the section entitled "Occupation." Individuals can be assessed based on this list.

Assessing Noise Risks

Living, working, and playing noise risks can be assessed using the EPA's rule of thumb (see page 265).

Acid Rain Assessments

A walk around the nearest pond and statue can provide information about the effects of acid rain (see page 265). There are no measures to date to assess the effects of acid rain on human skin and hair.

Assessment of Air Ions

Assessing the typical weather, proximity of bodies of water, waterfalls, mountains, frequency of showers (all neg-ion producers); use of synthetic fibers, smoking (active or passive), and time spent in hermetically sealed buildings or vehicles (all pos-ion producers) will give a gross ratio of pos-ions to neg-ions.

Light

The ratio of number of hours spent in full-spectrum light to fluorescent light will give a gross measure of well-being due to light source.

Color

Color can be used to stimulate or calm. An assessment of the client's needs in this regard will assist in choosing appropriate colors. Refer to the color intervention section for specific information.

ENVIRONMENTAL INTERVENTIONS

When discussing the environment, it is not unusual to hear a sigh followed by, "But everything causes cancer, so why worry?" The National Cancer Institute has developed a brochure entitled, "Everything Doesn't Cause Cancer" (1980), which may be helpful in these cases.

Points of interest in the brochure include:

- Many cancers can be prevented by reducing exposure to the carcinogens.

Table 50. Breath for Unity

Many of us never allow ourselves the luxury and potential well-being we could obtain from getting in touch with Mother Earth. In celebration of your unity with the earth:

- Go outside and find a bit of earth to stand on—your lawn or some grass in a park, sand, a forest, or seashore—somewhere where you feel contact with nature.
- Take off your shoes and socks.
- Undo tight, restrictive clothing.
- Look at the earth beneath your feet and imagine the tremendous energy source available to you.
- Inhale through your nose and visualize breathing in the earth's energy through your feet; imagine it rising up your legs and into your hip socket.
- Think of your feet as spreading and opening to the energy of the earth.
- Exhale through your nose, sending your breath from your coccyx down, down to the very center of the earth.
- Feel yourself beginning to exchange energies with the earth. Draw the earth's energy into your body and send back any darkness or negativity or problems you wish to be rid of.
- Repeat this breath until you feel one with the earth.

Copyright, 1980, Carolyn Chambers Clark, THE WELLNESS NEWSLETTER, 1(5):1. Reprinted with permission.

- Everything does not cause cancer if the dose is high enough. High doses of many chemicals are toxic, but they will not cause tumors. Other forms of toxicity, such as loss of hair or weight, various organic malfunctions, and even death, should not be confused with carcinogenesis.
- The risk of cancer may be increased when people are exposed to several carcinogens at the same time, e.g., smoking and working in an asbestos factory.

Environmental interventions include conservation of natural resources, protection from pollutants, and active plans to mold a life style and shape the environment to enhance wellness. The environmental dimension is only part of the whole wellness approach. Thus, interventions are planned to optimize nutritional, stress management, interpersonal, fitness, and self-care approaches.

Unity with the environment is difficult given the stresses and strains of modern life. Table 50, breath for unity, provides an opportunity for reestablishing environmental unity.

Table 51 provides information regarding protection from some environmental influences.

Table 51. Protection from Environmental Influences

Harmful substance/ occurrence	Protective measures
1. Hazardous Solid Wastes	Become involved in the assessment and legal processes to monitor solid wastes more carefully; ask to be on local EPA mailing lists for meetings and hearings; talk to state officials to find out state laws and how they will be enforced; subscribe to *Exposure* (The Environmental Action Foundation, 724 Dupont Circle Bldg., Suite 724, Washington, D.C. 20036); obtain a copy of the House of Representatives report on hazardous waste disposal sites and Hunt the Dump instruction packet from A. Blakeman Early, Sierra Club, 330 Penn. Ave., S.E., Washington, D.C. 20003.
2. Air Quality Ventilation	Install a heat exchanger (pulls in fresh air and blows stagnant air out); many air conditioners recirculate the same air; clean reservoirs and change filters in air conditioners; biocidal water treatment can minimize growth of microorganisms in cooling towers (Ager & Tickner, 1983). Have name placed on mailing list to receive *Indoor Air News* (Consumer Federation of America, 1424 16th St., N.W., Washington, D.C. 20036).
Gas stoves	Use electric stoves; gas equipped homes are linked with allergies and respiratory conditions (Randoff & Moss, 1980).
Smoking	Ask visitors who smoke to use the front porch for smoking; stay away from areas where others smoke; increase intake of vitamins C and A.
Formaldehyde	Avoid urea-formaldehyde foam; cover particle board with vinyl wallpaper and paint plywood furniture with low density paint; avoid permanent press clothing, plastic, adhesives, and other items if they seem linked with eye irritation, headache, cough, or skin rashes.
Other pollutants and toxic substances	Use recommended houseplants (see p. 268) to detect toxic substances; avoid using disinfectants, air "fresheners," insecticides, aerosols, floor waxes, and moth balls (Indoor air pollution and S. 1198 fact sheet, 1985).
3. Water Quality	Install activated carbon filter on drinking water tap or a line bypass system; change filters as product supplier suggests.
Soft water	Disconnect or never install water softener; check drinking water for sodium content; consider breast feeding infants; those at high risk for soft water in-

274

	clude those with congestive heart disease, hypertension, renal disease, cirrhosis of the liver, and infants (Keough, 1980).
Fluoridated water	Those at risk include people who eat large amounts of protein, calcium, vitamin D, take alcohol, and are over 50; increase magnesium intake; use natural fluoride foods including fish, tea, milk, and eggs (Garrison, 1985) and/or fluoride toothpastes to protect against dental caries.
4. Crowding	Redesign environment or use stress reduction techniques to decrease crowding effects.
5. Radiation	Use food substances that bind radioactive materials and help excrete them: sea kelp, apples, slightly unripe fruit, sunflower seeds, miso, calcium tablets or calcium-rich foods, B-vitamins, buckwheat, sprouted seeds, peanut or olive oil, raw leafy green vegetables, vitamin C tablets or vitamin C-rich foods.
x-rays	Avoid unnecessary x-rays; dental x-rays only every 3–5 years (American Dental Association) or every 6–10 years (other authorities); ask for thermography instead of x-rays; inquire about the reliability of the x-ray procedure; ask for specific dose that will be received; insist on hearing the benefits in detail; only have x-rays done by a specialist or in a radiology department by a certified technician using up-to-date equipment, small doses, and adequate body shields. Especially at risk are young women who suspect breast cancer, pregnant women, children, and unborn fetuses (Abrams, 1979; Epstein, 1978).
Smoke detectors	Avoid standing under a smoke detector; discard when cracked (Clark, 1982; George, 1985).
Luminous dials	Avoid wearing a watch with a luminous dial or sleeping next to a clock with a luminous dial.
Microwave relay high relay towers for telephone and television	Look for neighborhood towers; avoid buying a home or living near one.
Microwave ovens	Check yearly for leakage; avoid opening and closing unnecessarily or banging its sides.
Checkpoints at airports or department stores	Move speedily through checkpoints; stay far away from x-ray of luggage and pick up belongings only at end of ramp.
6. Consumer Products	Read labels and purchase only those products that enhance well-being; contact CPSC for guidelines (1111 18th St., N.W., Washington, D.C. 20207).
Alcohol	Avoid alcoholic drinks and increase intake of recommended vitamins and minerals when drinking.
Additives	Processed, junk foods contain high amounts of additives and are low in nutrient quality. Avoid saccha-

Table 51 *(continued)*

Harmful substance/ occurrence	Protective measures
	rin, foods with red dye #40 and synthetic coal tar dyes, certified colors, cosmetic food additives, and nitrites found in sandwich meats, salami, bologna, hot dogs, smoked meats and fish, and bacon (Epstein, 1978).
Aluminum cookware	Use iron, glass, or stainless steel cookware.
Cans with leaded seams	Choose food packaged in other types of containers; never leave opened cans in the refrigerator; place unused contents in a glass container and seal; increase intake of vitamins A, C, E, and selenium.
Benzene	Artists and hobbyists using products containing benzene can consider substitute products and increase their intake of vitamin C (Epstein, 1978).
Cadmium in artist and hobbyist materials	Increase selenium and zinc intake; correct any iron deficiencies; use substitute materials.
Cigarettes	Stop smoking to reduce risks of cancer of the larynx, lungs, esophagus, mouth, bladder, and heart disease.
Cleaners, aerosols, waxes	Use organic cleaners (brown soap and cold water will remove most stains); avoid aerosols and use paste rather than spray waxes and only in well-ventilated areas; wear gloves when touching strong chemicals; contact Women's Occupational Health Research Center, School of Public Health, Columbia University, 60 Haven Ave. B-1, New York, NY 10032.
Cosmetics	Avoid purchasing any products carrying a warning label, 2,4-toluene-diamine or 4 methoxy-in-phenylene-diamine, yellow #1, blue #6, and reds #10−13 (used in lipsticks and soaps primarily).
Estrogens	Use other forms of birth control; take additional magnesium if on "the pill"; refuse "morning after" pills (DES) offered in some clinics to disrupt pregnancy; use vitamin E for debilitating symptoms of menopause; take estrogens only at low doses for short periods of time (Epstein, 1978).
Hair dyes	Read labels carefully; write to manufacturers for information; medium and dark-haired people can use henna; streaking, tipping, or frosting are safer and should be used instead of dyes; use natural hair tints such as lemon juice and camomile tea.
Prescribed drugs	Be apprised of *all* risks before deciding to submit to treatment; read all inserts and relevant portions of the

	PDR; choose less toxic alternatives when possible, e.g., brown soap assists in healing many skin conditions; application of vitamin E (oil capsules) assists in healing burns, cuts, sores, etc.; use preventive methods (stress reduction, nutrition, color, reflexology, etc.) so drugs are not needed.
Seat belts	Wear seat belts and ensure that all those riding in the car do.
Toys	Choose age-appropriate toys; supervise play and maintain ground rules.
Pesticides	Use natural repellents or subscribe to *Lawrence Review of Natural Products* (P.O. Box 186, Collegeville, PA 19426); use dormant oil sprays (contact: David Pace, Organic Farm and Garden Center, Box 8082, Emeryville, CA 94608); plant marigolds and nasturtiums in the garden to deter insects; plant garlic or use as a spray on plant leaves; buy or feed ladybugs, praying mantises, wasps, birds, and toads; hang a bouquet of dried tomato leaves in rooms to repel mosquitoes, flies, and spiders; place dried lavender, cedar chips, or rosemary in bags to deter moths; sprinkle crushed catnip on ant trails; use citronella and lavender oil to repel biting insects; send for *Integrated Pest Management Systems Newsletter* for answers regarding home and garden pests (Rt. 1, Box 28A, Winters, CA 95694).
7. Occupation	Contact OSHA (Labor Dept., 200 Constitution Ave., N.W., Washington, D.C. 20210) regarding policies, laws, and programs. Demand informed consent regarding dangers and a surveillance program to follow up worker symptoms and treatment. Include occupational health in contract or collective bargaining agreements; serve on hospital planning committees to ensure future additions meet wellness and safety standards; report any hazards to appropriate superior or union representative in writing; keep a copy and send one to the appropriate agency if no action is taken; the law protects against firing for a workplace complaint. Workers (including nurses, dental assistants, x-ray technicians, and monitors at airport checkpoints) should wear a film badge; stand at least 6' away from x-ray source; wear lead shields; limit time with clients with radioactive implants; and use gloves/forceps and appropriate disposal procedures for contaminated items. Parents should inspect schools for asbestos and unsafe laboratory or physical education practices (Mancino, 1983).
8. Noise	Wear earplugs if exposed to loud engines; plan some time daily in a quiet, restful environment; ensure employers monitor noise levels; union representa-

Table 51 *(continued)*

Harmful substance/ occurrence	Protective measures
	tives have the right to observe monitoring and obtain records; by law, hearing protectors must be available to workers exposed to 85 DB or more (OSHA Standards, 1981).
9. Acid Rain	Wear protective covering on hair and skin when out in the rain; work with environmentalists to control the effects of acid rain.
10. Pos-ions	Spend time out of hermetically sealed buildings, preferably at the seashore or mountains; take a shower daily; walk amongst plants and trees daily.
11. Light Sunlight	Wear a sunscreen (PABA) and protective clothing when in direct sunlight; avoid long hours in the sun.
Fluorescent light	Choose full-spectrum fluorescent light if full-spectrum natural light is not available; if in a tightly sealed building during daylight hours, walk to work or park 20 minutes from work; go outside during lunch and breaks; avoid sunglasses; use Vitalites for desk or kitchen lighting.

Use of Color to Enhance Wellness

Table 52 shows use of color to heal. Colors can be worn or colored gel filters can be taped over the bulb of a lamp and placed 4'–8' away and used in natural, indirect light. Colored paper or fabric swatches can also be used.

The Effect of a Natural Setting on Wellness

A recent study examined the effect of environment on healing (Ulrich, 1984). The records of 46 post-cholescystectomy clients in a suburban Pennsylvania hospital were examined to determine whether assignment to a room with a window view of a natural setting might have restorative influence. Twenty-three clients assigned to rooms with windows looking out on a natural setting had shorter postoperative stays, received fewer negative evaluative comments in nurses' notes, and took fewer potent analgesics than 23 matched clients with windows facing a brick building wall.

Table 52. Use of Color to Heal

Color	Reported effect
Red	Invigorates, stimulates, energizes. Good for anemia, poor blood circulation, liver and heart conditions. Not suggested for use in highly emotional states.
Pink	Use for pelvic problems, hip and buttock tenderness. Stimulates caring and love.
Orange	Invigorates and stimulates feeling and endocrine action; stimulates confidence, respiratory action, relieves gas and sluggish digestion, drains infections, decreases menstrual discomfort. Wearing an orange scarf around the neck is useful for thyroid conditions.
Yellow	Stimulates the nervous system and brain activity. Increases receptivity for knowledge, self-confidence, appetite, enhances liver and gall bladder functions. Assists in dissolving arthritic deposits.
Lemon (yellow with some green)	Cleans mucus, activates the thymus gland, builds bone, speeds up the healing process of a cold. Relieves the body of muscular tension.
Green	Stabilizes and calms. Used for high blood pressure, hot flashes, menopause, infections, and resistance to healing. Stimulates the pituitary.
Turquoise	Reduces aches and pains, skin conditions.
Blue	Stimulates the pineal gland and deep sleep. Assists with fever process.
Indigo	Sedative. Reduces swelling and pain. Firms skin.
Violet	Muscle relaxant. Builds white blood cells and depresses the appetite.
Purple	Slows heart rate and reduces heart pain. Increases venous drainage during systemic congestion and excessive menstruation.
Scarlet	Stimulates heart rate and arterial action. Revives kidney and adrenal function.
All colors	Sunlight. The great healer for all conditions.

Source: D. Berkson, *The Foot Book*. New York: Harper and Row, 1977, pp. 204–206.

INTEGRATIVE LEARNING EXPERIENCES

Beginning Level

1. Assess the environmental factors influencing your level of wellness. Discuss these with a peer and devise an action plan (in writing with realistic dates for evaluating and rewarding progress). Refer to Table 51 for ideas.
2. Write to one or more of the wellness-oriented nursing organizations listed in the epilogue for further information.
3. Identify the specific environmental contributions for clients with the following conditions:

   A. Birth defects
   B. Spontaneous abortion
   C. Upper respiratory ailments/difficulty breathing
   D. Cancer risk
   E. High absenteeism
   F. High blood pressure
   G. Bone disease in clients receiving dialysis
   H. Neurological symptoms
   I. Skin irritation/rashes
   J. Asbestosis
   K. Loss of appetite, constipation, nausea, tremors, weakness, numbness, colic, and kidney disease
   L. Hearing loss, elevated blood pressure, tension, nervousness, fluid imbalances
   M. Fatigue, tension, hyperactivity
   N. Circulatory difficulties
   O. Cataracts

4. Investigate the use of color in your lifestyle and its effects. Devise a plan to use color as an environmental intervention.

Advanced Level

1. Collaborate with three clients to devise a plan to enhance their environmental wellness.

REFERENCES

Abrams, H. (1979). The "overutilization" of x-rays. *NEJ Med* 300(21):1213–1216.
Ager, B., and Tickner, J. (1983). The control of microbiological hazards associated with air-conditioning and ventilating systems. *Annals Occuptl Hyg* 27(4):346–358.

Bongard, F., et al. (1981). Fatal hospital-acquired burns. *JAMA* 252(20):2813.

Brown, H., Bishop, D., and Rowan, C. (1984). Drinking water safety. *Am J PH* 74:479.

Bryce, R., and Enkin, M. (1984). Lifestyle in pregnancy. *Can Phys* 30:2127–2130.

Clark, C. C. (1981). Reader queries: safe ways to control insects. *The Wellness Newsletter* 2(5):3.

Clark, C. C. (1982). Are you picking up harmful radiation? *The Wellness Newsletter* 3(5):3.

Clark, C. C. (1983). From the editor. *The Wellness Newsletter* 4(5):1–2.

Diamond, J. (1979). *Behavioral Kinesiology*. New York: Harper and Row.

Dickson, D. (1979). US academy denies threshold for radiation. *Nature* 279:90–91.

Diesendorf, M. (1980). Is there a scientific basis for fluoridation? A review of the report by the Royal College of Physicians. *Com Hlth Studies* 4(3):224–230.

Don, F. (1977). *Color Your World*. New York: Warner Destiny Books.

Epstein, S. (1978). *The Politics of Cancer*. San Francisco: Sierra Club.

Fagerstrom, K. (1984). Effects of nicotine chewing gum and follow up appointments in physician-based smoking cessation. *Prev Med* 13(5):517–527.

Forskningsroen, N. (1984). Passive smoking and the infant. *Tobaken Och Vi* 29(3): 7–9.

Fumigants used in the food industry. (1983). *Staying Alive Safety and Health News of the Food and Beverage Trades* 22:1–2.

Garrison, R. H. (1985). *Nutrition Desk Reference*. New Canaan, CT: Keats Publishing Co., p. 65.

George, A. (1985). Measurement of sources and air concentrations of radon and radon daughters in residential buildings. Paper presented at the ASHRAE Semi-Annual Meeting, June 23–27, Atlanta, GA.

Houck, C. (1979). Caution: artificial light may be hazardous to your health. *Review* March:27–34.

Indoor air pollution and S. 1198 fact sheet. (1985). Washington, D.C.: Consumer Federation of America, p. 1.

Is AJN relevant to nursing? (1980). *Nurse's Environmental Health Watch* 1(1):6.

Keough, C. (1980). *Water Fit to Drink*. Emmaus, PA: Rodale Press, Inc.

Liberati, L. (1982). *Lawrence Rev Natural Prods* 3(1):1.

Mancino, D. (1983). Creating a safe hospital environment. *The Wellness Newsletter* 4(5):3–5.

Mendelsohn, R. (1979). *Confessions of a Medical Heretic*. Chicago, IL: Contemporary Books, Inc.

Naeye, R., and Peter, E. (1984). Mental development of children whose mothers smoked during pregnancy. *Obstetrics and Gyn* 64(5):601–607.

NIH. (1980). *Basic Concepts of Environmental Health*. Research Triangle Park, NC: NIH Publication #80-1254.

OSHA standards: 1981 to 1984. (1984). *Exposure* 41:8–11.

Ott, J. (1973). *Health and Light*. New York: Simon and Schuster.

Rall, D. (1984). Toxic agent and radiation control: meeting the 1990 objectives for the nation. *Public Health Reports* 99(6):532–538.

Raloff, J. (1982). Noise can be hazardous to our health. *Sci News* 121:377–381.

Randolf, T., and Moss, R. (1980). *An Alternative Approach to Allergies*. New York: Harper and Row.

Regne, J. (1984). More than what you drink. *Exposure* 41:2.

Rosenfield, A. (1978). Forecast: poisonous rain. *Saturday Rev* Sept:16–17.

Sandler, D., et al. (1985). Cancer risk in adulthood from early exposure to parents' smoking. *Am J PH* 75(5):487–492.

Soyka, F. (1977). *The Ion Effect.* New York: Bantam.

Tedesco, P. (1982). ANA delegates take two strong environmental stands. *Health Watch* 3(2):1, 9.

Ulrich, R. (1984). View through a window may influence recovery from surgery. *Science* 224:420–421.

U.S. Dept. HEW. (1977). Statistics needed for determining the effects of the environment on health. Hyattsville, MD: Office of Health Research, Statistics, and Technology.

Voldman, E. (1983). Socially accepted drugs and pregnancy. I. Cigarettes and pregnancy. *Revista de Obstet y Gyn de Venezuela* 43(2):59–61.

Watchdog. (1981). *Exposure* 9(July):1.

9

COMMUNITY WELLNESS PROGRAMS

This chapter presents the following information:

- Justification for community wellness programs
- Assessing wellness program needs
- A survey of wellness programs in industry, hospitals, and clinics
- A community assessment tool
- A sampling of federally funded community wellness programs
- Suggestions for planning and implementing wellness programs
- Methods of evaluating wellness programs

JUSTIFICATION FOR COMMUNITY WELLNESS PROGRAMS

Common sense dictates that preventing illness saves money, yet the majority of the health care dollar is spent on treating illness, not preventing it. Over $387 billion (almost 10.6% of the gross national product) was spent on illness care in the United States in 1984. Corporations paid $77 billion of this bill. Cardiovascular disease costs the U.S. economy $80 billion annually. Drug abuse costs the economy $26 billion/year. The annual economic cost of cigarette smoking amounts to $47.5 billion. About 29 million workdays, representing over $2 billion in earnings, are lost each year because of coronary heart disease, hypertensive disease, and stroke. Cancer is the second leading cause of death in the United States and accounts for about 420,000 deaths a year. Tobacco's contribution to all cancer deaths is estimated to be 30%. Eighty-five percent of lung cancer deaths are due to cigarette smoking. An estimated 30 million workers (or 30% of the 100 million employed persons) are at increased risk of developing heart disease, stroke, and kidney disease because of high blood pressure. Data from three National Heart, Lung, and Blood Institute-sponsored demonstration projects show that workplace high blood pressure control programs are effective in controlling employee hypertension.

It has been estimated that the average one-pack-plus per day smoker, over a lifetime, may cost the company between $335 and $600 per year in extra expenses (absenteeism, illness care costs, etc.) as compared with an equivalent nonsmoking employee. The American Health Foundation estimates that if the company does not pay for time off to attend smoking cessation sessions, but does pay the majority of program costs, the average cost per quitter should be less than $200, assuming a quit rate of 50% after 1 year.

It has been estimated that a "typical recreational drug user" in the workforce is late three times more often than fellow employees, requests early dismissal or time off during work 2.2 times more often, has 2.5 times as many absences of 8 days or more, uses 3 times the normal level of sick benefits, is 5 times more likely to file a workers' compensation claim, and is involved in accidents 3.6 times more often than other employees. For every $1 invested in treatment in their program, General Motors can identify $3 in return for employees who recover fully. Phillips Petroleum Company reports that its program saves more than $8 million a year in fewer accidents, less sick leave, and higher productivity. Kimberly-Clark experienced a 43% reduction in absenteeism and a 70% reduction in accidents among a sample of employees who participated in a corporate drug and alcohol abuse program ("The Magnitude of the Problem," 1983).

A number of studies have provided information regarding how wellness programs reduce illness care costs or affect behavior positively. Shepherd et al. (1982) reported the influence of an employee fitness and lifestyle modification on illness care costs. They assessed use of illness care utilization for 534 employees of two life insurance companies. Claims were examined for the year prior to the program and the year in which an employee fitness and lifestyle change program was initiated in one of the insurance companies. Employees of the company with the fitness and lifestyle modification program had fewer hospital days and fewer claims of all types than employees of the control company. The fitness and lifestyle modification program benefited employees at all levels of participation in the program, suggesting an overall improvement of lifestyle rather than a specific effect of exercise. Total savings averaged $84.50 per employee per year.

A randomized controlled trial of antismoking advice for 10 years

(Rose et al., 1982) provided advice to 1,445 male smokers aged 40–59 at high risk of cardiorespiratory disease. After 1 year reported cigarette consumption in the intervention group (714 men) was one fourth that of the control group (731 men). At 10 years the reported reduction averaged 53%. Over 10 years death from coronary heart disease was 18% lower and mortality from lung cancer was 23% lower in the intervention group than in the control group. However, deaths from other types of cancer were significantly higher in the intervention group. The nonlung cancers seemed unrelated to changes in smoking habits.

Pillsbury Company's Be Your Best Program has offerings in three life style areas: (1) fitness and exercise, (2) nutrition and weight control, and (3) mental well-being and stress management. Twice a year the complete program, featuring assessments to determine health risk factors and education workshops, is offered to 200 employees. The most significant benefit is that employees who participate in the program submit fewer claims and that those claims submitted were less costly than claims made prior to involvement in the program. The program director estimates that for the year 1981–1982 there was a $3.63 return on every $1.00 invested in the program.

Some of the major difficulties in obtaining data to support wellness program efforts are: the time lag between starting the program and seeing an impact, difficulty in analyzing individual components of the program to distinguish cause and effect relationships, and self-selection of participants.

Although not focused on employees, a study completed by Vickery et al. (1983) provides support for the cost benefits of educating clients about their own care. A prospective randomized, controlled trial of self-care educational intervention conducted in an HMO showed statistically significant decreases in total medical visits and minor illness visits in three experimental groups as compared to the control group. The results were clearly linked to receiving books and a newsletter presenting self-care information. A telephone information service was available but was not used. Estimated savings in utilization were between $2.50 and $3.50 for each dollar spent on the educational interventions. The addition of a nurse counseling session to the written information was suggested as a way to further increase cost savings and appeared to be attractive to high utilizers of services.

ASSESSING WELLNESS PROGRAM NEEDS

All communities, schools, companies, and agencies can benefit from wellness programs. Many have already developed them; however, they may have been based on what the planners believed were important; a wellness view includes the client in the planning process. Some questions to ask and methods to use to begin to assess the wellness program needs have been suggested by Parkinson (1982, pp. 22–26):

- What are the sociodemographic characteristics of the population? (Determine age, sex, ethnic origin, occupation, employment status, education, and residence using a health history or risk-appraisal form.)
- What are the costs of health care, disability benefits, and insurance premiums for the population? (Determine number and cost, including any insurance claims, and average the rate by the number of people; determine the number, frequency, duration, and costs of incidental and disability absences.)
- What are the use patterns for health care by the population? (Determine what kinds of preventive and wellness issues are brought to health care providers, what chronic and acute conditions are being treated; talk with health care providers and obtain summaries of use patterns if possible.)
- What conditions or diseases are present or potential in the population? (Randomly sample the population or obtain a representative sample and use written questionnaires, phone interviews, or one-to-one interviews to obtain information; determine blood pressure, height, weight, lipids, blood sugar, and other information indicative of wellness state; survey current lifestyle habits (nutrition, exercise/movement, stress management skills, parenting skills, communication skills, knowledge of how to obtain wellness information, self-care skills, smoking, drinking, use of drugs and medications); if necessary, determine those at highest risk and plan programming accordingly)
- What wellness programs are currently available for the population? (Talk with providers of programs and participants or use questionnaires to obtain needed information; for certain populations, the media may publicize programs; in these cases, obtain information from the media or public relations department.)
- How effective are the current wellness programs in enhancing wellness? (Obtain evaluation information from program providers and interview or survey participants.)
- What wellness needs does the population identify? (Interview or survey the population or a representative sample.)
- What kinds of wellness programs does the population think should be included? (Interview or survey the population or a representative sample.)

- What are the levels of needs in the population—awareness, knowledge, change in attitudes, change in behavior, reduction in risk or reduction in disease or death? (If sufficient funds and time are available, all levels can be developed; if not, use interview, survey, and information collected from the results of answering the above questions to make a determination.)

Community Assessment

The Community Assessment (Table 53) gives information for assessing wellness in a community.

Table 53. Community Assessment

Who and What is the Community?

1. How is space distributed and used? (Buildings, crowded areas, natural and physical barriers to social interaction, parks, playgrounds?)

2. How safe and healthful are work and school environments? (Are smokers and nonsmokers segregated? Are junk food and cigarette vending machines highly accessible? Are alternatives offered? Is the use of stairways promoted? Are they accessible? Well lit? Is car pooling encouraged? Is flex time used to allow employees time to engage in wellness activities before work or during lunch? Are high quality child care services available for residents? Are buildings well ventilated and do they have adequate natural light and sufficient work/learning space?)

3. What are the cultural mix and stability of the population? (Are there one or more cultural groups living in harmony or in conflict, and how much acculturation and stress occur due to people who move in or out of the area?)

4. What are the age, sex, and family groupings? (Elderly population, single-occupancy commuter group, young marrieds with children, singles, a mix?)

5. What income levels are represented and to what extent? (Wealthy? Middle class? Poor people receiving governmental or charitable assistance for health care? Or a mix?)

6. What are the occupational levels? (Hard driving executives who leave the family's health concerns to their wives? Action-oriented population that learns by doing? A mix? What does the occupational level tell you about the population's education, health problems, problem solving patterns, and methods of learning?)

7. What community resources are available and where are they? (Where are the schools, hospitals, shopping areas, and clinics located in relation to available transportation? What self-help or supportive groups and services exist in the community? What facilities are there for wellness programs? What space could be developed to provide further wellness services? What skills or resources do the residents have that could be shared through a wellness program exchange? Is there any way to trade unused sick leave for a well day? Could unused sick leave be converted to cash? Do faculty, bosses, or town legislators support personal health promotion objectives? Can additional rewards or incentives be built into the current health/

Table 53. *(continued)*

illness insurance programs without taking away existing benefits? If there are company or school-subsidized cafeterias, could wellness-promoting foods be subsidized more than junk foods?)

How Are Needs Met?

1. Are needs met or prevented from being met by space, culture, age, sex, family, income, occupational level, or community resource factors?

2. What do the community's clergy, health care practitioners, welfare agencies, and clients know about what needs are not being met?

3. What do records of health services, worker's compensation claims, and accident and safety records tell you about how needs are met and what wellness needs are not being met?

4. What do questionnaire or survey methods tell you about what community residents say are the types of wellness activities they would participate in if offered?

5. What specific risk factors exist in this population and how are they being addressed or not?

6. How can family members of community residents be considered in planning wellness programs and used to provide needed support systems?

How Are Deviance and Disturbance Handled?

1. Are those with psychiatric/mental health difficulties rejected by the community? In what way?

2. How are homosexuals, delinquents, or those who abuse alcohol, drugs, or food treated by community members?

3. What political, educational, or social views lead to rejection of those who deviate from the norm?

4. Are there humane or highly institutionalized agencies available in the community to help deal with deviant members? What are they?

5. Does the community reject the idea of placing treatment facilities for its deviants within the community? How?

6. Is there a prevailing view that people who deviate from accepted behavioral patterns should be punished? How is this belief put into practice?

How Are Identities Developed?

1. How do families, faculty, administrators, etc. teach their members to act?

2. What kinds of religious/spiritual organizations or groups exist in the community and what is their prevailing view of human motivation?

3. What youth agencies/helpers are there and how do young people relate to them?

4. What kind of formal and special education programs are available and how are they used by the community?

5. How could already existing agencies or groups be used more effectively?

How Are Community Functions Accomplished?

1. Are community decisions made before adequate information has been obtained? What possible effect(s) might this have?

2. Are decisions made by default, based on the personal concerns of a few, or made by consensus? What are the consequences of this type of decision making?

3. Is communication fragmented and inefficient? How does such communication seem to affect the community?

4. Are communication messages based on a sense of community ("We're all in this together") or on stereotypes and the establishment of distance between groups ("It's us against them")? What are the effects of both types of communication messages?

5. How accurately do the local media convey information to the community?

6. Are there informal (rumor) communication channels?

7. Are problems solved informally with board and committee meetings used only to record earlier decisions? How might this affect the community or the decision-making process?

8. How are ad hoc, neighborhood, or block associations used in decision making?

9. How readily are newcomers accepted by the community?

10. Is leadership concentrated among a few groups or is it widely distributed in the community?

11. Are there wide vacillations in power or frequent changes in the power base that could affect health planning or treatment?

12. Where is power located, how is it perceived, and how is it used?

13. What overlapping areas and missing links are there in wellness services?

14. What segments in the community are receptive and hostile to outside influence?

15. Is there a sense of trust between community members and leaders?

16. Is there community disintegration? (Has a recent disaster, widespread ill health, extensive poverty, confusion of cultural values, weakening of religious affiliations, extensive migration of new groups, or rapid social change radically affected the community?)

What Are the Resistances to Change in This Community?

1. What factors in the system will be affected as a result of a change toward wellness?

2. What forces are operating to inhibit change toward wellness?

3. What information or experiences must precede the change toward wellness?

4. What new procedures or experiences will need to be developed as a result of a movement toward wellness?

5. Who is likely to suffer from the change?

6. How aware are community residents of the need for change?

7. Are community residents sufficiently involved in planning for the change?

Table 53 *(continued)*

8. What is the relationship between the change agent and community residents?

9. What past relationship between the change agent and the client might be influencing resistance to change now?

10. How open have community residents been to the introduction of change in the past?

11. How can free and open communication, administrative support of and reward for problem solving efforts, shared decision making, sufficient time to problem solve, written statements of what the change goals will be, professionalism, concern for long-term planning, cohesiveness among change agents, feelings of security among residents, timing, and resident confidence in ability to change be enhanced to lower resistance to change?

A SURVEY OF WELLNESS PROGRAMS IN INDUSTRY, HOSPITALS, AND CLINICS

In 1983 the author conducted a survey of 149 Fortune 500 company executives, 129 hospital and clinic administrators in the New York–New Jersey–Connecticut area, and 79 subscribers to *The Wellness Newsletter* (1983). Newsletter subscribers working as wellness enhancers were the most responsive (52.23% of the surveys returned); health care agency administrators returned 42.64%, and corporate executives returned 33.56%.

The most frequently offered programs were: lose weight, stop smoking, increase fitness, reduce stress, stop smoking, and lower blood pressure. As expected, wellness promoters provided the greatest number of wellness programs (except for avoiding injury at work and combatting alcohol and drug dependency). This is not a surprising finding since corporate and workplace wellness programs have been well established in these areas for some time. It is interesting, if perhaps predictable, that health care agencies provide so few programs; either this is a fertile field for wellness-prepared nurses or a highly resistive one.

In each setting, nurses scored high as providers of wellness programs; nurses were the most frequently mentioned providers by all three populations. This is interesting since many nursing programs do not currently provide wellness and preventive foci in their curriculums, yet nurses are expected by others to provide preventive actions.

Respondents were asked their reaction to a wellness educational degree component for nurses and employers' possible use of its graduates. Between 61% (health care agencies) and 95% (wellness promoters) thought it was needed. Perhaps more nursing schools should be developing wellness nursing tracks, minor subject concentrations, or entire curricula based on a wellness conceptual framework.

Respondents were asked their reaction to having wellness nursing students and graduates work for them. Wellness promoters were the most enthusiastic; nearly 80% would take students and more than half would hire graduates of such programs. Health care agencies were also quite willing; 72% would take students, but claimed that economic cutbacks might make it difficult for them to hire nurses with wellness skills. This is surprising since wellness is thought to reduce costs, but it may reveal lack of awareness of this concept (and, indeed, more than 25% responded that the cost benefits of wellness were not known to them), or possibly reluctance to move toward prevention and risk loss of an available population.

Many of the larger corporations already had active wellness programs implemented; some contract with outside resources such as YM-YWCAs and would not require additional staff. The small and/or highly diversified corporations also did not seem to need the assistance of wellness students or graduates. The medium-sized corporations seemed most eager to obtain consultation and would take students and later hire graduates of a wellness nursing program.

SOME FEDERALLY FUNDED COMMUNITY WELLNESS PROGRAMS

Currently, the federally-funded Center for Health Promotion and Education gives grants to states to focus on high-risk populations. Some of the current efforts are as follows:

1. The Detroit Health Department is conducting a program targeting 12- to 24-year-old females who receive obstetric, gynecologic, or family planning services. The primary target audience is women at risk because of drinking or smoking during pregnancy or use of oral contraceptives. Interventions are stages in clinics. Methods used include verbal, visual, and audiovisual communication, skills training, behavior modification, social contracting, and modeling. The level of risk is determined individually and each client is then assigned to one of four modules: *maintenance* to monitor clients who have quit smoking or drinking for at least 6 months; *coping* to help clients who have quit smoking or drinking within the past 6 months to maintain abstinence; *high-risk* to assist clients to reduce or quit cigarette smoking and alcohol, focused on women using oral contraceptives; *prevention* to help clients sustain nonsmoking and nondrinking. Clients are administered a pretest to

evaluate knowledge, attitudes, and beliefs and an assessment survey to determine risk factors. Clients complete a 7-day diary, social-contract forms, a cigarette-monitoring chart, learn relaxation techniques, complete a life-change test and a personal stress analysis form, and complete an assertiveness-training and values-clarification exercise (J. C. Hill, Detroit Health Department, 1151 Taylor St., Detroit, MI 48202).

2. Hocking Technical College in Ohio has developed a Community Health Education Center that serves a four-county area. The primary target groups are adolescents and their families, particularly ninth graders at risk for smoking and alcohol abuse. Approximately 800 students and 200 families are currently enrolled in the program. Secondary targets are civic groups, employees, elementary and secondary school teachers, health providers, and the general public. Services are provided in schools and homes, at community places, worksites, and on the campus. Skills training, simulation, cognitive learning, and direct communication via verbal and audiovisual media are used. Efforts to raise public awareness are conducted through the mass media. The school health curriculum focuses on smoking, alcohol, and stress, consisting of a 10-unit course emphasizing wellness and responsible decision making. Role playing, games, self-assessments, discussion, goal-directed projects, and films are used to enhance learning and induce change. Home visits are made by family health workers who assess families, develop lists of goals and priorities, and provide counseling. Consumer health efforts focus on small-group classes and workshops on weight maintenance, hypertension control, fitness, stress management, and smoking cessation. Each course has four to six units. Informational presentations are provided to civic groups. Newspaper articles and weekly radio broadcasts provide information via the mass media. Evaluation of the program consists of a life style questionnaire administered to each family before and after a minimum of four home visits, a questionnaire on smoking and alcohol administered to control- and experimental-group students, pre- and post-tests administered to participants in small-group classes and workshops, and an administrative planning tool used to predict future needs and alternatives and allocate resources. Results of the evaluation tools administered to 227 ninth graders indicate the program has made significant positive changes in students' alcohol knowledge, attitudes toward drinking, problem-solving skills regarding alcohol use, and attitudes and knowledge about smoking. Risk factors targeted for families and the community at large are smoking, inactivity, obesity, hypertension, and poor nutrition. Resource materials are used to address the risk factors. In the future the program will expand to offer services to business, industry, and possibly elementary schools (E. Bonaguro, Hocking Technical College, Route 1, Nelsonville, OH 45764).

3. The Education Services Center in Austin, Texas is targeting the students in grades 4–12 of one school district. Children of alcoholics constitute a specific subgroup within the primary group. Methods used include skills training, cognitive learning, direct verbal communication, and modeling. Students in grades 4–7 also use behavioral contracts. Personnel dealing with children of alcoholics learn cognitive skills and visual and verbal communication skills. Other school personnel, parents, and community representatives receive skills training, cognitive learning, modeling, simulation, and direct communication via visual, verbal, audio, and audiovisual media. The project consists of five components: 4th–7th graders participate in a survey of tobacco and alcohol use, attitudes, and knowledge; teachers' perceptions of students' use patterns are also surveyed. Students learn about decision-making processes and interview adults about their decision-making processes concerning alcohol and tobacco use. Students at the high school level receive a pretest, group development activities, analysis of the pretest, personal motivation sessions, activities designed to examine the smoking habit, discussion of ways to abstain, administration of a post-test, and a maintenance-building activity. The 9-hour program (teachers receive a 1-day training workshop to teach the segment) has been implemented in four high schools. The third component involves training for establishing peer counseling and student leadership. The fourth component involves training and technical assistance to 20 school personnel regarding the needs of children of alcoholics and of strategies for meeting those needs in school settings. The fifth component involves training and technical assistance to relevant committees in identifying and using community resources and implementing prevention programs. Data collected from the 4th–7th graders indicates the program has lowered the proportion of students who plan to use tobacco from 21 to 10% and raised the proportion of students who believe that tobacco use is harmful from 58 to 79%. Data from the four high schools indicate that all participants reduced their use of cigarettes by at least 33%, developed better self-images, and learned new information about the smoking habit. Two of the three schools have developed peer counseling and student leadership programs. The project uses a social contract curriculum developed by project staff for 4th through 7th graders, the Youth Smoking Cessation Program model developed by the American Cancer Society for high school students, and various resource and program development manuals, packages, and reports (C. Hull, Education Services Center, Region XIII, 7703 North Lamar Blvd., Austin, TX 78752).

4. The Utah Navajo Development Council has developed a program to combat alcohol and tobacco use for 350 5th graders on the 8,000-

square-mile Navajo Reserve in southeastern Utah. The school-based component involves simulation, skills training, and direct communication. Trained high school students act as peer role models and facilitators for the 5th grade curriculum. The 5th graders receive 12 lessons concerning alcohol and tobacco information, decision-making skills, resistance to persuasion, coping skills, and self-cultural awareness. The clinical- and community-based interventions provide informative material in the Navajo language on the nature of alcohol and tobacco, short- and long-term effects of use, parent-child relationships, promotion of preventive health, and coping skills. The program has been hampered by the loss of 20% of the peer facilitators during the first year and poor relationships between peer facilitators and teachers. Risk factors addressed include smoking, alcohol abuse, and other cancer and cardiovascular disease risk factors. The program plans to expand the school-based component to reach 4th and 6th graders. The preliminary impact of the program has been generally positive (G. Nelson, Utah Navajo Development Council, PO Box 908, Blanding, UT 84511).

5. A program in one Washington county targets students for preventing alcohol and tobacco use in grades 6–8. Interventions take place in schools and youth organization settings. Methods include cognitive learning, skills training, simulation, and direct communication. Eight sessions of small group work (8–10 people) use video equipment and make short television programs about alcohol, tobacco, peer pressure, and resistance to peer pressure. Participants are evaluated using pre- and post-tests and followup tests administered 2 and 6 months after the sessions. Results from the first project year indicate at the 2-month followup participants have a 41% increase in knowledge about drinking, a 28% increase in knowledge about smoking, and a decline in drinking. Video training sessions, log books, curriculum outlines, and lesson plans and evaluation instruments are used (J. Weiss, Project Health! Drug Abuse Council, 2730 Pine Street, Everett, WA 98201).

PLANNING AND IMPLEMENTING WELLNESS PROGRAMS

Worksite Wellness Programs

Parkinson (1982, p. 9) suggests that a worksite wellness program focus on all of the following: high blood pressure control, smoking control, drug/alcohol abuse control, weight control and nutrition education, exercise/physical fitness, early cancer detection, accident prevention/self-protective measures against environmental and other hazards in the workplace, and stress management.

Goldbeck (1984) contends that wellness programs at the worksite are not only focused on the individual but also the factors in the institution that decrease wellness, including emotional wellness. He states worksite wellness leaders face the following challenges:

- devising programs available to and adapted for dependents and retirees
- integrating wellness with the medical model of delivery without becoming subordinate to it
- keeping open to new research and innovation, including visualization to assist in cancer remission, etc.
- maintaining integrity when wellness clashes with the traditional rules of corporate behavior
- restricting the use of health risk appraisals, executive physicals, and other assessment tools to programs that assure education and followup

Factors Affecting the Success or Failure of a Worksite Wellness Program

Although a complete program is recommended, what is developed is based on expressed employee needs. A major factor in a successful program (or in implementing any kind of change) is the participation of those involved in planning and implementation. Employees can be contacted initially through questionnaires, surveys, or small group meetings to provide input. When the participants "own" the program, they will be motivated to participate in it. Many programs are beautifully planned by administrators but fail to gain acceptance because participants had no input and were not concerned with the same issues as the planners.

Canton and Monroe (1984) suggest that wellness planners must be cognizant of and learn to track and understand new work attitudes which include:

- dissatisfaction with the nature of work
- dissatisfaction with authority
- increased pursuit of leisure
- development and reinforcement of personal identity outside the workplace
- a shift from expecting work to provide security, power, and status to providing self-esteem, support, creativity, affiliation, autonomy, challenge, growth, learning, and well-being

- feelings of uncertainty, insecurity, and anxiety due to rapid societal changes
- an increasing role for women in leadership

Canton and Monroe (1984) add to the list of problems that cause failure in wellness programs and suggest ways for wellness nursing practitioners to anticipate and work through issues before they arise. Sources of failures are *organizational* (insufficient job design, improper work tasks, lack of supervision, insufficient administration, inadequate training, lack of career development, improper work roles, lack of power, or lack of authority); *program problems* (insufficient expertise of the persons in charge, inadequate quality of the program, improper program-environment-person fit, inadequate program goals and plan comprehensiveness, insufficient availability of resources, inadequate time available to implement the program, lack of practicality of the program design and strategies or inappropriate incentive systems); *people problems* (relate to the nature of program support by top-level management or participants, the values and norms of the organizational climate, degree of interpersonal conflict in the organization and competency of program facilitators); *systemic problems* (employees feel over/underworked, burdened/unchallenged, sexually or racially harassed or powerless or are continually exposed to hazardous working conditions or toxic substances; labor-management conflicts; profit motive receives more support than human resource development).

The Life Gain Program: An Example of a Systems Approach to Wellness

The design and implementation of a worksite wellness program should be conceptualized as part of an overall systems approach that enhances the quality of work life as well as increases productivity and reduces absenteeism and health care costs. When viewing the work system as a whole, work and anti-wellness factors are identified, existing problems are pinpointed, total organizational participation and support is encouraged, and long-term benefit and followup are planned for.

When planning programs from an open systems view, interventions are based on:

- involving relevant people in a meaningful way in the planning process
- choosing powerful incentives and stating them clearly so employees will be motivated to participate
- involving employee families in programs
- encouraging employees to be responsible for wellness behaviors

- using innovative and creative approaches to relevant problems
- ensuring confidentiality
- ensuring a positive effect on teamwork, trust, communication, productivity, cooperation, and power
- affecting long-term attitudinal and behavioral changes
- choosing attainable and realistic program goals
- planning followup for each phase of the program
- choosing a convenient location and program length
- designing an evaluation plan prior to initiating the program
- ensuring program goals reflect a consensus of participants
- completing a needs assessment of the population at risk
- training facilitators adequately
- emphasizing free choice, participation, open communication, trust, and experiential learning
- blending individual and organizational tasks, goals, and needs
- developing a realistic timetable
- addressing the personal, occupational, familial, social, and environmental aspects of well-being
- deciding whether a prepackaged or individualized program best meets the system's needs
- identifying and intervening in resistances to introduction of a wellness program
- addressing ethical issues
- addressing labor and management issues
- identifying ways to connect wellness programs to other employee assistance programs
- ensuring an adequate budget

When two or more people share goals over time, a culture develops. Many negative norms pervade work cultures. Common sense implies that everyone wants to be well and if the appropriate information and tools are provided, people will change toward wellness. In many work cultures (including hospitals) there are pervasive feelings of helplessness and powerlessness. The culture (or "system") is conceptualized as an amorphous mass that influences the worker while it eludes change. "This pervasive feeling that we cannot do anything about it is one of the most important initial obstacles that challenges any change program" (Allen & Kraft, p. 77).

The Normative Systems approach called Life Gain (Allen & Kraft, pp. 77–78) assists employees to work on both individual and cultural variables to effect change. Small groups work together to design and modify their cultural norms until commonly shared goals are found. Through the work group members become aware of the cultural norms of the groups to which they belong and see its impact on them. They also learn they have a choice and that norms can be chosen that sustain and support them and lifestyle changes. The method has been used effectively to change delinquent subcultures into responsible groups, supermarkets from objects of crime and pilferage to places for honesty and openness, communities that litter to clean communities, businesses from mediocrity and low productivity to places where the norm is excellence and high productivity, and police-neighborhood relations from violence to friendship and respect.

The Life-Gain System for organizational and community change includes the following four phases:

- *Start-up:* obtain leadership commitment; analyze/set goals; develop task forces to tailor a program around the specific needs of the organization/community; collect baseline data to measure progress
- *Involvement:* workshops exposing participants to alternatives and participation in wellness self-assessment procedures and goal-setting procedures; workshops not begun until a supportive environment has been well established among the change agent team members; participants identify the particular norms influencing their wellness and work together to systematically change the norms that get in the way of achieving their goals; a buddy system is used for verifying progress after the workshop; modeling of wellness behaviors by leaders is an effective motivating factor; in corporate environments, the modeling effect is most effective when workshops are started with the highest level of management first
- *Initiating change:* general support groups, specialized support groups, self-help programs, task-force programs; participants freely choose groups to which to belong; information and resources are presented, but the group members select which are right for them; printed and audiovisual self-help information is available to participants; as a reinforcement mechanism, graduates of the workshop are invited to join organizational task forces created in the start-up phase; skill training in behaviors relevant to each dimension of wellness is available; incentives including awards, citations, public praise, and money are given as reinforcements; intrinsic rewards from participating are fun and the pleasure of well-being
- *Sustaining change:* family members become involved in the program; reinforcement of one's own change process occurs when participants reach out to help family members; evaluation data are gathered to discern how well the program is accomplishing its objectives; individuals receive feedback on their progress in small short report meetings, newsletters, and bulletins; the Organiza-

tional Support Indicator measure is readministered regularly to note organizational progress toward providing more supportive environments for change; an active alumni organization brings in new information in programs; regular renewal meetings are held; a range of communication devices are available to help participants keep abreast of new wellness information and maintain improvements

Prior to implementing any major program, a pilot or small sample run-through is recommended (Brennan, 1983). Such an approach can head off any major problems, fine tune the program, and reveal if learning methods are appropriate and if proper data are being collected.

Reducing Smoking at the Worksite

Employers are beginning to realize the impact of smoking on the health and productivity of smokers and nonsmokers. Absentee, accident, and hospitalization rates are all at least 50% higher for smoking employees than for nonsmokers. Employers have been held legally responsible for at least part of the disability costs for smoking employees who contracted smoking-related illnesses and for claims of adverse effects from nonsmoking employees (Behrens, 1985, p. 5). Other costs borne by employers due to smoking include: excess office maintenance, increased depreciation of office equipment and furniture, increased insurance costs, increased ventilation needs, lower employee morale, decreased productivity, and increased risk of fire (Behrens, 1985, p. 7).

Two recent studies illustrate that smokers and nonsmokers are concerned about smoking at the worksite. In one survey 75% of smokers and 87% of nonsmokers favored either designated smoking areas or a total prohibition of smoking. These numbers are impressive when compared to a recent Roper report revealing that 53% of the total population and 58% of smokers were unaware that smoking is the probable cause of many heart attacks, and 59% of the population and 63% of smokers did not know that there is irrefutable evidence that smoking causes most cases of emphysema (Behrens, 1985, p. 6).

A growing body of court cases and legal opinions support employee rights to a smoke-free work environment and employer rights to hire only nonsmokers and ban smoking at the workplace. In Fuentes vs. Workmen's Compensation Appeals Board, 1976–1977, a smoker successfully sued his employer for one-third of the disability due to emphysema because the employer permitted him "to inflict harm on himself" by smoking during working hours. Moral and economic incentives abound for banning smoking at the worksite, and legal precedents provide further encouragement to support smoking restrictions and bans.

Nonsmokers have begun to sue for their right to a smoke-free working environment and win. In one case the court found that "The right of an individual to risk his or her health does not include the right to jeopardize the health of those who must remain around him or her in order to properly perform the duties of their job" (Shimp vs. New Jersey Bell, 1976).

It is the consensus of legal opinion that employers are fully within their constitutional and legal right in banning smoking at the workplace unless the right to smoke is specified in a union contract. According to Behrens (1985, p. 8), "There appear to be no legal grounds for the claim that smoking at work is a 'right.' "

Initially companies, agencies, or hospitals may ban smoking in specific areas. This intervention can only be considered a first step because such a policy makes smoking the norm; that is, smoking is acceptable everywhere except in areas designated as NO SMOKING. The next step in banning smoking is to identify the organization as NO SMOKING with the exception of those areas designated as SMOKING areas. This places the onus on the smoker to seek out the smoking area rather than forcing the nonsmoker to seek out a nonsmoking area for clean air.

A number of companies have successfully implemented total bans, including Provident Indemnity Insurance, Austad's Company, and Radar Electric. To be effective, the chief executive officer must be behind the policy 100%. Pro-Tec, Raven Press Ltd., and Independent Press, among others, have instituted policies of not hiring smokers.

Worksite smoking programs use cover topics, such as: the psychology of quitting, breaking addictive behaviors, using support systems, coping with smoker's nerves, smoking and nutrition (including weight gain), maintaining the nonsmoking behavior, and exercise as a substitute for smoking. Some of the successful cessation techniques that have been used are: cold turkey, gradual weaning, rapid smoking, hypnosis, and biofeedback. Group classes, small groups, self-help materials, computer-assisted instruction, and one-to-one counseling have been employed. Popular options for session lengths range from a 5-day intensive format to weekly sessions over 1 or more months. Some organizations have found including spouses and other family members useful due to the social support provided. Most programs utilize a combination of print material, audiovisuals, demonstrations, skills training, lectures, and/or group discussions. Smoking cessation programs are most successful when linked with strong smoking policy, incentives to quit, environmental changes, and a broad-based health promotion or wellness program (Behrens, 1985, pp. 13–14).

Some incentives that have been used successfully to help smokers quit include:

- Offer nonsmokers a differential rate or discount on health and life insurance.
- Offer free or reduced-rate cessation programs at the worksite.
- Pay for a portion of the cost of cessation programs taken in the community.
- Provide cessation programs on company time or on shared time with employees.
- Offer cessation programs for family members.
- Offer cash payments to quitters after 6 or 12 smoke-free months.
- Incorporate disincentives for quitters who revert to their smoking habit.
- Hold drawings for prizes for quitters.
- Provide equal incentives to long-term employees and new hires who do not smoke.
- Reward nonsmokers who "adopt a smoker" and encourage the smoker to quit.
- Participate in the "Great American Smoke Out".
- Select your own 24-hour period and encourage smokers to quit for the day.
- Distribute carrot sticks and sugarless gum to help quitters make it through the day smoke free.
- Hold a stop smoking fair with local vendors from all types of community stop smoking programs.
- Conduct stop smoking competitions among volunteer teams of employees or with neighboring companies with prizes.

The nurse may coordinate or provide the program or can use community resources including church programs, Red Cross, YMCA-YWCA, Cancer Society, Heart Association, or Lung Association. Whether in-house staff or community resources provide the program, involvement of employees in developing a smoking policy and program will facilitate its development and increase its chances for success.

Some suggestions for including employees in a smoking cessation program are (Behrens, 1985, pp. 26–27):

- Survey employees to determine their smoking in general, in worksite restricted areas, and opinions about offering cessation programs at work.

- Appoint an employee committee representative of smokers and nonsmokers to make recommendations about the content of the policy and/or the implementation plan and timetable.
- Have a representative of top management hold all-staff meetings to explain the proposed policy and program, to hear input, but to remain committed to limit smoking.
- Consider offering cessation programs on neutral turf if the atmosphere is highly charged in response to company policy.
- Hold meetings with all levels of management and listen to their comments, offer support, and make suggestions concerning negotiating disputes with employees.
- Meet informally with employees to ask advice from informal leaders and request assistance from a respected employee in dealing with an especially hostile fellow worker.

A recent approach to smoking cessation is the use of nicotine chewing gum. In a study of its use in the general population among people who had not taken the initiative to stop smoking, there was a decline in success rates to 6% for all three groups (acupuncture, nicotine gum, and no treatment). The studymakers concluded that nicotine gum would be more effective when used in special smokers' clinics than in general practice (Clave & Benhamou, 1984).

Another study showed that nicotine gum when combined with long-term followup appointments resulted in a 1-year abstinence rate for 27% of the clients (Fagerstrom, 1984). Although nicotine gum may be useful for some smokers, especially heavy smokers, it may not be of great benefit to light smokers who may require other interventions (Glantz, 1984).

Employers are beginning to hire with a bias toward nonsmokers. Thus, the ability to stop smoking is becoming an economic as well as a wellness issue. A survey of managers in the Seattle area showed that 53% were already giving preference to nonsmoking applicants. Since the U.S. Supreme Court has verified smoking as a legal criteria for hiring, discrimination against smokers does not violate equal opportunity statutes and will probably be used as a reason for not hiring in the future (Weis, 1984).

Wellness on the Campus

Opatz (1985) points out that the philosophy of student development which has emerged in colleges and universities includes the notion that human development is continuous; occurs when change is anticipated and planned for; is most effective when an integrated approach is taken; and is enhanced when students, faculty, and staff work collaboratively to promote it. More recently the idea of *intentionality* (helping students determine their own needs and direct their own development) has been put forth. These ideas parallel and support the concept of wellness.

The first formally established wellness program on a university campus was developed at the University of Wisconsin at Stevens Point in 1972. Other schools have since adopted the model. The program was developed and is directed by the University's Student Life Division. Wellness has been defined as the overall mission of the division. The following areas have adopted the model: health service, counseling center, residence life, student life activities and programs, university centers and business operations; and wellness curricula have been adopted in physical education, health education, nutrition, and psychology.

Fred Leafgren, Assistant Chancellor for Student Life, suggests 11 strategies for coordinating and enhancing wellness:

- *Establish* administrative leadership (including personal involvement in the process) and support. Key staff are selected and trained to implement and coordinate wellness programs.
- *Inventory* existing programs to identify those programs presently providing wellness services and minimize overlap and duplication.
- *Identify* staff who are interested in modeling a wellness life style and encourage their participation in a wellness committee.
- *Identify* students already interested and committed to a wellness life style and encourage their participation in the planning process.
- *Bring* all existing personnel resources (faculty and non-student affairs administrators) together for brainstorming and goal setting early in the planning process.
- *Involve* all student affairs units in a partnership for wellness program implementation.
- *Ask* each academic department to inventory its programs and services and identify those that may be related to wellness, if only tangentially.
- *Inform* students and faculty about the program and available opportunities. Use a regular publication, assessment tools, etc.
- *Establish* priorities for wellness goals and activities.
- *Provide* adequate training for professional staff and students involved in implementing the program.
- *Evaluate* wellness programs for comprehensiveness and effectiveness in assisting students in their development as persons.

Many facets of the program at the University of Wisconsin are unique and creative. Entering freshmen are given the option of a traditional physical examination or a Lifestyle Assessment Questionnaire (LAQ).

Over 90% choose the LAQ. This approach introduces the student to wellness before stepping in the door. Students receive the results during group interpretation sessions in the residence halls conducted by trained residence staff. The results are filed in the student's file and used as a basis for wellness programs early in the school year.

The Student Health Center shows self-care videotapes in the waiting room, and numerous printed self-care materials are available. When students complain of symptoms, e.g., a cold, rather than being referred to a professional, they go to The Cold Clinic where they find a self-assessment program directing them to examine their throat, take their temperature, and fill out a prescription form to take to the pharmacist. Moving even further toward wellness, such a clinic might provide instruction for nutritional, stress management procedures (imagery, etc.), and fitness/movement procedures to reduce or remove symptoms and treat the original conflict/issue.

The wellness coordinator is responsible for the publication of a wellness newsletter, the food service nutrition programs, the development of wellness information materials, and the training and supervision of student Lifestyle Assistants. Approximately 10–15 students are hired each year to initiate programs for fellow students, including aerobic dancing, weight reduction, stress management, and fitness assessments.

The wellness program has had a positive effect on the campus environment. Alcohol consumption is closely regulated and smoking policies protect the rights of the nonsmokers; smoking is allowed only in designated areas and in many of the Student Life Offices there is no smoking at all. The Food Service contract is negotiated to include provision for high quality fresh fruits, vegetables, and whole grain foods. All entrees are labeled for fat, carbohydrate, and protein content. Cooks and food preparers are taught the basic principles of nutrition and new methods of cooking.

The Nursing Division at the University of Tampa is just beginning to establish a wellness milieu. Students in the wellness nursing course self-assess their wellness and choose wellness goals and a peer facilitator to work with during the semester. Each student learns how to help another student explore the beliefs and motivations behind the wellness goal chosen, identify actions needed to accomplish the goal, establish rewards for movement toward the goal, divide responsibilities for goal attainment, and evaluate movement toward the goal. Having an ongoing relationship with a peer facilitates movement toward the goal by providing structure and encouragement. Students who used graphs, journals, or other written measures to show progress and structure movement stated they were more satisfied with the outcome.

Working on their own development and perceiving how it "feels" to be a client provides a valuable experience for students to use when working with clients. The second part of their clinical experience in the wellness nursing course provides opportunities for students to work with simulated and/or real life clients practicing all of the wellness dimension interventions.

Wellness concepts and the wellness conceptual model are interwoven in other nursing courses. In nursing research students have been involved in developing wellness oriented research questions and in reviewing wellness oriented research. In family nursing, students learn family systems theory and family wellness assessments and interventions.

In a pilot program in community health nursing students had the option to participate in more traditional community health clinical experiences or to use the campus as community. They used Table 53, Community Assessment, to assess the University of Tampa campus. The clinical objectives were to assess the campus, identify wellness needs, develop and implement wellness programs based on identified community needs, and evaluate the effectiveness of implemented wellness programs. Four students worked as a group to complete the objectives and write up a report of their work. Students used questionnaires and personal interviews to obtain further data regarding specific programs students were interested in participating in. Perhaps due to insufficient time to publicize and validate findings, programs were not well attended; since data were collected anonymously and not coded, it was not possible to follow up and obtain further information regarding nonparticipation.

Community Health Nursing students worked with their instructor (the author) to provide monthly noon luncheon wellness presentations. Each student chose a wellness dimension of interest and coordinated that presentation. One finding of the group was that there were many wellness resources and duplications and suggested a wellness coordinator should be appointed to coordinate wellness on the campus.

Students talked to the Food Service Director and offered to work with the dietician, they developed a program with Dormitory Resident Advisors to provide wellness information for dorm residents, began work on a campus wellness resource center, and participated in a Health Fair sponsored by the Student Health Service. Additionally, they talked to many administrative and faculty people, communicating about the wellness thrust of the nursing program, and developed a wellness contact list of key staff, faculty, and administrators.

Throughout the nursing program students will continue a wellness journal, plotting their movement toward wellness. Many classes are begun with a relaxation exercise to assist students and instructors to relax and focus on learning. Faculty are planning to identify their own wellness goals and work with a peer to facilitate the process. Faculty and students will both use wellness journals to plot their progress.

EVALUATION OF WELLNESS PROGRAMS

Evaluation issues should be considered when programs are planned. The assessment/intervention/evaluation process is continuous and interactive. In order to design a program that will ultimately be effective, client needs must be assessed. The Windsor et al. (1984, pp. 59–60, 70) list of planning problems has been adapted below.

Evaluation Planning Begins When Program Planning Begins

1. What are the dimensions of the problem of interest—clients with diagnosed disease or relatively well people with unwell life styles—and what is the prevalence of the problem? What is expected to be different as a result of the program?
2. What specific behaviors must clients learn or acquire or strengthen to enhance wellness?
3. What resources are needed for wellness to be enhanced?
4. What kind of support services are needed to enhance wellness?
5. Which behavior changes can and should be measured, how, and when?
6. What wider changes in conditions and situations are expected; which ones can and should be measured, how, and when?
7. What approaches will best achieve the desired effect and how can they be monitored for quality and efficacy?
8. What organizational and logistical arrangements are needed to support the program, including orientation and training of personnel?
9. What kind of budget is needed and how can it be obtained?

Most, if not all, of the questions need to be asked of "experts" *and* clients.

Types of Evaluation

Program evaluation is used to improve program planning, development, or administration. It describes accomplishments, problems, and processes, reducing uncertainty in day-to-day decision making.

Evaluation research determines the effectiveness of a program model or tests a theory; it focuses primarily on the potential effects of a new program. When designing an evaluation program, it is useful to ask, "Do I want information as the program proceeds to feed back and improve it?" (if so, use formative evaluation procedures), or "Do I want to withhold feedback and evaluate only after the program is finished?" (if so, use summative evaluation procedures). Moberg (1984, p. 3) suggests that formative approaches are most relevant to prevention programs.

There are three levels of evaluation to consider: process, outcome, and impact. At the process level, activities of the program are considered (number and types of clients and staff, resources expended, services provided). Program monitoring systems measure effort, the program's capacity for success, and document level of activity. All prevention programs should establish a program monitoring system (Moberg, 1984, p. 3).

A monitoring system enables an accurate count of how many people were served during the year, what services were provided, and what the characteristics of the clientèle are. This kind of information indicates whether the intended population is being served and whether program content needs to be altered to meet the population being served. Consumer satisfaction surveys, participant observation, and open-ended interviewing can provide additional monitoring information.

Outcome evaluation examines the attainment of program objectives (change in participant behavior, attitude, knowledge or level of problems). Smoking prevention programs would have successful outcomes if a meaningful percentage of participants did not smoke in the future; smoking cessation programs would have successful outcomes if a meaningful percentage of participants continued not smoking for a prescribed period of time—the longer, the more successful. Cost benefit analysis (minimize costs while maximizing benefits) is another outcome measure.

Impact evaluation examines the total effect of a program, including its "spinoff" effects. Impact evaluation of an alcohol abuse prevention program might examine whether the program has reduced the incidence of alcohol abuse among youth in a community, whether there are fewer drunk driving incidents, or whether more alternatives are being used.

Attempting to examine all three levels in one evaluation effort is unrealistic and inappropriate. A level is chosen depending on resources, information needs, and accountability requirements.

Steps in Planning Program Evaluation

The following steps are useful in planning program evaluation (Moberg, 1984, pp. 7–9):

1. Identify and organize a key users group composed of an evaluator, key staff, and, if possible, clients.

2. Identify and refine relevant evaluation questions by asking diagnostic questions: What is the assessed need of the participants? What is the conceptual model the program is based on? What benefits, goals, and objectives are anticipated? What kinds of interventions are planned? What is the target population? What resources are available? Who needs information about the program and why? What data are essential for internal and external reporting? What data are currently available? What are the major issues being faced by the program? What is the political, value, and cultural context? What standards or regulations must the program comply with? Has the program model been tested elsewhere?

3. Specify program goals and objectives. Write down general goals, then list possible indicators of goal achievement. Select the best indicators and translate the indicators into measurable objectives, e.g., by the end of the program, clients will role play a 10% increase in the number of socially acceptable ways to refuse a cigarette; by 8/5/87, 90% of students will identify the wellness resource center as a viable alternative to physician visits.

4. Select evaluation methods and data collection instruments appropriate to evaluation questions. Questions to ask include:

- Should evaluation be prestructured (fixed) or vary according to the data (dynamic)?
- Are we most concerned with past participants (retrospective) or future ones (prospective)?
- Should we focus on the total program (holistic) or on specific parts of it (component)?
- Should specific hypotheses be tested (inductive) or will we develop generalizations based on the data (deductive)?
- Should groups receiving the program be compared to similar groups who do not get the program (experimental or quasi-experimental design) or look only at program participants?
- Should data be quantitative (56 participants . . .) or qualitative (the process of participating in wellness activities was . . .)?
- Should data come from existing records, observations, interviews, or questionnaires?
- Should a sample of participants be chosen (volunteers, representatives, randomly) or the entire population be examined?
- Should we ask open-ended or structured questions to obtain data?
- Should we use single-item indicators or multiple-item scales?

5. Develop an evaluation plan, including:

- A statement of the evaluation question(s);

- A description of what data will be collected from whom using what instruments;
- A listing of who will be responsible for each evaluation task;
- A statement of conditions under which data collection will take place and methods for standardizing data collection;
- Plans for regulating the flow of evaluation data, summarizing it, and analyzing it;
- Plans for protection of subjects (obtaining informed consent and limiting access to identifying information);
- Time frame for data collection, analysis, reporting, and checkpoints with key user's group;
- Plans for use of the findings, including a statement of level of certainty which can be placed in the findings given the research design.

6. Pilot test the evaluation system to ensure respondents understand the questions, are willing to respond, that data are coded and interpreted consistently, that data collection time allowances are accurate, and that data collectors understand the format.

7. Implement the evaluation plan ensuring that data forms are turned in and briefly examined shortly after completion; build in sanctions to enforce this.

8. Summarize and interpret the data. If the sample is small enough and of a quantitative (numbers) nature, hand tally and pocket calculator can produce frequency distributions (e.g., number of males who participated), cross tabulations (number of males vs. females who stopped smoking), or means (e.g., mean age is achieved by adding the ages and dividing the total by the number of participants). More sophisticated and/or statistical analyses may require consultation. Qualitative analyses could include reproducing the data without comment, developing organizational categories, developing case studies, or developing typologies (e.g., isolating and categorizing the essential characteristics of successful types of participants). Throughout this process, the key user's group should be involved and provide feedback that is implemented.

9. Disseminate and use the findings. Sharing findings with other wellness programs will assist in legitimizing specific models, refining hypotheses, and improving practice.

Selecting Evaluation Tools

When selecting an existing instrument, ensure *items reflect relevant concepts*, the instrument *is the appropriate length* (too long will create resistance in participants; too short will not be reliable), and *is reliable* (consistent between persons, over time, and/or internally) *and valid*

measures what it claims to measure; one consideration is determining
whether the instrument has face validity—by looking at it, on the face
of it, it looks as if it measures what it purports to measure) with a
population similar to yours; look for a discussion of these issues
accompanying the instrument.

Two (or more) methods of measurement are usually better than one.
For example, if a quantitative measure and statistical methods are employed, a hypothesis may be refuted (resulting in a return to square
one), but an interview with participants may still reveal useful information. Contrarily, if a post-test measure of student nurse wellness peer
facilitators reported their peers demonstrated more assertiveness after
their work together and interviews with the peers independently found
movement in the direction of more assertion, confidence is added to the
conclusion that peer facilitation affects assertive behavior in the population under study.

When choosing a method, determine its feasibility by asking, "Are
there sufficient resources available to conduct the proposed evaluation?"
including budget, time (to conduct the evaluation, reasonable to expect
from a client, and to carry it out in the proposed time frame), expertise,
computer or data entry services, clerical time, duplicating equipment
time, and relevant to the developmental phase of the program (an
impact study is not appropriate for a beginning program that is only 2
years old). At this point, statistical and computer specialist consultation
can be sought if necessary.

Validity Considerations in Selecting an Evaluation Design

In addition to considering the reliability of an instrument, the *internal
validity* (extent to which an observed effect can be attributed to an
intervention) is of importance. Eight factors can affect internal validity

1. *History* (unplanned internal or external events that affect the population under study, e.g., a new law banning smoking in schools
   interferes with a study of the effects of a smoking cessation program on smoking in school);
2. *Maturation* (normal growth and development changes, e.g., children grow out of heart murmurs);
3. *Testing or observation* (participants change their behavior because of
   being watched while being interviewed or taking a test);
4. *Instrumentation* (changes in the characteristics of the measures introduce bias; e.g., some observers are well-trained and others are
   not);

5. *Regression* (selection of a treatment or comparison group based on a very high or low level of a characteristic, e.g., those who score very high on a pre-test are recruited for a weight management course);
6. *Selection* (as groups or individuals are selected or volunteer, the group(s) is not representative of all smokers, or all overweight clients, etc.);
7. *Attrition* (10% or more dropouts introduces bias into the outcome of a study);
8. *Interactive effects* (any combination of the above).

Instrumentation, selection, and attrition are the most frequent compromisers of evaluation results (Windsor et al., 1984, p. 131). Therefore, it is important to protect the results from these eight factors. A major protection is choice of evaluation design.

Program Evaluation Designs

Windsor et al. (1984, pp. 132–138) discuss five major evaluation designs:

1. *One Group Pretest and Post-test:* although it is tempting to infer that significant increases or decreases in scores on the post-test are due to an intervention, they could as likely be due to other factors, especially if there is a great deal of time between the pretest and post-test, or if maturation, historical factors, or regression interfere.

2. *Nonequivalent Control Group:* by adding a comparison group, the effects of history, maturation, testing, and instrumentation will be lessened. It is essential to make groups as comparable as possible. One way is the peer-generation method: participants are asked to identify a non-participant friend of the same age and sex.

3. *Time Series:* this design is usually used when a trend is being studied; up to 50 data points are used to assess an effect; the principal threat to internal validity is history; this design does not provide definitive evidence about the impact of an intervention unless it is replicated.

4. *Multiple Time Series:* outcomes are studied at differing points for a group receiving the intervention (treatment group) and for a group not receiving it (control group).

5. *Randomized Pretest and Post-test with Control Group:* this experimental design produces strong control over threats to internal and external validity (increased confidence in generalizing findings to other settings and populations with similar characteristics *if* there is confirmation that the two groups are equivalent; this can be obtained by examining each of the effects of the threats to internal validity for both groups).

In many settings, it may not be ethical or feasible to withhold treatment from a control group; in some cases the intensity, duration, methods, materials, or frequency can be varied for the control group; when a new program is being established, the old method of treatment can be administered to the control group and the new program to the experimental group.

Determining Sample Size

When quantitative designs are used, the sample size is crucial to ensure sufficient statistical power in data analysis. The appropriate size for groups is determined prior to an intervention. *Statistical power* is the probability of rejecting a null hypothesis if it is false (Type I error). The null hypothesis asserts the two groups (treatment and control) are not significantly different.

To determine the efficient sample size, parameters must be defined. Statistical significance (α) is usually set between .01 and .05. Next, the β level, or probability of accepting a null hypothesis when it is false (Type II error), is computed. β should be equal to $1 - 4\alpha$; if $\alpha = .05$, $\beta = 1 - 4(.05)$ or .80 (Windsor, 1984, p. 139). Finally, the current median level of expected effectiveness is calculated. A search of the literature or an examination of ongoing program data should reveal the expected effectiveness of a particular program. For example, the literature indicates that the self-initiated cessation rate for smokers is approximately 10% ($p = .10$). A reasonable expectation of impact for a smoking-cessation program at a 6- to 12-month followup is about 30% cessation, or 0.30. Standard size statistical tables can then be consulted to find how many participants are needed for each group to test the significance of a difference (Windsor, 1984, p. 139).

Problems in Program Evaluation

In addition to the obvious problems of evaluation such as lack of sophistication of the researcher, there are other problems that may be encountered. Frequently it is difficult, if not impossible, to meet the criteria for experimental control that would lend greater confidence to findings. School-based programs are the exception; it is relatively easy to randomly select classrooms for treatment.

Issues of interest to employers, such as productivity and morale, are difficult to measure with any degree of confidence. Yet management may demand that researchers relate results to "the bottom line" (profits) in order to continue funding wellness programs. The costs associated with researching the benefits of wellness may be considerable. The evaluation process itself is not considered profitable and therefore the wellness nursing practitioner may have difficulty convincing management that they should invest in data analysis.

INTEGRATIVE LEARNING EXPERIENCES

Beginning Level

1. Use the case study of the Block family below to make recommendations for wellness nursing interventions regarding nutrition, fitness/exercise, stress management, positive relationships, environmental wellness, and self-care.

The Block family lives in a small house with little privacy from their neighbors or one another. The windows have heavy curtains that allow little light or air in. *Jim Block*, the father, age 42, is a management consultant for a large corporation. He is overweight, "out of shape," travels a lot, and seems emotionally and physically removed from the rest of the family. He once mentioned that he doesn't want to be like his father and die of a heart attack. *Wanda Block*, the mother, is 40 years old. She is just beginning to pursue her own life and has enrolled as a freshman at the local college; she feels guilty about being away from the twins so much and having to leave the house before breakfast. She smokes cigarettes continually and drinks coffee whenever you visit. *Mrs. Suzanna Block*, Jim's mother, age 60, has diabetes. She came to live with her son's family when her husband died last year. She alternates between being depressed and telling her daughter-in-law how to run the household. There are angry scenes at dinner between Wanda and Mrs. Block. *Gregory Block*, one of the twins, is 10 years old. He is doing poorly in school. His mother calls him "the bad one." He subsists on chocolate bars and cokes. You noticed him standing on the corner near school talking to the local drug dealer. *Glenda Block*, Gregory's twin, does the food shopping for the family and cooks some meals; these consist of hamburgers, cokes, french fries, and store bought cakes and cookies. *Ramona Block*, age 17, is unmarried and lives at home with her 6-month-old infant, Randy. You saw Ramona in a hot embrace with her date in a car near the house. *Randy Block*, age 6 months, was born with multiple physical defects. Ramona pays little attention to Randy; he is being raised by his grandmother.

2. Complete a community assessment using Table 53, pp. 287–290.

Advanced Level

1. Develop and implement a smoking cessation program with three clients or a group of clients. Summarize your results using p. 108.
2. Develop a blueprint for the assessment, implementation, and evaluation of a wellness program in a hospital, school, or corpora-

tion, including your justification for such a program. Expand your nursing role by approaching administrators in three hospitals, schools, or corporations and discussing the feasibility of adopting your plan.

REFERENCES

Allen, R., and Kraft, C. (1984). The importance of cultural variables in program design. In *Health Promotion in the Workplace*, M. O'Donnell and T. Ainsworth, Eds. New York: John Wiley & Sons.
Behrens, R. (1985). A Decision Maker's Guide to Reducing Smoking at the Worksite. Washington, D.C.: U.S. Department of Health and Human Services.
Brennan, A. (1983). How to set up a corporate wellness program. *Management Rev* May:41–47.
Cancer risks found for hospital workers. (1982). *WOHRC NEWS* 4(4):1,6.
Canton, J., and Monroe, T. (1984). The importance of worker involvement in program design. In *Health Promotion in the Workplace*, M. O'Donnell and T. Ainsworth, Eds. New York: John Wiley & Sons, p. 58.
Clavel, F., and Benhamon, S. (1984). Nicotine chewing gum in general practice. *Brit Med J* 289(6454):1308.
Glantz, L. (1984). Nicotine chewing gum not for all smokers. *Clin Pharm* 3(3):236.
Goldbeck, W. (1984). Forward. In *Health Promotion in the Workplace*, M. O'Donnell and T. Ainsworth, Eds. New York: John Wiley & Sons, p. viii.
Moberg, D. (1984). *Evaluation of Prevention Programs: A Basic Guide for Practitioners*. Madison, WI: WI Clearinghouse.
National Cancer Institute. (1980). *Everything Doesn't Cause Cancer*. Washington, D.C.: NIH. NIH publication 80-2039.
Opatz, J. (1985). Wellness in colleges and universities. In *Proceedings of the Ninth Annual Community Health Nursing Conference: Maximizing Wellness in a High Tech Age: Focus for Community Health Nursing*, M. Assay, Ed. Chapel Hill, NC: Department of Community Health Nursing.
Parkinson, R. (1982). *Managing Health Promotion in the Workplace*. Palo Alto, CA: Mayfield Publishing Co.
Shephard, R., et al. (1982). The influence of employee fitness and lifestyle modification program upon medical costs. *Can J PH* 73(4):259–263.
The magnitude of the program. (1983). *Program Summary of a Conference on Worksite Health Promotion and Human Resources*. Washington, D.C.: Health and Human Services, p. 25.
Vickery, D., et al. (1983). Effect of a self-care education program on medical visits. *JAMA* 250(21):2952–2956.
Weiss, W. (1984). Giving smokers notice, going public with policies against hiring smokers. *Management World* July:44,41.
Windsor, R., et al. (1984). *Evaluation of Health Promotion and Education Programs*. Palo Alto, CA: Mayfield Publishing Co.

10

RESEARCH AND
WELLNESS THEORY

This chapter discusses the following topics:

- The content of nursing research
- Turning illness-oriented research questions into wellness-oriented ones
- Research methods especially suited to wellness theory
- Research providing support for wellness theory
- Developing relationship statements and testing theoretical relationships

Planning and carrying out wellness-focused nursing research implies the reader already has a working knowledge of conventional research methods. Nursing research from a wellness focus also implies a wellness framework from which to practice. Without it the research that will be produced may be more illness-oriented than wellness-oriented or more medically-oriented than nursing-oriented. This chapter attempts to provide the reader with information necessary to begin generating wellness nursing questions, suggests some methods that may be most useful in studying wellness-oriented questions, supplies a report of some evolving research to support wellness theory, and suggests some wellness relationship statements that can be used to test the theory.

THE CONTENT OF NURSING RESEARCH

According to the American Nurses' Association Policy Statement (1980), nursing is focused on the diagnosis and treatment of human responses to health problems. Barnard (1982) reviewed nursing texts and found that they were predominately oriented toward the diagnosis and treatment of health problems, not *human responses* to health problems. Some human responses nursing could focus on more directly are: self-care, self-esteem, destructive relationship issues, lack of knowledge, sexuality, activity, pain and discomfort, and strain from parenting.

From a wellness perspective, examples of the kind of nursing questions to ask and research might be:

- What is the type of pain experienced during a sore throat?
- Is imagery or therapeutic touch more useful for this kind of pain?
- What is the effect of confronting irrational beliefs in relationships with others?
- What changes in self-esteem occur when a parent produces an infant with a disability?
- Is value clarification or journal writing a more effective self-care measure for low self-esteem?
- What is the effect of beliefs about the meaningfulness of life on wellness activities?

TURNING ILLNESS-ORIENTED RESEARCH QUESTIONS INTO WELLNESS-ORIENTED ONES

There are a number of ways to turn illness-oriented research questions into wellness-oriented ones. One way is to focus on a well population. Although it is possible to use a problem orientation with a well population, it is easier to see how to structure questions to focus on wellness concerns. An example of research focusing on a well population appears in the section "Research Providing Support for Wellness Theory" later in this chapter.

Another way to turn illness-oriented questions into wellness ones is to begin to relate problems or human responses to the dimensions of wellness. For example, instead of focusing on the pain or illness experience of otitis media, the focus would be on the prevention and minimization of pain using self-care strategies. Some questions that might be asked are:

- What is the relationship between level of exercise and otitis media?
- What is the relationship between positive expectations about the outcome of otitis media and healing?
- What is the effect of eating additional amounts of high vitamins C, A, and zinc-containing foods on the otitis media process?

- What is the effect of progressive relation and healing imagery measures on the otitis media process?
- What is the effect of color, full spectrum light, or noise on the otitis media process?
- What is the effect of peer or family supportive communication on the otitis media process?

A variant of this procedure is to take some of the indicants of whole person wellness (Figure 2, Chapter 1, p. 5) and begin to formulate them into research questions, especially those related to manageability, comprehensibility, and meaningfulness. Antonovsky (1984) has been developing a model based on the sense of coherence as a determinant of health. His work has relevance for wellness research because he has begun to examine health as a process, not merely as the absence of disease. Additionally, he conceives of the process as one of moving toward greater order and meaningfulness; this idea, too, is relevant for wellness.

His model is most relevant for the wellness dimension of stress but can be expanded to encompass other dimensions. Antonovsky's "sense of coherence" is formed from a cluster of attitudes that he calls:

- comprehensibility (perceiving stimuli as making cognitive sense as information, as opposed to finding them unpredictable, random, noisy, and chaotic);
- manageability (having resources at one's disposal either directly under one's control, or having access to resources controlled by dependable others);
- meaningfulness (feeling life makes sense in emotional terms so that some life problems are viewed as worth investing energy in).

Using Antonovsky's (1984) concept of coherence, the following wellness-oriented questions could be formulated:

- What is the relationship between the belief in the ability to influence the level of fitness either directly or with the help of others and fitness activities?
- What is the relationship between believing the solution to life problems is worth investing energy in and preventive nutrition?
- What is the relationship between believing one is able to make sense out of new and risk-requiring situations and attempts to form positive relationships with others?

The Intersystems Wellness Nursing Model (Figure 1, Chapter 1, p. 4) could also be used to generate wellness-oriented research questions. For example:

- The more the nurse serves as a wellness role model, the more likely the client will be to move toward a wellness orientation.
- The greater the movement toward a wellness belief system, the more wellness-oriented behaviors will be exhibited.
- The more the client participates in wellness self-assessment, the greater the movement toward wellness.

Another idea is to use the conceptual framework developed by Mehl (1981), a proponent of a holistic approach to research. He pointed out the fallacy of thought that underlies the medical model in which an adverse factor or factors is believed to "cause" an illness or disease. Such a model ignores why one particular, unique human being becomes ill; until recently this kind of question has been defined as irrelevant because it is outside the paradigm. Psychoneuroimmunology, a new field spawned from the interrelationship of three disciplines, promises to address some of the most important questions in the area of understanding the mind/body link (O'Regan, 1983). However, until these links are established and accepted by traditional medicine, many "scientific" studies will continue to address parts of bodies or organs and to infer effect on the whole person.

Because of the uniqueness of individuals, Mehl questions whether randomization procedures used in quantitative research are valid. If each person has a unique position in time and space, how can randomization of space/time units be appropriate? A holistic model, such as wellness, is based upon the significance of the individual. Theory construction is systematic, is based on the assessment of factors affecting individuals, and does not require that the same factor affect every individual in exactly the same way to be considered significant (Mehl, 1981).

Using this method, a nurse researcher might begin with a detailed description of the life of individuals with a life problem, such as diabetes: childhood events, stresses pre-illness, spiritual beliefs, life events, emotional changes, paralleling changes in their illness and their general world view. Only after one individual's pathway to diabetes is understood would the nurse researcher begin to look for similarities and differences among different individual pathways. Theory might be formulated for each individual regarding how diabetes functioned in his or her personal system. Continuing with the research, it would be important to observe if diabetes changed for each person as factors changed.

Using Mehl's model, an example of a wellness-oriented question might be: What are the interactions of exercise on the development of client Jones related to diabetes, spiritual beliefs, life events, emotional changes, paralleling changes in her view of diabetes and her general world view, stresses and ability to use stress management procedures, positive relationships with others, preventive nutrition, and amount of full-spectrum light exposed to?

According to Mehl (1981), a holistic approach to research begins with a description of all possible factors in the life of an individual with a particular disease or problem leading to an understanding of which combinations of factors affect that particular disease or problem. Only then would other individuals be studied and similarities and differences be noted. Theory would then accumulate regarding the many possible individual pathways of development of the problem.

This kind of approach emphasizes the interactive nature of variables rather than the isolation and proof of one effect. It is also congruent with a systems approach that focuses on interactive factors and in which there are many paths to one outcome; in systems terms, this is referred to in systems theory as *equifinality* (Putt, 1978).

Mehl (1981) is also supportive of the emphasis on the meaning and quality of life so essential to a wellness model. He discusses the importance of value clarification by the individual and support of that person's right to decide on his or her own values. Additionally, Mehl gives precedence to observation and description of client behavior over statistical procedures.

Another method of turning illness-oriented research questions is to search current research reports for ideas. For example, in looking through abstracts of research on mind and immunity, the following studies were found: Achterberg and Lawlis (1977) found that blood chemistries tended to reflect ongoing or concurrent disease states in those with cancer; that there was a statistical relationship between psychological variables and blood chemistries; and that psychological factors were predictive of subsequent disease status. The researchers concluded that blood chemistries offered information about the current status of disease, whereas the psychological variables offered future, and perhaps preventive, insights. Some questions this research might raise about nursing research are:

- What is the nurse's role in assisting clients to identify the feelings that are interfering with their wellness or supporting their disease?
- What feelings are interfering with this client's healing processes?
- How can client feelings about disease be used to prevent further development of the disease?

A study by McClelland et al. (1980) focused on the need for power and its relationship to illness. The researchers noted that previous research reported that individuals high in the need for power, high in inhibition, and high in power stress were more likely than other individuals to report more severe illness. The McClelland study found that the high power group had above average urine excretion of epinephrine and below average concentrations of immunoglobulin A in saliva. They interpreted the findings as consistent with the hypothesis that when a strong need for power is inhibited, there is an immunosuppressive effect making individuals more susceptible to illness. From a wellness perspective, the following questions might be asked:

• Which clients most need to maintain a sense of power and control over themselves and/or their disease process?
• How can the nurse identify these clients readily?
• What interventions would be useful in increasing immune responses in these clients and in clients in general?

A number of researchers have noted the correlation between inability to express anger and poor prognosis in cancer (Bageley, 1979; Bieliauskas et al., 1979; Borysenko, 1982; Morris et al., 1981). Such studies may raise the following issues from a wellness perspective:

• Which clients are suppressing angry feelings?
• What effect is suppressed anger having on their lifestyle and/or disease process?
• What nursing interventions can be used to enhance anger expression?
• What is the effect of anger expression on well-being and/or ability to heal?

RESEARCH PROCEDURES FOR HOLISTIC, COMPLEX PROCESSES

Studying wellness requires research procedures that allow the researcher to examine holistic, interactive processes. Two kinds of research approaches are especially suited: qualitative research and action research.

Qualitative Research

Qualitative research taps the context and meaning of observed behaviors. Qualitative research is most à propos for the discovery of theory and understanding. Its scope is holistic; its methods emphasize interactions of variables (Mullen & Iverson, 1982).

Recently, more and more researchers in fields with a traditional quantitative (numbers) emphasis, such as psychology, sociology, educational research, and others have shifted to a more qualitative paradigm. This shift is in line with a trend toward holism. Qualitative data are well-grounded in real world observations and contain rich descriptions and explanations of processes. Quantitative data tend to isolate findings and make analysis difficult if one does not find what one is hoping to find.

For example, a pair of nursing students were searching for correlations between anxiety, loneliness, and grade point average in their classmates. They did a multiple regression correlation (used to understand the effects of two or more independent variables on a dependent measure), but there was so much variance unaccounted for that all they were able to conclude was that there was no significant relationship between the three. What if they had gathered some qualitative data such as interviewing a focused sample of students with low or high grade point averages to find out other variables that the students thought might be involved? Their discussion of findings would have been much richer and they would have untangled more of the puzzle of the relationship of the variables.

Swanson and Chenitz (1982) point out that nursing exists in the social world, yet frequently uses quantitative, laboratory methods of the basic sciences in its research designs. Quantitative research often does not have meaning for the practice world of nursing because researchers isolate variables to a single dimension to look at direct relationships between them. Such an approach overlooks the highly complex and diverse nature of nursing and frequently falls short of providing direction for nursing interventions (Swanson & Chenitz, 1982).

Additionally, it provides little understanding of the context that gives meaning to actions. Noting that the family planning literature on male contraception has large theoretical gaps, Swanson and Chenitz (1982) set out to find out what prevented men from using contraceptives, rather than to simply count men and their contraceptive use. She found that the "hassle" of using contraception was mentioned frequently by the man she was interviewing. One of the major advantages of a qualitative method is that it allows the researcher to analyze data while collecting it. This quality permitted Swanson to further explore the concept of "hassle" and found that if contraception did not fit into their lifestyles, they did not use it.

As she continued her study, Swanson began to interview couples and found that lifestyle factors influenced contraceptive use.

Although contraceptive use appears to be a simple matter, it embodies a complex activity which is influenced by many social, sexual, and physical variables. How one feels about one's self, one's partner, what is acceptable sexually, is convenient, valued, approved by others and tolerated by institutions are but a few factors represented by "contraceptive" use. (1982, p. 244)

The grounded theory method of qualitative research has been written about by a number of nurse researchers, but never with such lucidity as by Stern (1980). She studied stepfather families and their integration into an existing family. She began by conducting intensive interviews with 30 stepfather families from a variety of social classes and ethnic groups. She also observed the families interacting and coded all data according to their main substance, eventually clustering them into categories. Two of the categories noted were family rules and enforcement techniques.

As Stern moved to the second phase of concept formation, she began to develop a conceptual framework that represented integration from the family member's point of view. The framework chosen was discipline because the topic elicited strong emotional responses when discussed with families.

During the next step, concept development, categories were linked together to define key variables, e.g., categories of teaching, accepting, and copying were included in the larger category of affiliating actions or those actions that seemed to bring the stepfather and child closer together. As relationships became clearer, Stern returned to the literature and formulated the question, "Under what conditions do the variables discipline and integration co-exist?" (p. 22). She returned for another look at the data to clarify this relationship. She found that integration and discipline occurred together only when affiliating actions were also present. This is the point at which statement synthesis (Walker & Avant, 1983, p. 83) occurred; a statement about the relationship between phenomena under observation was made by Stern. Her thinking became consolidated and she proposed the term "integrative discipline" as the core variable that explained integration of stepfathers into families around the issue of child discipline.

Stern continued refining the concept by coding data in terms of theoretical ideas. She wrote memos to herself as she coded data. Memo writing is a useful technique in qualitative studies. The researcher writes a sentence, paragraph, or a few pages about a momentary idea that occurs while looking at data.

Memos are always *conceptual* in intent. They do not just report data, but they tie different pieces of data together in a cluster, or they show that a particular piece of data is an instance of a general concept. (Miles & Huberman, 1984, p. 69)

Finally, memos were reorganized and used to produce a research report. The final report presented theoretical outcomes substantiated by examples from data.

Action Research

Action research is the use of research methodology to solve problems. Social change can be brought about at the same time that there is a valuable contribution made to nursing science. An underlying assumption of action research is that members of our organization are better able than anyone else to define their problems and propose solutions for them because they are best acquainted with their own situations. This assumption implies that it is desirable, and even necessary, for clients to possess decision making skills (Cunningham, 1976).

Clients are assisted to define the problem as they see it and then to generate hypotheses. They learn to specify and define terms, decide on a way to measure change, decide how change will be implemented, decide how to interpret data to see if they support or refute their hunches or hypotheses, and infer generalizations (Corey, 1953, p. 29).

In action research, hypotheses are ways of stating objectives; they predict the consequences of carrying out actions and move participants toward those actions (Corey, 1953, p. 133). An overriding theme is that people are more likely to change "if they participate in exploring the reasons for, and means of, change . . . The action training and research process releases the interpersonal energies that are stifled in most authority-bound systems" (Gardner, 1974).

Action research tends to enhance the position of the individual and to diffuse sources of power. Clients are given freedom, meaningful activity, opportunity to participate, recognition of their worth, needed decision making and problem solving skills, and growth and security opportunities (Gardner, 1974). Each of these seems likely to enhance wellness also.

> The quality of life is enhanced as indicated by: satisfied clients, timely delivery of goods or services, visibility of activities to the wider citizenry, participation is within the range of societal norms, and there is choice whether goods or services are wanted. (Gardner, 1974, p. 108)

There may be language barriers between nurse researchers and clients and interviews or mailed questionnaires may be inappropriate, because each group has its own perspective and understanding of the major parameters of the problem areas. The nominal group may be the best way to help all involved understand the problem (Van de Ven & Del-becq, 1972).

For example, participants studying the problem of obtaining wellness services in a community would be asked to list the subjective (personal feelings and emotions that were barriers to attaining wellness services) and objective (organizational or environmental difficulties which interfered with movement toward wellness) barriers. The next steps are as follows:

1. 15 minutes for the participants to silently generate ideas.
2. In round robin, each person shares one problem and each is written on a large pad of paper by number alternating between subjective and objective columns. No ideas are discussed or critiqued, but participants are encouraged to write new ideas as they are stimulated by others' ideas.
3. 30 minutes to discuss, clarify, elaborate, dispute, or add new items; no items are eliminated.
4. 15-minute break.
5. The group ranks the priority of items, choosing the 10 most critical elements, writing one each on a 3×5 card and ranking them in order of importance.
6. A spontaneous discussion follows in which participants can reclarify, elaborate, defend, or dispute the preliminary vote. Some problems are now redefined at this point.
7. The priority of items is changed by individuals as they rerank them on their own sheets, assigning a value of 100 to his or her most important item and values between 0 and 100 to the other items.
8. The researcher collects the final ratings and reports the votes to the group. A 20-minute discussion period follows.

The *nominal group process* technique allows for multiple individual inputs simultaneously while keeping participation balanced. The method also controls variance; a major source of error or variance can arise when there is incongruence between the researcher and/or practitioner system and the client or user system. The nominal group reduces incongruence.

Cunningham (1976) suggested that participants in action research begin to generate action hypotheses that describe the possible actions that could be taken to solve a problem and the necessary resources to implement them. In developing an action research plan, the action researcher helps the participants to allot time into segments and to outline the activities to be done in each time segment, noting how responsibilities will be assigned. The action researcher facilitates the transfer of information and decisions to the participants, and serves only as a watchdog or conscience for the group (Cunningham, 1976).

Traditional research is judged for value in terms of the amount of dependable knowledge it adds to that which has already been recorded and is available to anyone who wants to be familiar with it. The value of action research is "determined primarily by the extent to which findings lead to improvement of the practices of the people engaged in the research" (Corey, 1953, p. 13).

The issue of random selection (so difficult to attain in the real world) is not a problem because the action researcher only wants to discover generalizations that will help them work more effectively together on the same situation as that in which the studies were conducted (Corey, 1953, p. 14).

Traditional research can dehumanize those being studied because the data that have been collected may never yield any benefit for them. Sanford (1970) suggests that the best thing to do for social systems such as colleges and universities is to study them. He came to this conclusion after interviewing students during their college years and reporting the findings to the entire campus. He found that the reports had a "significant impact" on the student culture (p. 11).

At Berkeley, Sanford decided to teach students about higher education by having them study one another. They interviewed one another, after preparing a comprehensive interview schedule, thus learning what were the significant research questions. As a group they acquired a lively sense of community, shared purposes, dissatisfactions, and ideas about what needed to be changed. "A process of change was set in motion. The student body as a whole proceeded to organize itself and to institute a new system for governing the school" (p. 12).

Sanford (1970) found that faculty did not act on student recommendations because they had not been studied. Eventually students began studying and interviewing faculty and feeding back results to them.

Sanford (1970) suggested that action research questions should be practical, general, and open-ended, e.g., how to improve teaching, how to change features of the academic culture, how to promote the development of individual faculty members.

There is a dearth of research by nurses using action research methods. Shea (1978) reported an action research project to help nurse managers solve the problem of whether they needed a director of nursing or whether a community mental health center could be run by a nursing committee.

Although there are few nursing research projects in the literature using an action research approach, it has significant implications for wellness nursing. A wellness perspective implies the consumer of ser-

vices is responsible and deeply involved in the wellness process. Therefore, an action research approach that involves clients in the study of
their own wellness processes would be relevant.

Action research might raise some of the following questions:

- How well are we accomplishing our wellness goals?
- How might we make our work more expeditious?
- How do we feel about ourselves and what we are accomplishing?
- What should we accomplish in the next wellness group meeting?
- How can wellness programs be improved?
- What kind of assistance would help us develop our potential?
- What are the problem areas in wellness programs that should be
  changed?
- What is the planning process we used to develop wellness pro-
  grams?
- What hypotheses about wellness can be formulated?
- What is the best way to introduce change to facilitate wellness
  behaviors?
- What tools should be used to identify our progress?
- What reactions to our wellness programs do our family members
  have?
- What reactions to our wellness behaviors do our supervisors at
  work have?

RESEARCH PROVIDING SUPPORT
FOR WELLNESS THEORY

One of the main issues in wellness practice is how the nurse assists the
client to move toward wellness. It is relatively easy to teach wellness
procedures. What is difficult is facilitating clients to regularly engage in
wellness. One of the roads to bridging the difficulty is understanding
what facilitates and prevents clients from engaging in wellness behaviors. Therefore, this study is presented as an example of how nurse
researchers may begin to develop wellness theory.

To begin moving in this direction, the author began a study of nursing
students and their reports of what facilitated and prevented them from
engaging in wellness behaviors, using qualitative methods. A semistruc-
tured questionnaire was developed based on the wellness dimensions
and was revised based on feedback from the students. Results were fed
back to students to assist them in understanding factors that affect their
participation (as a group) in wellness activities.

Fifty-five students participated in various phases of the study. As questionnaires were completed, they were analyzed by the researcher for common categories. During the first phase of the study, the issues that were identified as preventing students from engaging in wellness behaviors included: time, fear, guilt, low self-esteem, cravings, overeating, negative environment, lack of motivation, giving up, isolating oneself, being depressed, and inconvenience. Factors that were identified as encouraging participation in wellness activities were:

- someone with good communication skills who listens ("encourages me to discuss what's bothering me;" "Is patient"); gives feedback ("tells me I'm appreciated"; "helps me confront issues"; "points out my progress toward goals"; "points out my potentials");
- is persistent ("reminds me of my goals"; "doesn't nag"; "reassures me I can be honest"; "reminds me how good it will feel if I exercise, etc."; "pushes me to do more");
- encourages ("asks me to list what I do well"; "asks me how I'm doing on my goal"; "talks calmly");
- provides information ("gives me educational materials"; "reinforces benefits of wellness"; "tells me how other people have coped"; "suggests helpful activities");
- has a sense of humor (laughs and makes wellness fun);
- shares wellness activities or role models wellness;
- provides touch ("shows they care with touch"; "gives me a hug when I'm low"; "gives me a massage when I'm tense");
- activities are convenient or affordable;
- when own success is acknowledged;
- when important to others' wellness activities ("when I know he depends on me to go jogging with him, it's easier to get up").

Further isolating categories, the following skills were identified:

- time management
- assertiveness
- access to wellness information/knowledge
- change skills, especially those assisting in attitude change

An additional factor, which held across the board, was the presence of a peer who provided support and a problem-solving, accepting, assertive relationship; in some, but not all, cases, the presence of caring touch was identified.

By examining the data again, the relationship between peer facilitator and self-esteem became clearer. It appeared that what the peer facilitator provided for those with low self-esteem was an external source of self-esteem; someone who "cares enough to devote time to me and who shows me it's O.K. to care about myself and take time to do this."

Other relationships became evident. A patterning of self-esteem, a well thought out plan or wellness goal, regularity in working toward it, feedback from a peer, from oneself, or one's body fell into a set of promoting conditions for each respondent. These conditions did not seem to be phases, but rather interacting variables. There was always action toward pursuing a wellness goal, but depending on the participant it was irregular, unplanned, mechanical ("I do it because I think I should"; "Someone else thinks I should"), or positively reinforcing ("I want to do it because I know I'll feel good during or afterwards").

The issue of self-esteem and wellness is paradoxical. Earlier research has shown that people who regard themselves highly are more likely to set aside time for wellness activities than those with low self-esteem, and that self-esteem or self-concept is enhanced through participation in physical fitness activities (Hanson & Nedde, 1974; Sidney & Shephard, 1976; Sonstroem, 1978). Some unanswered questions include:

- How can those who need external motivation to participate in wellness activities be identified?
- What is the individual mix of self-esteem, plan, regularity, and feedback that leads to wellness?

According to Borba and Borba (1982), indicants of low self esteem include: fearfulness and timidity, aggressiveness (bullying, bragging, derogating others), expectations of failure, reluctance to express feelings, and difficulty making decisions. In re-examining the data, the nursing students who reported evidence of one or more of these indicants did have difficulty regularly pursuing a wellness goal unless they had a peer facilitator who provided structure for pursuing the goal and positive feedback and ongoing encouragement.

Using the data from the 55 nursing students, additional relationship statements were developed based on further reading and thought, including:

- Participation in regular wellness activities exists when (a) the person has learned the benefits of participation and receives self-reinforcement to participate, or (b) the person has a peer to encourage, share, initiate, remind, push, etc.
- If the person has low self-esteem (tends to label oneself as "lazy" or lacking in persistence to engage in wellness activities), then a peer who provides regularity, encouragement, and positive feedback leads to increased participation in wellness activities.

- If the person has inconsistent belief systems so that thoughts, feelings, and actions are not supportive of one another, there will be less participation in wellness activities unless peer support is provided. (Breaks in belief systems were identified when participants responded with comments such as "I should . . ." and/or "I'm lazy" and then reported irregular participation in wellness activities. Consistent belief system was indicated when a participant stated, "I want to . . ." or "It makes me feel confident and strong" and then reported regular participation in the wellness activities.)

Figure 21 shows the interaction of variables that appear to facilitate or prevent nursing students from engaging in wellness behaviors.

Another issue in wellness nursing is the elusiveness of wellness. If wellness has to do with quality of life, it is important to explore this concept further. To do so, the author asked 20 nursing students the following questions:

1. In your opinion, what does the phrase "quality of life" mean? (Be as specific as you can; give any examples of how you measure your quality of life.)
2. What specific things do you think increase your quality of life?
3. What things can you do to enhance your quality of living?
4. What things do you think others can do to enhance your quality of life?
5. Is there anything else that might increase your quality of life?

Results provided support for the wellness dimensions presented in Chapter 1. Examples of responses providing support for each dimension are found in Table 54.

DEVELOPING RELATIONSHIP STATEMENTS AND TESTING THEORETICAL RELATIONSHIPS

According to Chinn and Jacobs (1983, pp. 96–97), theories can only be tested when a translation is made from the theoretical to the concrete.

The activity of testing of theoretical relationships involves three subcomponents: (1) formulating the specific statement of relationship, often a hypothesis, (2) determining the operational definitions necessary to validate the statements, and (3) validating the statement through systematic methods.

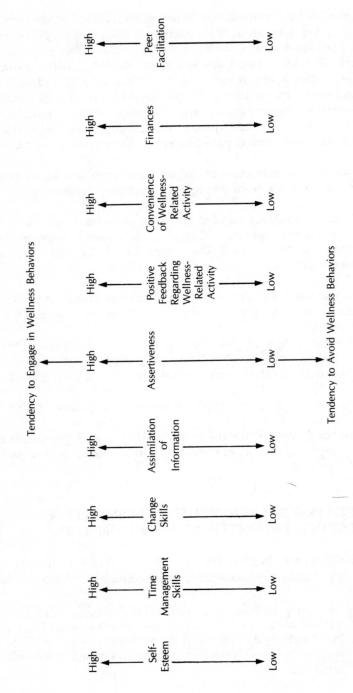

Figure 21. Variables facilitating and preventing nursing students from engaging in wellness behaviors.

Table 54. Examples of Quality of Life Responses and Wellness Dimensions

Fitness Dimension: Regular exercise; healthy body

Nutrition Dimension: Eating appropriately

Belief Systems and Relationship with Self: Feeling confident; feeling good about myself; sense of accomplishment; maximizing potential; existing as a total being; mind/body/spirit; positive outlook; setting goals; being kind to myself; self-awareness; sense of humor; peaceful; self-acceptance

Stress Management: Stop worrying; put things in perspective; learn not to react to pressure; 7–8 hours of sleep; taking time out for myself

Relationships with Others: Sharing laughter and fun; being understood; being liked; being appreciated; firm spiritual base; being supported; being accepted; caring and being cared for; being able to compromise; standing my ground; giving to others; being open to others; sharing opinions and criticisms; noncompetitiveness; being respected; sharing experiences; being reliable; encouraging others; listening without being critical; being a role model; allowing independence

Environment: Peaceful; recharges me; allows privacy and sufficient space; pleasant; allows choice; encourages learning; presents a challenge; is aesthetically pleasing; safe; allows full participation; is organized; is clean and nonpolluted; provides the proper amount of stimulation; allows pride in possessions

To accomplish the first subcomponent, empirical indicators must be substituted for abstract concepts. Some possible relationship statements for testing wellness theory might be:

1. When fitness goals are written, there is a greater likelihood that action toward fitness will follow.
2. When fitness goals are systematically evaluated, there is a greater likelihood that new fitness goals will be set as previous ones are met.
3. When fitness goals are attained, there is a greater likelihood that movement toward wellness in other dimensions will occur.
4. When preventive nutrition goals are attained, there is a greater likelihood that movement toward wellness in other dimensions will occur.
5. There is an inverse relationship between time spent specifying fitness goals and time needed to act on them.
6. There will be a positive relationship between frequency of wellness goal facilitation and progress toward goal attainment.
7. The more the nurse serves as a wellness role model, the more the client will move toward wellness.
8. The more the nurse resolves his or her inconsistent belief systems, the more helpful he or she will be to the client's ability to move toward wellness.

9. The greater the movement toward a wellness belief system, the more wellness behaviors will be exhibited by the client.
10. The more the client participates in self-assessment, the greater the movement toward wellness.

INTEGRATIVE LEARNING EXERCISES

Beginning Level

1. Develop research questions from a wellness perspective based on your area of clinical practice focused on:

   A. A well population
   B. The dimensions of wellness
   C. Antonovsky's concept of coherence
   D. The Intersystems Wellness Nursing Model
   E. Mehl's conceptual framework
   F. A search of current research reports or publications

2. Write in your journal regarding what motivates you to engage in wellness behaviors.
3. Write in your journal about what quality of life means to you.

Advanced Level

1. Complete 1 above.
2. Look at the list of questions you developed in number 1 and decide which could be approached from a qualitative and/or action research method. Give a rationale for your choices.
3. Use a survey or questionnaire to elicit responses from 10–30 well people about what encourages and discourages them from engaging in wellness behaviors. Compare your responses to the ones found from a nursing population.
4. Interview 10–30 well people about what "quality of life" means to them. Compare your answers with those found in this chapter.

REFERENCES

Achterberg, J., et al. (1977). Psychological factors, blood factors and blood chemistries as disease outcome predictors for cancer patients. *Multivariate Experimental Clinical Research* 3:107–122.

Antonovsky, A. (1984). The sense of coherence as a determinant of health. *Advances* 1(3)(Summer):37–50.

Bageley, C. (1979). Control of the emotions, remote stress, and the emergence of breast cancer. *Indian J. Clin. Psychol.* 6:213–220.

Barnard, K. (1982). Determining the focus of nursing research. *Mat Child Health Nursing* 7:299.

Bieliauskas, L., et al. (1979). Psychological depression and cancer mortality. *Psychosom Med* 41:77–78.

Borba, M., and Borba, C. (1982). *Self-Esteem: A Classroom Affair*. Minneapolis, MN: Winston Press, pp. 2–3.

Borysenko, J. (1982). Behavioral–physiological factors in the development and management of cancer. *Gen Hosp Psychiatry* 4:69–74.

Chinn, P. L., and Jacobs, M. (1983). *Theory and Nursing*. St. Louis: C. V. Mosby.

Clark, C. C. (1984). What encourages and prevents students from engaging in wellness activities. *The Wellness Newsletter* 5(6):3–4.

Clark, C. C., and Shea, C. (1978). *Nursing Management*. New York: McGraw-Hill.

Corey, S. (1953). *Action Research to Improve School Practices*. New York: Teachers College Press.

Cunningham, B. (1976). Action research: toward a procedural model. *Human Rels* 29(3):215–238.

Dunn, H. L. (1977). *High Level Wellness*. Thorofare, NJ: Charles B. Slack.

Gardner, N. (1974). Action training and research: something old and something new. *Public Admin Rev* March/April:106–115.

Hanson, J. S., and Nedde, W. H. (1974). Longterm physical training effect in sedentary females. *Journal of Applied Physiology* 37:112–116.

McClelland, D., et al. (1980). Stressed power motivation, sympathetic activation, immune function and illness. *Journal of Human Stress* 6:11–19.

Mehl, L. (1981). *Mind and Matter: Foundations for Holistic Health*. Berkeley, CA: Mindbody Press.

Miles, M., and Huberman, A. (1984). *Qualitative Data Analysis*. Beverly Hills, CA: Sage.

Morris, T., et al. (1978). Psychological response to breast cancer: effect on outcome. *Lancet* 2:785–787.

Mullen, P., and Iverson, D. (1982). Qualitative methods for evaluative research in health education programs. *Health Education* May/June:11–18.

Nursing, a social policy statement (1980). Kansas City, MO: ANA.

O'Regan, B. (1983). Psychoneuroimmunology: the birth of a new field. *Investigations* 1(2):1–2.

Putt, A. (1978). *General Systems Theory Applied to Nursing*. Boston: Little, Brown.

Sanford, N. (1970). Whatever happened to action research? *Journal of Social Issues* 26(4):3–23.

Sidney, K. H., and Shephard, R.J. (1976). Attitudes toward health and physical activity in the elderly. Effects of a physical training program. *Medicine and Science in Sports* 8:246–252.

Sonstroem, R.J. (1978). Physical estimation and attraction scales: rationale and research. *Medicine and Science in Sports* 10:97–102.

Stern, P. (1980). Grounded theory methodology: its uses and processes. *Image* 12:20–23.

Swanson, J., and Chenitz, W. C. (1982). Why qualitative research in nursing? *Nursing Outlook* 30(April):241–245.

Van de Ven, A., and Delbecq, A. (1972). The nominal group as a research instrument for exploratory health studies. *American Journal of Public Health* 62(March):337–342.

Walker, L., and Avant, K. (1983). *Strategies for Theory Construction in Nursing*. Norwalk, CT: Appleton-Century-Crofts.

EPILOGUE

IN SEARCH OF WELLNESS NURSING PRACTICE

By the end of the 20th century, most people believed that physical disease was a symptom of some underlying emotional, mental, social-psychological or spiritual pathology . . . the relationship between stress and illness had at last been comprehended by the 1990s. Employers were expected to take responsibility for eliminating stress-ful or "dis-ease" producing environments . . . By 2010, most of the old hospitals were gone . . . typically converted into health education and fitness centers . . . by the 21st century, the traditional health care providers who remained primarily defined their role as evaluating their clients' level of wellness . . . A typical late 20th century client entering into a wellness contract with a healer or self-help group was usually asked what threats, losses and gains their sickness represented to them. The majority of chronic illnesses were treated by helping the client alter his or her lifestyle . . . By the early 1990s most people accepted the fact that the body was its own finest laboratory and children were taught techniques which allowed the body to follow its best adaptive course when they were ill . . . Values—the client's and the provider's—are now an explicit part of any discussion of wellness strategy . . . The need for a disease care system and the concept of patient have faded. The ideal future is one where the wellness system empowers people to transform themselves. (American Council of Life Insurance, 1980)

If futurists are to be believed, nurses need to take heed and prepare for practice outside the hospital environment. The writing is already on the wall for hospitals—DRGs, cutbacks in Medicare and Medicaid and recent reimbursement rule changes, nurse–physician conflict, malnutrition in hospitalized clients (Butterworth, 1974; Mendelsohn, 1979, p. 74), known degree of unreliability in laboratory tests and other procedures (Mendelsohn, 1979, pp. 3–10), unknown and unmonitored drug interactions (Table 31), unnecessary surgery (Mendelsohn, 1979, pp. 49–65), iatrogenic or hospital-induced illnesses (Mendelsohn, 1979, pp. 67–83).

The beginning of a wellness nursing practice can occur in a hospital setting, but it will probably be a fragmented practice. It will mean looking the other way about all the events listed above (and more) that occur daily; it will mean not talking with clients because it is not supported by most administrators. It will mean discharging clients sooner— which is probably a good idea, given the iatrogenic possibilities in the hospital—to keep pace with DRGs. It will mean remaining safe and secure in a protected, if hostile, environment.

But positive signs are there—a quiet revolution is brewing! (Luck and Kellman, 1985). Nurses are escaping from hospitals. Several new national nursing organizations show promise: Nurses in Transition (P.O.B. 14472, San Francisco, CA 94114), the American Holistic Nurses Association (Box 116, Telluride, CO 81435), Nurse Healers Professional Associates Cooperative (Box 7, 70 Shelly Avenue, Port Chester, NY 10573), and Nurses Environmental Health Watch (655 Avenue of the Americas, New York, NY 10010).

Practicing wellness nursing in a holistic fashion will mean breaking out of the hospital–physician–drug company-controlled anti-wellness environment. It will be frightening at first, but it will enhance nurses' wellness by enhancing self-confidence and mastery.

Luck (1985, p. 245) points out that prior to 1910 nurses practiced independently and preventively in the community; with the advent of a regulated medical profession, hospitals or "Temples of Doom" (as Mendelsohn refers to them, 1979) were created. But hospitals are only a passing fad according to futurists, so there *is* hope.

Wellness nursing practice offers other sources of hope. Many nurses have feared private practice because by diagnosing and treating they were under the gun (in some cases) for "practicing medicine without a licence." But wellness nursing does not focus on illness and does not replicate medical practice; medical practice and wellness nursing practice are complementary. Physicians are educated to work with illness; they are not educated to be wellness practitioners. As long as nurses work in the manner suggested in this book, there is no way they can be accused of practicing medicine. This differentiation is underlined by the nurse–client contract in wellness nursing in which the client is ultimately responsible for his or her own body and decisions regarding it.

What nurses must do is overcome their fear of "being out there alone" without a large system as a buffer. This fear (and lack of self-confidence) is probably what keeps people in other fields (as well as nurses) from striking out in private or group practice. Once this fear is confronted, the rewards can be heady.

For those nurses who have tried private practice or have confronted their fears and choose to stay in the hospital environment for as long as it survives, other measures are possible. One of the major problems with nurses is their inability or refusal to support one another. If someone attacks a physician, physicians close ranks and protect each other. If someone attacks a nurse, there are few, if any, nurse supporters who will support that nurse. Often nursing administrators will side with physicians or hospital administrators to maintain the status quo. This must stop if the hospital environment is to be humanized. One way this can begin is by initiating the LifeGain system in hospitals. It will probably have to be started by nurses themselves since it is unlikely they will be given funds to humanize their working environment.

"Our hope for the future is that new directions in wellness are a vehicle for greater human happiness, health and consciousness" (American Council of Life Insurance, 1985, p. 404).

REFERENCES

Gleit, C., & Tatro, S. (1981). Nursing diagnoses for healthy individuals. *Nursing and Health Care* October, 2(8):456.
Tatro, S., & Gleit, C. (1983). A wellness model for nursing: Promoting high level wellness in any setting through independent nursing functions. *Nursing Leadership* March, 6(1):5–9.

A NOTE ON NURSING DIAGNOSES AND WELLNESS

Looking at the accepted nursing diagnoses, it is clear that some new ones may need to be developed to encompass wellness nursing practice. For example, where does one fit the following: resistance to change, lack of positive experience or reward, need for external source of self-esteem, need for feedback, need for goal setting, need for prioritization of goals, lack of consistent value system, empathy deficit, and assertiveness deficit?

The term noncompliance (an accepted nursing diagnosis) may not be appropriate for a wellness viewpoint. First, wellness nursing allows the client *choice*; what is viewed as noncompliance by the nurse may be an alternative choice from the client's point of view. Second, noncompliance does not fit the conceptual framework of hypnosis and other procedures that work at a subconscious level; the therapeutic term *resistance* might be more apt.

Another issue that arises in mind/body change processes is that of transitory physiological reactions that occur on the way toward mind/body/spirit integration. Possibly developing a nursing diagnosis of the need to integrate transitory reactions would suffice.

As nurses become more proficient in assisting clients to enhance their self-healing processes, a diagnosis of self-healing process deficit or need may be developed. Time management is another issue not addressed by current nursing diagnoses; an additional nursing diagnosis of inappropriate time management could be developed. Finally, a nursing diagnosis for hardiness, such as hardiness deficit, could be developed.

There are some nursing diagnoses relevant to nutrition, including: nutrition, alterations in, less than body requirements, and more than body requirements. One that may be needed in the future is: nutrient malabsorption, drug-induced.

Some nursing diagnoses that may need development for fitness and healing include: conditioning deficit; body awareness deficit; body organization deficit; lack of right/left cerebral balancing; and self-healing process deficit.

Some nursing diagnoses that may be appropriate for environmental concerns are: potential for chronic disease; full-spectrum light deficit; noise pollution; and privacy deficit.

Gleit and Tatro (1981, p. 456) have redefined nursing diagnosis to include wellness:

> A nursing diagnosis is the statement of an individual's response that is healthy or actually or potentially unhealthy and which independent nursing interventions can help to reinforce or strengthen in the direction of optimal health. The diagnostic statement should also identify essential factors related to the healthy or unhealthy responses.

Based on this definition,

> . . . the first clause of the diagnosis will be expressed as a positive behavior (based on the client's strengths) that the client is currently engaged in to promote high level wellness. Because the first clause is behaviorally stated, it may be incorrectly interpreted as a prescription rather than a behavior that the client is engaged in to promote wellness. (Tatro & Gleit, 1983, p. 7)

Examples of how wellness nursing diagnoses might look based on Gleit and Tatro's work follow:

- Walking briskly for 20 minutes 3 times/week related to a knowledge of aerobic fitness benefits.
- Practicing progressive relaxation for 15 minutes twice a day related to stress management benefits.
- Eating fresh green, yellow, and red vegetables daily related to preventing cancer.
- Wearing seat belts when riding in a car related to personal safety.
- Participating in weekly family meetings related to encouraging positive interpersonal relationships among family members.
- Completing weekly journal entries related to developing consistent belief systems.

REFERENCES

American Council on Life Insurance. (1985). Comprehensive report of the cooperative commission on wellness. In *The New Holistic Handbook, Living Well in a New Age,* S. Bliss et al., Eds. New York: Viking-Penguin, pp. 402–404.

Butterworth, C. (1974). The skeleton in the hospital closet. *Nutrition Today* (March/April):4–8.

Luck, S., & Kellman, S. (1985). A quiet revolution: holistic nursing. In *The New Holistic Handbook, Living Well in a New Age,* S. Bliss et al., Eds. New York: Viking-Penguin, pp. 244–248.

Mendelsohn, R. (1979). *Confessions of a Medical Heretic.* Chicago, IL: Contemporary Books, Inc.

INDEX

Abdomen, directions for examining, 217
Acid rain, 265,272,278
Action research, 323–326
Acupressure,
  assessments, 231
  evaluations, 107–108
  interventions, 248–251
Aerobic dancing, 194
Aerobic exercise
  assessments, 183–185
  definition, 183
  evaluation, 107–108
  regimes, 189–192
Aerobic walking technique, 190–192
Affirmation, 48–50
  case study, 50
  concepts, 48
  evaluation, 107–108
  interventions, 48–50
Age and responsibility for wellness, 31
Aggressiveness and nutrition, 147–148
Air quality, 259–260,268–269,274
Allergies, self-hypnosis for, 92
Aluminum
  and Alzheimer's disease, 149
  and ALS, 150
Alzheimer's disease
  and aluminum, 149
  and calcium, 149

American Hospital Association, 10
American Nurses' Association, and environmental resolutions, 264–265
Amino acids, 145–147
Anger
  and exercise, 201
  and stress reduction, 81–105
Antibodies, 212
Anxiety
  and exercise, 200–202
  and stress management, 81–105
Arthritis, and exercise, 198
Assessment questions, client, nursing history, 39–40
Assertiveness, 62–78
  assessments, 65
  and criticism, 67–70
  definition, 62
  evaluation, 65, 107–108
  "I"-messages vs. "you"-messages, 62
  and stress, 63
  techniques for enhancing, 63–78
Attrition in exercise programs, overcoming, 199–200
Autogenics, 95–97
Awareness through movement,
  interventions, 186,187–189, 196–197
  theory, 170–171

Back exercises to prevent back pain,
  191–192
Baseline data, 32
Bedridden clients, and exercise,
  195–197
Behavior
  countable, 32
  goal-directed, 33
  and lead, 151
  and nutrition, 113–162
  reinforcer, 33
  rewarding, 33
  shaping, 34
Behavioral kinesiology
  assessments, 216–218
  and balanced energy, 205
  evaluation, 107–108
  and indicator muscles, 206
  interventions, 235–238
  and thymus, 206–207
Biofeedback, 86–87
Blocks to listening, 28
Body/mind interactions, and fitness,
  200–202
Bonding, infant massage
  and, 246–248
Bow pose, in yoga, 238
Breast, self-examination directions,
  215
Breathing, 85–86
Boundaries of wellness theory, 14

Campus wellness programs, 302–306
Cancer and environmental wellness,
  258
Cancer and preventive nutrition,
  beta-carotene, 122
  dietary guidelines for reducing
    risks, 141
  vegetarianism, and, 140
  vitamin C, 122
  vitamin E, 139
  selenium, 139
Calcium
  and Alzheimer's disease, 149
  and eclampsia, 149–150
  and hypertension, 120–121

and osteoporosis, 148–149
Cardiovascular disease and preventive nutrients, 141–142
  complex interrelationships, 145
  dietary fiber, 144–145
  EPA, 144
  essential fatty acids, 143
  fat soluble vitamins, 147
  garlic, 147
  habits associated with, 142
  high density lipoproteins, 142
  hydrogenated fats, dangers,
    143–144
  inositol, 126,147
  lecithin (phospholipids), 144
  polyunsaturated to saturated fat
    ratio, 143
  serum cholesterol, 142,145–146
  total fat, 142–143
Cat stretch, in yoga, 240
Center for Health Promotion, 8
Center for Prevention Services, 8
Center for Work and Mental
  Health, 8
Cerebral hemisphere imbalance,
  217–218
Change,
  assessing resistance to, 30
  decreasing resistance to, 30–39
  evaluating the effect of, 30
Chi, 206, 210
Children, exercise and, 199
Chlorination, potential hazards of,
  260
Cholesterol, serum, 142,145–146
  and vitamin C, 146
  and soybeans, 145–146
Chromium, and diabetes, 150–151
Clark health/wellness belief scale,
  40–42
Cobra pose, in yoga, 238
Cognitive complexity, 14
Cohen and Mills, theory, 167–170
Color, and environmental wellness,
  267–268,272,278–279
Community wellness programs,
  283–313

assessing need for, 285–287
in clinics, 290–291
community assessment, 287–290
evaluating, 306–313
federally funded, 291–294
in hospitals, 290–291
in industry, 290–291
justification for, 283–285
planning and implementing,
     294–306
Compliance, irrelevance of, 2
Coping skills training, 100–102
Construct, wellness as, 11
Consumer products and environ-
     mental wellness, 262,270–
     271,275–277
Contracting process, 34–36
Contralateral movement, 169
Crowding, and wellness, 269–
     270,275

Depression, and exercise, 201–202
Detection tests and prevention, 215
Destructive behavior, self-hypnosis,
     92
Developmental movement, 167–185
assessments, 177–178
interventions, 185
theory, 167–170
Diabetes,
and chromium, 150–151
and exercise, 197–198
Dietary goals, 116–119
Dietary guidelines for reducing can-
     cer risks, 141
Differentiation of self, 12,20–25
interventions, 25
levels/assessments, 22–25
theory, 20–24
DRGs, 10
Drug-nutrient interactions, 151–153

Eclampsia, and calcium, 149
Effleurage stroke, in massage, 241
Ellis, Albert, 98
Empathy, 58–62
evaluating, 107–108

helping clients develop, 61–62
levels of, 58–61
Endorphins, 201
Energy, 1, 205,217,230,238
Environment, 13
Environmental wellness, 258–282
and acid rain, 265,272,278
and air quality, 259–260,268–
     269,274
and American Nurses' Association,
     264–265
assessments, 268–272
and cancer, 258
and color, 267–268,272,278–279
and consumer products, 262,270–
     271,275–277
and crowding, 269–270,275
evaluations, 107–108
interventions, 272–279
and ions, 265–266,272,278
and light, 266–267,272,278
and noise, 265,272,277–278
and occupation, 262–265,271,275
and personal space, 261
and radiation, 261–262,270,275
and smoking, 260,274
and solid waste, 274
and water quality, 260–261,269,274
EPA, 144
Essential fatty acids, 143
Evaluation,
of community wellness programs,
     306–313
of individual wellness programs,
     107–108
research, 306–307
sample size determination, 312
selection of tools, 309–310
validity considerations, 310–311
Evolutionary process and wellness,
     5,11
Exercise,
and anxiety, 200–201
and arthritis, 198
and attrition rates, 199–200
for bedridden clients, 195
and bone mineral loss, 198

Exercise, *(cont.)*
  and children, 199
  for debilitated clients, 195–197
  and depression, 201–202
  and diabetes, 197–198
  and endorphins, 201
  and imagery, 200
  and low back pain, 191
  and memory loss, 198–199
  preparation for, 200
  and relaxation, 201
  and weight loss, 158

Facilitator of wellness, nurse as,
  2,17,35
Family, theory and interventions,
  20–30
Fat soluble vitamins, 147
Feldenkrais, Moshe
  interventions, 185,187–189,
    196–197
  theory, 170–171
Fiber, dietary, 144–145
Fight-or-flight response, 81
Fitness,
  assessments, 177–185
  interventions, 190–199
  record, 219–222
  theoretical frameworks for, 167–
    176
Fitness interventions
  aerobics, choosing appropriate, 190
  for arthritis, 198
  for bedridden clients, 195
  for children, 199
  conditioning, 189–192
  for depression, 201–202
  for diabetes, 197–198
  developmental movement, 185
  Feldenkrais, 185,187–189,196–197
  for flexibility, 193–194
  keeping back fit, 191–192
  for low self-esteem, 201–202
  shoes, choosing appropriate, 190
  walking technique, proper, 190–
    191
  for memory loss, 198–199

  for stress reduction, 106
Flexibility,
  assessments, 181–183
  interventions, 193–194
Fluoridated water, potential dangers
  of, 261
Friction stroke, in massage, 241

Garlic, and lowered cholesterol, 147
Growth plates, exercise and, 199

Hardiness, 105–107
Hatha yoga, 209
Healing,
  environment and, 278
  imagery and, 47
Health belief model, 30–31
Health education, compared to well-
  ness nursing, 7
Health hazard/health risk appraisals,
  38–39
Health, compared to wellness, 3
Health promotion model, 31
Heart disease, and soft water, 260
Heel cord flexibility, 183
Hidden agendas, 77–78
  overcoming, 78
  types, 77
Holmes schedule of recent experi-
  ence, 82
Homolateral movement, 169,236
Homologous movement, 169,236
Human field assessments, 222,230
Hydrogenated fats, dangers of,
  143–144

Imagery, 43,45–48
  to enhance healing, 47
  and movement, 187
  movie of the mind, 46–47
  to prepare for an upcoming
    situation, 46
  to solve problems, 46
Immunity, and copper and zinc, 151
Immunoglobulin A, 212–213
Incentives, for smoking cessation,
  301

Infant massage, 246–248
Inositol, 126,147
Integrated learning experiences
  assertiveness, 78–80
  centering, 53–56
  community wellness, 313–314
  differentiation of self, 53–56
  empathy, 78–80
  environment, 280
  exercise and movement, 202–
    203
  introduction to wellness theory,
    15–18
  nutrition, 159–161
  research, 332
  self-care and touch, 255–256
  stress management, 107–111
  value clarification, 53–56
Internal locus of control, 40,42–43
Intersystems wellness nursing
  model, 4
Ions, positive and negative, 265–
  266,272,278
Itching, self-hypnosis for, 92

Kneeling pose, in yoga, 239
Krieger, Dolores, 207–208
Kurtz, and Prestera's body message
  theory, 171–176

Laboratory tests, reliability of, 229
Lead,
  and behavior, 151
  and sudden infant death, 151
Lecithin, 144
Liangzui point, in acupressure, 251
Lifegain program, as a systems
  approach, 296–299
Light, 266–267,272,278
Lion pose, in yoga, 239
Locus of control, 40,42–43
  and EPIC model, 42–43
  and internality-externality, 40–42
Locust pose, in yoga, 239
Lymph nodes, directions for examin-
  ing, 216
Lymphocytes, 211

Massage,
  assessments, 231
  evaluations, 107–108
  interventions, 241–248
McClelland, David, 212–214
Memory loss, and exercise, 198–199
Meridians, 210
Midlife crisis, 31
Minerals, and RDAs, and functions/
  sources, 131–135
Motivation, intrinsic, 2
Mountain pose, in yoga, 239

Neck and eye exercises, 239–240
Neurolinguistic programming,
  anchors, 53
  case study, 53
  context reframing, 50–53
  evaluating, 107–108
  interventions, 53
  representational systems, 51–52
  resources, 53
  speaking the client's language, 52
  theory, 50–53
Noise, and environmental wellness,
  265,272,277–278
Nursing diagnoses and wellness,
  88,337–338
Nursing interventions,
  abdominal muscles, weakened,
    191–192
  aggressiveness, 62–68
  air or water pollution, 274
  allergies, 92, 250
  Alzheimer's disease, 149
  amenorrhea, 250
  amyotrophic lateral sclerosis
    (ALS), 150
  anemia, iron deficiency, 250,279
  anger, 62–78
  anxiety, 28–30,81–105,200–202,
    238,244–248,250,279
  appetite suppressant, 279
  arm or leg jerks, 124
  arm or leg soreness, 249
  arthritis, 198,240,250,279
  asthma, 92,97,238,251

Nursing interventions, *(cont.)*
  backache, 125,251
  back pain (pregnancy), 238–240
  bad breath, 124,232
  bedwetting, 93
  bloating, 124
  blushing, 97
  bonding, 246–248
  bone aches, 148–149,198,279
  bones, brittle, 148–149,198,279
  bradycardia, 132–133, 279
  brain damage, 133,186
  breathing difficulty, 125,250,279
  brown spots on hands and feet,
      125
  bruising, 126
  bulemia, 250
  calves, tender, 123,127
  cancer, 122,132,134,139–141,
      207–208
  cardiovascular disease, 141–147,
      185–200
  cellulitis, 250
  circulation, poor, 238,241,243–
      245,250,254,279
  colds, 92,250,279
  congestions, systemic, 279
  constipation, 238–240,250
  convulsions, 250
  coughing, 97,250
  cramping, menstrual or meno-
      pausal, 124
  criticism, dealing with, 67–77
  deadlines, missing, 102–105
  decisions, difficulty making, 26–28
  depression, 125,201–202
  dermatitis, 124–125
  diabetes, 96,131,150–151,197–
      198,232,238,240
  distention, 250
  dizziness, 250
  dysmenorrhea, 125,250,279
  ear ringing, 250
  eclampsia, 149–150
  edema, 250
  electrolyte imbalance, 250
  endocrine disorders, 185

  energy, trapped, 244–248
  eyes, bloodshot, 123
  eyes, burning/itching, 123
  eye irritation, 232
  eyestrain, 232,239–240
  fatigue, 125,232,238,250–251,279
  fears, 85–105,123–124
  feet, burning, 123
  fever, 250,279
  flatulence, 239,250,279
  flexibility, lack of, 240
  fractures, 131–133,250
  frostbite, 250
  fusion, emotional, 30
  G-I disorders, 123,232
  gall bladder dysfunction, 279
  goals, lack of, 34–38,43–53
  gums, bleeding, 126
  hands and feet, tickling sensation,
      125
  headache, 86–87,232,250–251
  healing, inadequate, 47,279
  hearing loss, 250
  heart, pains, 125,232
  heat rash, prickly, 124
  hemorrhoids, 144–145,250
  hot flashes, 279
  hypertension, 86–87,120–121,250
  immune deficiency, 235,279
  inconsistent beliefs/behavior,
      40–53
  indigestion, 232,238,241,250,279
  infection, 124–126,250,279
  infertility, 250
  inflexible spine, 232,240–241
  insomnia, 239,250,279
  itching, 92,124,250
  jet lag, 250
  kidney injury, 250,279
  legs, swelling, 123,232
  lips, chapped, 123
  lips, sore, 125
  liver, sluggish, 238,250,279
  low back pain, 188,191
  lungs, weakened, 232,239
  memory loss, 124,279
  menopause, 124,279

menstruation, excessive, 279
mouth, sore, 125
movement, ineffective, 186
muscle pain, 125
muscle spasm, 250
nausea and vomiting, 125,207–208,232,250
neck and shoulder tension, 187,232
nonproductivity, 85–105
obesity, 92,240,250
osteoporosis, 148–149,198
ovaries, 238
overwhelmed, feeling of being, 85–105
pain, 86–87,250,279
peptic ulcer, 250
peristalsis, 237–238
phobias, 85–105
powerlessness, 62–78,85–105
premenstrual tension, 150
rapport, establishing, 58–62
respiratory problems, 250,279
rights, standing up for, 62–78
saying no, 63–66
sciatica, 250
sea sickness, 250
self-esteem, low, 48,63–69,98–102,201–202,247
self-talk, negative, 98–102
seizures, 250
sexual harrassment, 62–78
sexual nonperformance, 123
shock, 250
sinuses, 86,250
skin, rough and dry, 279
skin irritation, 279
smoking, 92,233–235,299–302
sore throat, 239
spinal flexibility, 240–241
stiff neck, 187, 249–250
stress, environmental, 274–278
stress, overreacting to normal, 123
stuttering, 86–87
sudden infant death, 151
suspiciousness, 124
swelling, 279

swollen joints, 250
tachycardia, 92–93,123,132–133, 207–208,279
thoughts, repetitive, 85–105
thyroid, regulate, 240,279
tics, 124
time, insufficient, 102–105
tooth decay, 124
tongue, red, 124
tremors, 124
underweight, 250
unsatisfactory relationships, 58–105
upcoming situations, preparing, for, 46
urinating, difficulty, 123
uterus, 238–239,250,279
varicose veins, prevention, 240
weight gain, 154–159
Nursing process, 2
Nursing research, wellness
developing problem statements, 316–320
lifestyle factors and contraceptive use, 321–322
progressive relaxation, 87–90
self-reports of what facilitates and prevents nursing students from engaging in wellness behaviors, 326–329
step family integration, 322–323
therapeutic touch, 207–208
and wellness theory, 315–332
Nutrition,
and aggressiveness, 147–148
and Alzheimer's disease, 149
and amyotrophic lateral sclerosis, 150
and cancer, 122–23,139–141
and congestive heart disease, 141–147
and diabetes, 150–151
and eclampsia, 149–150
and drug interactions, 151–153
food myths, 115–116
foods to eat to enhance wellness, 136–138

Nutrition, *(cont.)*
  guidelines for reading information, 115
  low salt, 120–121
  and osteoporosis, 148–149
  and premenstrual tension, 150
  signs of balanced eating, 114
  suggested dietary goals, 116–119
  supplementation, 119–122
  vitamins and minerals, 119–122

Occupation and environmental wellness, 262–265,271,277
Orem, Dorothea, 13
Osteoporosis
  and calcium, 148–149
  and exercise, 198

Pain, self-hypnosis for, 93–94
Painful feelings, imagery for, 48
Polyunsaturated fat, 143
Prana, 207
Premenstrual tension, 150
Preparing for upcoming situations, and imagery, 46
Primary prevention, 205,215
Problem-solving, imagery, 46
Psychoneuroimmunology, 211–214

Qualitative research, 320–323
Quality of life and wellness, 331
Questionable screening procedures, 229

Radiation, 261–262,270–275
Reflexology, 210–211
  assessments, 232–233
  evaluations, 107–108
  interventions, 251–255
Refuting irrational ideas, 98–100
Reinforcer, token system, 33
Relaxation,
  assessments, 82–85
  evaluations, 107–108
  interventions, 43–44, 85
  tapes, 44
  theory, 43

Reliability, 214
Research,
  designing wellness research questions, 316–320
  factors facilitating and preventing wellness behavior, 326–329
  fitness, 197–199,200–202
  nursing content, 315–316
  nutrition, 120–122,139–151, 154–159
  procedures for, 306–313,320–329
  progressive relaxation in nursing, 87–90
  quality of life, 331
  stress reduction, 82,88–90,93, 101,105–106
  touch and healing, 207–209,212– 214
  and wellness theory, 315–332
  worksite wellness, 284–285,290– 291,293–294
Right brain, 45
Rights, standing up for, 62–78
Rotter, and internal locus of control, 40
Running,
  shoes, 190
  walk-jog program, 189–190

Salt, and blood pressure, 120–121
Screening, health,
  as a preventive measure, 215,225– 229
  pros and cons of stress testing, 184–185
  questionable procedures for, 230
Selenium, and cancer, 139
Self-assessments,
  assertiveness, 65
  empathy, 59–60
  fitness, 179–180
  nutrition, 123–126
  sexual communication, 223
  stress level, 83–84
  wellness, 36–40
Self-care, 8,13,214–228
Self-esteem, and exercise, 201–202

Self-examinations,
  abdomen, 217
  breast, 215
  fitness, 179–180
  lymph nodes, 216
  thyroid gland, 218
  vaginal, 224
Self-hypnosis, 90–95
Self-responsibility, for wellness, 39
Self-talk, 21,98,102
Senate select committee on nutrition
    and human needs, 113
Setpoint theory, 157–159
Shoulder stand, in yoga, 240
Situps, 191–192,199
Smoking,
  and environmental wellness,
    260,274
  self-care, 233–235
  at worksite, 299–302
Solid waste, 274
Soybeans and amino acids, 145–146
Spinal movement, 168–169
Spinal twist, in yoga, 240
Stay well program, blue shield, 9
Sternomandibular joint, 217
Stress management,
  assessments, 81–85
  hardiness, 105–107
  interventions, 85–105
Stress testing, pros and cons, 184–
    185
Structural assessments, 178–180
Subsystems, 1
Sugar consumption, and behavior,
    148
Sun salutation, in yoga, 241–242
Swimming, 192,199
Systems model, 11
  for community change (Lifegain),
    296–299
  input, 14
  interface, 13
  output, 4

Tapotement stroke, in massage, 243
Telereceptive assessments, 222

Therapeutic touch,
  assessments, 208,222,230
  evaluation, 107–108
  interventions, 237–238
  theory, 207
Thought stopping, 97–98
Thymus gland,
  and balanced energy, 206–207
  and behavioral kinesiology, 205–
    207
  and indicator muscles, 206
Thyroid gland, directions for exam-
    ining, 218
Tiantu point, in acupressure, 251
Time management, 102–105
Triangle pose, in yoga, 240
Type A behavior, 213

Uddiyana pose, in yoga, 240
Unruffling the field, 208

Vaginal self-examination, 224
Value clarification,
  evaluation, 26
  interventions, 27
  theory, 26
Vegetarianism, and protection
    from,
  cancer, 140
  diabetes, 140
  heart disease, 140
  high blood pressure, 140
  obesity, 140
  osteoporosis, 140
Vibration stroke, in massage, 243
Vitamins and minerals,
  deficiency signs, 123–127
  food sources, 123–138
  functions, 123–135
  RDAs, 128–135

Walk/jog program, 189–190
Water quality, 260–261,269,274
Weight loss,
  and exercise, 158
  recommendations, 154–158
  theories, 156–159

Weight maintenance, 152–160
    and environment, 154
    by extension course, 152
    and peer support, 152,154
    and setpoint theory, 157–159
    and time calorie displacement,
        156–157
    and weight loss, 154–160
Wellness belief scale,
    theory, 40
    use, 40–42
Wellness model, 2,14
Wellness nursing
    defined, 1,2,6,11
    evaluation of, 107–108
    intersystems model for, 4
    practice, 334–336, *see also;* commu-
        nity wellness, environmental
        wellness, exercise and move-
        ment, nutritional wellness,
        positive relationship building,
        research, self-care, stress man-
        agement

Wellness self-assessment,
    compared to HRA, 38–39
    evaluation of, 107–108
    example, 36–38
    uses of, 38–39
Wellness theory, 6,7,14,315–332
Whole person wellness, 6
Worksite wellness programs,
    294–299

Xuehai point, in acupressure,
    251

Yoga, 208–209
    assessments, 229
    evaluation, 107–108
    interventions, 238–241
Yuyao point, in acupressure,
    251

Zinc, and immunity, 151
Zusanli point, in acupressure,
    251